How Superstition Won and Science L

JOHN C. BURNHAM

Rutgers University Press
New Brunswick and London

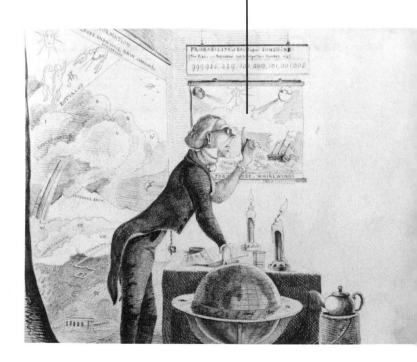

HOW SUPERSTITION WON AND SCIENCE LOST

Popularizing Science and Health in the United States

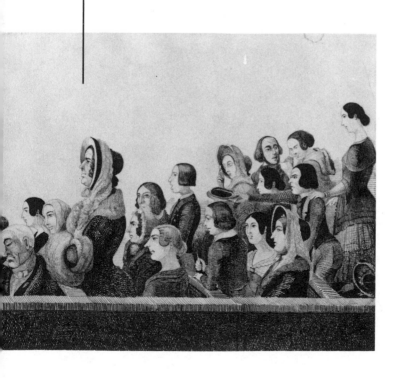

Library of Congress Cataloging-in-Publication Data

Burnham, John C. (John Chynoweth), 1929–
  How superstition won and science lost.

  Includes index.
    1. Life sciences—Social aspects—United States—
History. 2. Social medicine—United States—History.
3. Medical misconceptions—United States—History.
4. Psychology—Social aspects—United States—History.
5. Science—Social aspects—United States—History.
6. Journalism, Scientific—United States—History.
7. Superstition—United States—History. I. Title.
QH333.B87 1987   509.73   86–31360
ISBN 0–8135–1238–7
ISBN 0–8135–1265–4 (pbk.)
British Cataloging-in-Publication information available

Copyright © 1987 by Rutgers, The State University
All Rights Reserved
Manufactured in the United States of America

Second paperback printing, September 1988

Lyceum lecture on the weather: James P. Espy at Clinton Hall, 1841. Artist unknown. Courtesy of the Photo Library Department of the Museum of the City of New York.

To
science teachers of the United States
(for their role in fostering civilization)

and to
Marjorie
(for personal reasons)

Contents

List of Illustrations

Acknowledgments

Chapter 2 is based on "Change in the Popularization of Health in the United States," *Bulletin of the History of Medicine*, 58 (1984), 183–197, with the kind permission of Caroline Hannaway, editor of the *Bulletin of the History of Medicine*, and the Johns Hopkins University Press. Another version of chapter 3 was presented as a centenary address at the meetings of the American Psychological Association in 1980. An abstract of the whole argument was presented as a lecture in the Science, Technology, and Society Program series at Michigan Technological University in 1983.

Parts of chapter 2 are based on research carried out under a grant from the National Library of Medicine (NIH Grant LM 02539). The book as a whole was supported through perquisites regularly furnished by The Ohio State University, including a Faculty Professional Leave during which much of the revision was undertaken. Substantial support was also furnished by Marjorie A. Burnham.

Many colleagues have made valuable suggestions for improving this book. I am very grateful to them. Several have read the manuscript and offered suggestions with a generosity far beyond the call of ordinary collegial duty, and I would like to list their names as a recognition, however inadequate, of a really extraordinary service: Donald de B. Beaver, Hamilton Cravens, Frederick D. Dahlstrand, Bruce V. Lewenstein, Jane M. Oppenheimer, David J. Rhees, John L. Rury, and Michael M. Sokal. My great regret is that I have been unable to carry out all of their suggestions and meet all of their objections.

How Superstition Won and Science Lost

Introduction

Recently I was traveling aboard an airliner on which the head flight attendant provided amusing variations to the usual announcements required on domestic carriers. Indeed, the attendant's performance suggested that he was practicing to become a standup comedian. At the end of the flight, after we had by chance made an unusually tense, bouncing landing, our wiseacre announced on the public address system, "Once again, ladies and gentlemen, science has triumphed over the forces of superstition and darkness, and we have landed safely in Chicago, Illinois."

The good natured and appropriate laughter that greeted this well-timed satire indicated that people aboard the aircraft were familiar with a commonplace, the modern morality play in which science defeats superstition. The laughter also reflected the fact that the passengers may have felt for a moment some uncertainty about the ultimate victory of science. But, as in the conventional popular stereotype, all ended happily, and the ending included the victory of science.

That conventional story is the subject of this book. My findings, however, do not confirm the stereotype.

It may well be that the evolution of scientific ideas is progressive. But the courses of both the popular and social histories of science often vary from that of pure science. The account that follows explores some of the events that contributed to a certain cognitive dissonance as the popularization of science and health developed a history that differed from the history of scientific ideas and institutions. In following out my inquiry, I have not only utilized a wide sampling of materials from the past but have tried to include the findings of a number of different kinds of scholars whose work illuminates aspects of the subject.

People often assume that just as in laboratory and field research, so in the field of popular enlightenment, the fight of science against superstition was won by the forces of rationality and naturalism—at least won in

3

the highly technical society of the postindustrial United States. But the record shows that changes in the way in which science and health came to be popularized in fact ultimately reduced and frustrated the cultural impact of both science and scientists. Therefore I have designed this book to make a point: when everyone presumed that superstition and mysticism had been relegated to the past, and popularizers of science had turned to other concerns, two things happened. First, a functional equivalent to superstition arose. It was a functional equivalent because it played the same cultural role as superstition in an earlier day, and it could be recognized because it was just that against which popularizers of science had pitted themselves from the beginning: superstitious thinking and exploiters of superstitious beliefs, that is, both irrationalism and the agents of irrationalism. The second thing that happened was that popularizers eventually ceased waging a negative campaign against superstition in any form, for after all they no longer recognized it in the new guise. The consequence was that the cultural force of the popularization of science not only changed but diminished decisively.

At the opening of the nineteenth century, when popularizing began, many Americans tried to diffuse knowledge of the various areas of science as they were conceptualized then: natural philosophy, natural history, moral philosophy, and hygiene. By the late nineteenth century, naturalism—explaining everything as a product of nature—was the triumphant motif in popularization and showed up particularly in the quite explicit campaign against mysticism and superstition to which I have alluded; people at the time understood both the positive presentations of science and the negative, antisuperstitious, aspects of popular naturalism as the major aspect of the warfare between science and religion.

It was during the twentieth century that certain relentless institutional changes weakened and finally rendered largely ineffectual the traditional elements that had once energized and guided the popularization of science and health in the United States. The crucial transformation came when popularizers reduced the meaning of their material by isolating the products of research from the process and spirit of doing naturalistic science.

The triumph of superstition also was signaled by the retreat of broad, well-educated missionaries of science from the field of popularization and their replacement by those who were influenced by the mass media or actually worked in journalism, public relations, and advertising. In the process, science in the realm of the popularizers changed from a coherent view of nature, including humans, into choppy, unconnected "facts."

Such were the major streams of historical development that emerge clearly from a general survey of the main features of the record of popularizing.

To elucidate the patterns of change, I have turned to three areas of science: health, which implicitly included much medical science along with hygiene (in the broad, old-fashioned sense); psychology, which shared characteristics with not only hygiene and medicine but the natural sciences (as well as the behavioral–social sciences group) and was a science in its own right; and the mainline natural sciences. Events in the three areas were not always perfectly parallel, or at least the timing differed a little, but all three did converge at critical points. Indeed, it was my discovery of this convergence that led to the writing of this book. The patterns showed up more starkly in the health and psychology areas, but the parallels in the natural sciences were the more curious because of the complex and traditional context in which they appeared.

What emerges from these materials is not only the changing patterns of popularization of science and health but, particularly, an account of the traditional negative aspect of popularization to which I have alluded, namely, combatting error (one newspaper health column of the 1930s was actually called "The Debunker"). The history of scientific ideas and even scientific institutions enters into the narrative only secondarily, in a supporting role, and even the popular history of ideas is incidental; other scholars have offered and will offer much more exhaustive histories of popularization than this one. But all scholars working on the subject have in mind a particular phenomenon. Even at best, the ideas in popularization were by definition relatively simple, and philosophical coherence on a modern technical level is not relevant. I have therefore tried to treat the popularizers fairly, in their own terms, and in terms of their context, American culture.

Readers should find the themes of this essay familiar. Generations of thinkers have recognized the difference between popularized science that is "interesting" and that which is amazing and was for a long time known as "Gee Whiz!" science. Interesting science fits into a general world view and extends one's vision. Gee Whiz! science excites irrelevant emotions but does not extend one's horizons nor disturb one's mysticisms with a reasoned viewpoint. In fact, it may reinforce them. And popularization of either kind of science, interesting or Gee Whiz!, turns out to be intimately connected with the struggle between enlightenment and superstition.

As the narrative that follows reveals, then, it is an error to read back into the past the idea that we can reduce the traditional formulation of scientific enlightenment versus superstition to an amusing and insignificant cliché. For a century and a half, regardless of the terms that were used, the struggle between science and superstition—even in its later, largely masked form—was an important determinant of American culture. Assembling main lines of evidence, and particularly reports from generations of observers and participants, helps explain the haunting paradox of how that culture ended up so little influenced by science when the products of both the natural and health sciences so profoundly shaped everyday life and great events alike.

The main lines of evidence are patterns in popularizing that lead to a conceptualization of events that is resolved only in the concluding chapter. The chronological eras so fundamental to my account are based not so much upon the content of popularization but upon who the popularizers were, what they were trying to do, the forms that they employed, and the institutions through which they had to work. It is a complicated story, but I found that however textured the detail, the patterns still showed through.

Although popularization of science and health began only in the nineteenth century, as I shall explain in the first chapter, it had a distinct and identifiable history from the beginning. Therefore I present three separate narratives of the popularization of health, psychology, and the natural sciences, not only to establish the remarkable parallels between them but also to show the coherence of the history with which I am concerned. In each area the tension between science and superstition evolved in a pattern that in the actual events serves to suggest the full meaning and complexity as well as the validity of my thesis. So, too, do events suggest how persistent, if intricate, was the meaning of science in the realm of popularization as well as the many-layered way in which the functions of superstition moved from folk beliefs to artifacts of the consumer culture.

The bulk of my narrative concerns the ways in which popularizers attempted to adapt to changing cultural conditions. It was these attempts, as I show in chapters 2 through 5, that form a coherent story. But the story also shows that transmission of knowledge was never neutral. From the narrative and the patterns in it emerge conclusions and explanations that also form a unit and in so doing show how superstition won. The patterns, as I have suggested, lead to a series of conclusions:

In the traditional struggle between science and superstition, scientific naturalism and reductionism on the popular level contained a definite negative program against error.

This negative program against error was particularly effective in the last part of the nineteenth century but during the twentieth century became attenuated and derailed.

The reason that superstition was able to win was that the form that it took changed, and hardly anyone recognized it for what it was.

The new form that superstition took appeared as the standards of the world of journalism and advertising or what came to be known as the media.

The media world was nonnaturalistic and like superstition was actively competitive with the traditional world of popularized science.

In the media world the elements of sensationalism and disjointed segmentation of information were exactly the elements of superstition that earlier popularizers of science had attacked with skepticism and naturalism.

So completely did the new obscurantism of sensationalism and isolated fact dominate the media world that magical thinking and even conventional superstition were widely tolerated.

Scientists who believed in science as a calling rather than an occupation tended increasingly to withdraw from popularizing during the twentieth century, leaving the field to media personnel and educators.

In America's specialized society, specialists in popularizing, chiefly journalists, increasingly took over the function of presenting science to lay audiences.

Except in clearly labeled consumer or environmentalist crusades, the insensitivity of mid-twentieth-century popularizers to commercial interest and exploitation represented a major departure from traditional popularization and opposition to error and superstitious authority.

Nineteenth-century proponents of a scientific outlook assumed that their message was moral as well as intellectual. They linked belief in natural order with a lifestyle emphasizing service and self-denial as well as the courageous pursuit of reality. The confrontation between science and superstition therefore had aspects of cultural conflict. Indeed, one of the persistent problems of popularizers has been mobilizing the forces of curiosity to overcome the pain of the effort that understanding requires. The world of consumer culture, as recent historians of the subject have emphasized, involved self-indulgence, most transparently in the world of advertising. In that world, the intellectual aspects of popular science did not flourish. In the sense that most audiences of the popularizers chose a self-indulgent approach to the world, Americans willingly capitulated to the new superstition. But the agents of the world of the media were not just passive. Like the leaders of superstition in bygone centuries, they were attempting to assert their authority against the authority and world view of the popularizers of a reductionistic-rationalistic science.

It would be less than candid not to admit that what I found as I looked at the record of popularizing surprised me. In this book I shall carry my readers through the same series of discoveries that I made, starting with health and psychology and proceeding through the natural sciences, exploring the changes in institutions, in personnel, and in content of what was always known as popularizing.

But in the first chapter, which follows immediately, I also share another discovery: little has been written to develop the background that my narrative requires. The history of superstition is available only in the most fragmentary way, and scholarship on the recent periods, which would help conceptualize that part of my subject, is in disarray. Popularization is also a field little tilled, and the few modern treatments of the popularization of science are scattered and unsystematic. I start out, therefore, with an exploration of three difficult concepts: popularization, superstition, and, at least in a preliminary way, science. Popularizing, as I have suggested, in itself renders clean, philosophical definition and conceptualization irrelevant, and much of the book consists in fact of an attempt to show what in practice science—as well as popularization and superstition—meant in American culture. It is in the absence of the usual support from the literature that I have gathered together in the opening chapter enough historical background to launch my narrative. That background includes my fundamental finding that the struggle against superstition was an integral part of the act of popularizing science.

Chapter 1
Superstition and the Popularizing of Science

IN THE LATE nineteenth and early twentieth centuries, science took on a special meaning in American public discourse. With evangelical enthusiasm, many "men of science," as they were called, attempted to popularize a positivistic, reductionistic view of the natural world—and of human beings.[1] In popularizing, they not only had positive content to teach but typically viewed their mission in terms of the negative program to which I have alluded in the introduction. What they opposed was superstition and fanatical mysticism, belief in which produced consequences that were socially and morally undesirable.

For a number of decades, the fervent disciples of science carried with them—to a substantial extent—parts of the intelligent and influential American public. To stand for science did carry social and moral meaning, along with a world view, or what people then often called, somewhat grandly, "a philosophy of life."[2] This book is an exploration of how that Victorian tour de force in popularization of science gradually gave way to the recrudescence of superstition and mysticism in a new guise in the consumer culture. In the course of that change, what it meant to be a scientist changed, and what the act of popularizing meant changed also—to a large extent without anyone's having noticed it.

Contemporary Superstition

Few Americans of the late twentieth century doubted that superstition was effectively dead in their modern secular society. Even earlier in the

9

century, serious discussions of superstition were classified under "folk-lore"—that is, some quaint and unthreatening beliefs restricted to primitives, either those who lived abroad or those sheltered in some colorful side eddy of a tolerant and pluralistic culture.

Social scientists of a few decades ago documented with empirical research the decline of superstition. College students, for example, in 1925 showed a high rate of superstitious misconception, an average of over 30 percent believing in one list of common notions. But as early as 1952 only 6.5 percent among a comparable group showed belief, and the basis for many of these traditional ideas, such as those left over from phrenology or those passed on as someone's experience, had simply disappeared. The survey showed that students no longer believed, for example, that "certain lines in a person's hand foretell his future."[3] Such ideas, which represent conventional superstition, now belonged to the past.

There was, of course, the so-called occult revival of the 1960s and 1970s, featuring astrology, witchcraft and satanism, parapsychology, and Eastern mysticism. Under the microscope of the sociologist, however, the occult revival as a serious resurgence of superstition simply evaporates.[4] The occult turned out to be largely a playful interest, the practitioners contemptuous equally of science and religion so that they could freely kid around with either or both. Moreover, the death of conventional superstition is easily demonstrated by the following thought experiment. Generations earlier, a story that a house was haunted would have caused people in the area to avoid it fearfully. In recent times, such a rumor would have attracted people to see if they could flush out and tease the spirits. Despite the tendency of so-called witches and other occult believers to organize, real credulity of the traditional variety had ceased to be important.[5]

The overt superstitions that persisted among educated young people also changed in nature. Very likely in their new guise these superstitions may have had a prevalence comparable to those of earlier days. But, again, actual beliefs were not as serious as those of previous times, for the new ones tended to be explanations of bad luck, rather than attempts to control good luck, and they were personal, rather than general for the group—a particular piece of one's clothing, say, rather than the weather. Altogether the challenge to objective scientific laws was greatly muted, so much so that for practical purposes science appeared to be safe in a context no more momentous than a sheepish affection for a lucky scarf.[6]

That superstition in the sense of witchcraft, magic, and charms was no longer potent in the late twentieth century is therefore a fact altogether easily documented. Superstition as opposed to science, however—that is, superstition in the sense of a broader mysticism and unhealthy credulity—raises other questions. The term generally covers much more than specific magical folk beliefs; rather, thinkers have used "superstition" to stand for a whole set of phenomena that are exactly what science, ideally, is not, including bigotry, prejudice, and indoctrination, as well as mystery and personal manipulation of occult forces and, in general, exaggeration of the importance and power of subjective thoughts and feelings. It was only as part of another antiscientific movement, therefore, that the inconsistent foolish beliefs of the occult revival may have had any substantial significance in the culture.[7]

Functional Superstition

In the 1920s Bronislaw Malinowski pointed out that superstition and magic are functional in a society, and other sociologists have added that any magic will therefore stand until some stronger magic replaces it. Because primitive beliefs are functional, they maintain themselves and are hard to displace.[8] In American society, then, as in any society, the struggle between superstition and science has been fierce only when the one threatened the function of the other—which is, once more, not the case with lucky scarves.

Shifting the perspective to functional superstition, or superstitious thinking (not to mention even more undisciplined magical thinking), shows how, despite appearances and reassurances, the forces of obscurantism and darkness were not dead in the United States of the late twentieth century. Most Americans, for example, treated technology as if it were magic. Indeed, the mechanical way in which an action can bring about a result is a distinguishing feature of magic. The magical or miraculous nature of each technological and medical innovation appeared in the rhetoric of advertising, to say nothing of journalism. As early as 1922, Chester H. Rowell referred to "the daily miracle of the applications of physical science," and he went on to observe, "We accept these wonders, not because they are reasonable, but precisely because they are magical."[9] In print or film or life, the person who pushed a button did not have to know why the subsequent event occurred, whether it was obliterating a city with an atomic weapon or starting a motor. For generations, children typically grew up throwing switches without any way of thinking other than the magical to explain what happened. In an age of mass media and advertising (see chapter 6), most people did not have any occasion to advance further, to seek a level of explanation more advanced than the magical, that is, explanations that would be on some level natural. Technology may have been manmade magic, but mystery still effectively supervened. A person did not need to know how a frying pan lining came to have certain nonstick properties in order for the person to have a naive faith that if one paid the price, the vessel was charmed by a wizard in a white coat in some factory. So removed was technology from comprehension that large parts of the population read or watched various grades of science fiction, a genre in much of which old-fashioned fairy stories were reissued with mysterious elements reincarnated with technical names.

It is true, of course, that routinization of technological miracles removed them from the category of active magical thinking, although the potential always remained. But technology was not, historically, the aspect of civilization that battled against superstition. That honor belonged to science, and particularly to the popularization of science.

The Warfare of Science against Religion

In the late nineteenth century and for some decades after, educated Americans conceptualized the battle in terms of the warfare between religion and science, rather than between superstition and science. In recent years, some historians have tried to show that no such warfare existed, essentially on the grounds that science and good religion did and do not conflict and that the forces on either side were themselves divided.[10] In the actualities of popularized science in the United States, however, science and at least parts of religion were in conflict. "The antagonism between Science and Religion has become a commonplace of literature," observed psychologist James Thompson Bixby in 1876. In 1907 a writer in the *American Catholic Quarterly Review* could still state with assurance, "The new spirit of scientific inquiry . . . looks upon religion much as a cat does upon a dog, as its natural enemy." Psychologist Horace B. English as late as 1926 identified the problem as a clash of epistemologies and testified,

"The conflict between science and religion is real." Many other observers of the public arena regretted the conflict, but they never doubted that it existed.[11]

Combatants on each side fought in print and in the lecture hall for the loyalty of the reading and thinking public, and the correspondence of leading publicists of the earlier period such as E. L. Youmans is filled with accounts of actual verbal confrontations with religious figures, particularly outside of the larger cities. As late as 1958 in the face of antivivisection and antifluoridation campaigns, among others, the president of the Ohio Academy of Science repeated the traditional formulation: "We have often read about the war between religion and science. If viewed in an objective way, it has been rather the intolerance of man of new ideas, the opposition of a fixed medieval theology to a growing and changing science."[12]

In the last decades of the nineteenth century, two Americans, John W. Draper and Andrew D. White, actually wrote accounts of this warfare, classic histories that were known and discussed on both sides of the Atlantic and which bear much responsibility for the perpetuation of the "military metaphor." They and their antecedents help reveal how in the warfare between science and the forces of obscurantism, religion and superstition became confusingly entangled on the same side, setting the stage for advertising to co-opt this entire complex in the age of the mass media.[13]

Development of a Naturalistic Viewpoint

In ancient times, it was common for thinkers to explain events by invoking magic. The first noticeable change in the West came in the eighth century B.C., when Hesiod provided a sustained explanation that did not include magic. Subsequently, in a similar set of explanations, the pre-Socratic Milesian philosophers left out the gods. To later people, these philosophers' accounts of why thunderstorms and earthquakes occurred seemed quite as fantastic as other sixth- and seventh-century B.C. explanations that did involve gods and magic, but the Milesians introduced a new force that explained why things happened, namely, nature—a nature, moreover, that was not capricious. Although nature, that new force, was therefore merely competitive in explanatory power with traditional religion, the idea of natural causes nevertheless grew apace. Chroniclers of these events almost invariably cite, as the clearest example, the down-to-earth observation from the Hippocratic treatise on epilepsy, the sacred disease, "It is thus with regard to the disease called Sacred: it appears to me to be nowise more divine nor more sacred than other diseases, but has a natural cause from which it originates like other affections." [14] Here, in classical times, was a paradigmatic opposition: skeptics, inspired by a belief in naturalistic explanation, cast doubt on common, typically magical, notions, and the arena of discussion was, then, that of popular belief.

Religion per se was not necessarily unfriendly to natural explanation and the rationalism that came to accompany it. In the coming religion of late classical times, Christianity, the Bible condoned prophecy, it is true, but at the same time the Bible interdicted spells and charms. Moreover, the Christians developed a rational theology, and as they tried to convert all of Europe to their beliefs, institutional representatives necessarily found that they had to supplant all local gods, magic, and superstition.

Practical realities in an expanding church, however, to some extent subverted the consistent rationality of theology. Church officials started out forbidding local beliefs and practices, but what happened instead was that magic and superstition, rather than being prohibited, were often absorbed into church practices, and fine points of theology were forgotten in the haste to appeal to simple folk and attract souls into the church. This practical dilution of rationality proceeded to the point that when the Protestant Reformation began, the Protestants could and did separate religion and superstition sharply and attacked the Roman church for the superstitious and magical elements that had crept in over the centuries. By the seventeenth century, both the Roman and the reformed churchmen were trying to purify their domains by rooting out paganism in general, and superstition in particular. And this last development took place, of course, just as science was acquiring a distinctive identity. [15]

The Protestants had an advantage because they were already riding the crest of a popular movement, a from-the-bottom-up skepticism concerning sacraments and other ecclesiastical events—until, in Leslie Stephen's words, "Protestantism inevitably became a screen for rationalism." Americans of the seventeenth and eighteenth centuries worked within a Protestant tradition, and they found that Protestantism, especially that tinged with Calvinism, offered a God who could not be bought or controlled by a person's actions. Superstition had no place in such a system, for theologians held that God's providence determined every event, leaving no role for either chance or magic. By 1820, according to James Turner, Americans largely believed not in an unpredictable Jehovah but in a natural-law God. And they were joined by skeptics, who could chime in with the preachers in citing vulnerable places in Roman practices. This unwitting alliance between skepticism and Protestantism lasted into the nineteenth century and beyond in the United States.[16]

Early Protestants of course carried a large burden of credulousness themselves, and everyone knows about New England witchcraft, at the least. But in the New World, medieval and Renaissance superstitions and outdated sciences did not flourish as well as in the Old World, and social and religious leaders were relatively successful in the eighteenth century in smothering out both superstition and other outmoded beliefs that were competitive with either rational religion or rational science.[17] The major liability of Protestantism was a popular stream of literal Biblicism that in the nineteenth century often elicited the label of superstitious dogma.

This venerable cultural context clarifies the significance of the so-called warfare between science and religion in the United States. It was the accretion of superstitious practice and the way that it persisted conspicuously in parts of Europe that provided a factual basis upon which the two nineteenth-century Protestants Draper and White concentrated when they used the military metaphor. Draper was concerned especially with the civil and social power of ecclesiastics, whom he portrayed as figures protecting and expanding their influence among the credulous. White, who was concerned with all "dogmatic theology," targeted particularly obscurantist practices and extravagant statements of literal Biblicists. Both authors favored rationalism and freedom of inquiry, and both cited Galileo and Darwin as martyrs to conservative, traditional, and generally dogmatic religionists who when not overtly superstitious at least allied themselves with the forces of magic, legend, anti-intellectualism, and obscurantism. For practical purposes on a popular level, magic, legend, anti-intellectualism, superstition, and obscurantism were all one to positivistic thinkers of the late nineteenth century. Some of this mindset was suggested by the neurologist William A. Hammond in 1883 when he noted that despite an "inherent tendency in the mind of man to ascribe to supernatural agencies those events the causes of which are beyond his knowledge . . . ,[yet] as his intellect becomes more thoroughly trained, and as science advances in its developments, the range of his credulity becomes more and more circumscribed, his doubts are multiplied, and he at length reaches that condition of 'healthy skepticism' which allows of no belief without the proof." [18]

Skeptics

Popular partisans of science in this way came to draw on both a positive skepticism, that is, one based on natural forces, and a negative skepticism. [19] In every society, some individuals are more credulous than others. In the West, even in the eras and areas most dominated by magic, superstition, and witchcraft, certain individuals scoffed more or less openly at the faith that set the tone for the local culture. Some knew, for example, how unjust was trial by combat, how silly the charms. By the sixteenth century, Sir Philip Sidney could say succinctly as well as frankly of the soothsayers employed by members of the upper class, "Of these Soothsayers very few say sooth." [20]

All of this skepticism grew over the centuries, as has been suggested, and disbelievers often spoke out, so that by the late nineteenth and early twentieth centuries, popular science writers could cite a whole pantheon of heroes who had held out against witchcraft, like Weyer, or advocated rationalism in science and medicine, like Bacon and Harvey. A late-twentieth-century specialist in systematic doubt summarized the stance: "Skepticism is not, despite much popular misconception, a point of view. It is, instead, an essential component of intellectual inquiry, a method of determining the facts whatever they may be and wherever they may lead. It is part of what we call common sense. It is a part of the way science works." [21]

Skeptics flourished especially in the Enlightenment, when a number of able thinkers produced literary works embodying disbelief and doubt, works that continue to be delightful to read. This genre flourished not only in the world of Rabelais and Montaigne but in that of Hobbes, and in the New World as well. Elihu Palmer, for example, who in the late eighteenth century was dismissed from two American pulpits because of his Deist beliefs, sought truth "upon the ground of evidence, and not of authority," observing that "there is more honor, and much more utility in the relinquishment, than in the retention of errors." [22]

Palmer was an able forerunner of Victorian-era skeptics such as Robert Ingersoll and Mark Twain, whose functional descendants continued to insist that science provided a better basis for morals than did religion. "One of the most striking phenomena of the nineteenth century," noted biologist Albert P. Mathews of the University of Chicago in 1909, "was the great rise of science and the loosening of religious ties coincident with a marked improvement in general morality." It was such moralistic skeptics as these who were as capable of fervor as any religionist.[23]

If religion set the tone, still the Enlightenment skeptics set the terms within which American popularizers of science contended against superstition. A particular contribution of Enlightenment writers was their connecting undesirable emotionalism, usually called fanaticism, with credulity. Condillac spoke cautiously of fanaticism as the "enthusiasm of one who substitutes or adds his own visions to the true spirit of religion," and in the *Encyclopédie* Jaucourt noted that "even atheism . . . never destroys natural feelings, never attacks either the laws or customs of a people. . . . An atheist values public order out of the love of his own tranquility; but fanatical *superstition* overturns empires.[24]

The most famous Enlightenment skeptic, Voltaire, expressed in his writings the concepts and values that identified superstition and made it reprehensible and even socially deviant, and in America later generations followed such thinking in condemning superstition because (1) superstition involved defective reasoning about the natural or inexplicable; (2) for reasons of cupidity, self-interest, and profit, certain people (and Voltaire tended to include priestcraft of all kinds) encouraged superstitious belief; and (3) superstition represented the surrender of a whole point of view, that is, rationalism, with the implication that the standards of the emotional, unreasonable, even fanatical masses might triumph and destroy civilization as well as "overturn empires."[25] To these elements—hardheaded truthfulness, condemnation of exploiters of credulity, and fear of unreason—opponents of superstition generally added one more characteristic of their stance: opposition to, or at least ambivalence toward, authority. It was this skepticism about authority that was so strikingly missing when the authority lay in advertising and the mass media in the mid-twentieth century and after.

Authority

In any culture, superstition involves the idea that some assertion has validity. In the United States in the late nineteenth century, the person who asserted the truth of a superstition typically learned that truth from a parent or other authority figure. By the mid-twentieth century, however, the authorities for such superstitious belief as there was overwhelmingly consisted of television and peers.[26] This pattern was not merely that of the United States in modern times; in all ages there was, first, the authority of the source and, second, the fact that the belief received no reinforcement from a logically systematic context.[27] Because a superstition was and is an isolated belief, without systematic relation to other beliefs, authority was (and is) necessary to bolster it. And, further, to be against superstition can mean opposing not only beliefs but also the authority supporting the beliefs, as in Voltaire's contending that people supported credulity for dishonorable reasons; indeed, argument against superstition quickly tends to become ad hominem.

The position of superstition with regard to authority can therefore become complex. Given that the basis for superstition is authority, as opposed to reason or system, isolation distinguishes superstitious belief, whether it is isolated from a theological framework or a scientific one. But when one or both of those rationalistic frameworks, science or rational theology, is dominant in a society, superstition will then represent dissent, or even rebelliousness, as it may have in early medieval times and as it did in the late twentieth century. The American critic Theodore Roszak, for example, found in 1980 "a vast popular culture . . . still deeply entangled with piety, mystery, miracle, the search for personal salvation," a popular culture dissenting from the dominant "secular humanist establishment." The assault in the 1960s and 1970s on the social position of professionals involved both what Roszak referred to as "hunger for wonders" and an angry warfare against a whole style of life in which rationalism and science were inextricably associated with the upper part of the social hierarchy and with civilized behavior. Civilized upper-class people of course embodied the authority that held mysticism and superstition to be ways of thinking "which are not in accord with natural phenomena," as one 1932 formulation had it.[28] The playful nature of the occult revival of recent decades obviously accords well, too, with the suggestion that modern occultists' motives tended as much toward opposing authority as supporting thoroughgoing mysticism.

One of the major elements in the attempts of advocates of both theology and science to suppress magic and pseudoscience was therefore the clash for which there were venerable antecedents, indeed, a universal pattern. Whereas church fathers opposing superstition in seventeenth-century France, for example, were defending Aristotle and orderly thinking, within a century David Hume in England was expressing his contempt for popular supernaturalism by noting that philosophy was "the sovereign antidote to superstition and false religion."[29] Well before the nineteenth century, then, innumerable examples confirm that superstition rested upon sources of authority that were either not dominant or that opponents of superstition were attempting to undermine or discredit. That is, either superstition deviated from dominant social standards, or the enemies of superstition tried to label superstitious beliefs socially deviant.[30]

Superstition as Deviant

By the nineteenth and twentieth centuries, opponents of superstition regularly described credulous people in conventional terms that signaled a different and inferior status, typically, as noted above, exotic, weak, or primitive (perhaps in an earlier stage of intellectual and spiritual evolution). Thus the author of a zoology textbook of the 1920s, Horatio Hackett Newman, patronizingly noted, "We must not judge [the ancient] forefathers of zoology too harshly, however, for they were beginners, and in many ways, scientifically speaking, mere children. All of their ideas were beclouded by superstition, legend, and folklore. In this respect they were in no way different from the mass of unscientific-minded people today." Typically, credulity was associated with a low place in the social hierarchy; only the ignorant and contemptible held such crude beliefs. So a physician in 1916 connected faith in quack cures with "an unwholesome fear of God and the unseen" and "a heathenish conception of religion" that bred credulity. Or superstition represented anachronism or primitivism, either discarded belief or belief by people who had not yet progressed to civilization. Or, finally, it was childish and immature. An educator, Fletcher Dresslar, in 1907 characterized superstitions as "remnants of our psychic evolution," the result of "child-like conclusions." Social scientists in the twentieth century found that rural children tended to be more superstitious than their presumably more advanced urban equivalents. Finally, in addition to identifying superstitious belief with what was deemed lower-class, primitive, childish, backward, and uncivilized, writers came to connect magical thinking with pathological psychological processes, symptomatic of the other kind of social deviance, illness. Thus a writer of 1889 who acknowledged that superstitions still existed in the scientific age referred to such "superstitious beliefs and usages which are *in* our day but not *of* it."[31]

The low social status attributed to superstition ironically gave rise in the late nineteenth and early twentieth centuries to a phenomenon that bedeviled the fight against superstition in the popular arena: journalists found it newsworthy, in the traditional man-bites-dog formulation, to note any occasion on which a high-status person followed folk superstition: whenever a businessman or teacher or political or social leader indulged in charms or the occult or even the mystical, the story appeared prominently in the media, confounding the best efforts of reasonable people to discredit such notions, particularly when a major technique was to discredit them as socially unacceptable in the modern world. Members of the press in 1930, for example, were obviously delighted when the postmaster general refused to walk under a ladder.[32]

Twentieth-century opponents of superstition found in their own experiences concrete justification for their view that superstition represented a primitive stage in human social development. They succeeded, in fact, in showing how it was possible to use education to eradicate superstitious ideas, that is, to cause children, at least, to become more civilized and mature—and mentally healthy. Indeed, scientific progress was recapitulated in the experience. Dresslar in 1907 believed that "education must not stop short of the habit of scientific method and scientific feeling. A student at work in a laboratory learns soon that nature tells no falsehood and that her laws are inexorable." Within a few years, other educators were showing in experiments that both laboratory and textbook teaching were effective in "the elimination of superstition"—that is, both the substitution of a new authority (the textbook) and teaching scientific method by demonstration (the better magic) worked, and the students were protected from error.[33]

In all eras, campaigns to label superstition socially unacceptable and to substitute a new authority opened the door for skeptics and advocates of naturalistic explanation to extend their list of publicly discredited authorities—including theologies. When at the turn of the seventeenth century Francis Bacon set out a program for modern science, he utilized the Renaissance tradition of doubting authority not only to question superstition but to question even scholasticism and religion. Enlightenment skeptics continued to delight in lumping mysticism and superstition together and then tying both to almost any religion. Religionists therefore found that their opposition to superstition could be dangerous. Every Victorian village atheist knew that confusing superstition with all religion—that is, declaring religiosity to be as deviant as credulity—was an easy way to win an argument. "The Christian of to-day," wrote the famous agnostic Robert Ingersoll in 1890, "wonders at the savage who bowed before his idol; and yet it must be confessed that the god of stone answered prayer and protected his worshipers precisely as the Christian's God answers prayer and protects his worshipers to-day."[34]

When the warfare between science and religion was declared overtly, in those terms, in the late nineteenth century, the outcome remained in doubt. But by the 1920s, according to contemporary journalist Frederick Lewis Allen, the authority of science was dominant. Allen quoted the great liberal preacher Harry Emerson Fosdick:

> Is it scientific? That question has searched religion for contraband goods, stripped it of old superstitions, forced it to change its categories of thought and methods of work, and in general has so cowed and scared religion that many modern-minded believers. . . instinctively throw up their hands at the mere whisper of it. . . . When a prominent scientist comes out strongly for religion, all the churches thank Heaven and take courage as though it were the highest possible compliment to God to have [astronomer Arthur] Eddington believe in Him. Science has become the arbiter of this generation's thought, until to call even a prophet and a seer scientific is to cap the climax of praise.[35]

This is striking testimony about changing authority among the well educated, but, as will become evident below, in the field of popularization, religion was a distraction. Superstition continued to be the real issue because it helped to define, in a negative way, what "science" stood for. A rational theology did not.

The Religion of Science

The aggressive campaign against superstition that flourished in the United States for a century before World War II was distinctive. In 1939, for example, there was a "Maze of Superstitions" at the New York World's Fair, so set up that fairgoers literally as well as symbolically got lost if they took a wrong turn on the basis of choosing any of a series of common false beliefs in the field of health.[36] Where, in the seventeenth century, leaders of both religion and science had fought ignorant credulity, in the wake of the later Enlightenment the battle, as has been suggested, was secularized, and the forces of science tried to preempt all rational belief and hold the field alone against the forces of darkness. Especially after the Darwinian controversies began in the 1860s, literal Biblicism helped push many religious groups into alliance with obscurantism, particularly as the legions of science enjoyed some popular success and pressed their claims more boldly in attempting to win all of the public. As the entomologist Roger C. Smith observed in 1920, "Prevalence of natural history super-stitions and misinformation in countries and communities is in inverse ratio to the amount of reading" done by the inhabitants.[37]

The partisans of science were identifiable to a substantial degree. They were largely scientists themselves, or amateurs who would in that day pass as scientists. Not all, or even most, of the scientific population en-listed directly in the open warfare against superstition and ignorance; they found that just "doing science" took most of their energies. But in large part the ranks of combatants were filled by men, and sometimes women, who knew the laboratory or the field first-hand, or who, at the very least, taught scientific subjects.[38]

In the nineteenth century, as will be described below, educated people all over the United States for decades heard the most prominent scien-tists, even Louis Agassiz himself, explaining the natural world in natu-ralistic terms—sometimes in a pious context, but with explanations that were, for their day, scientific. These same leaders of science and medicine wrote for the periodical press and published popular books. Frequently newspapers published verbatim transcriptions of entire lecture series, or, at the least, extensive summaries. It has been customary to comment on this extraordinary propensity of American scientists of that century to popularize science. In the necessary complexity of human affairs, many issues were involved, some connected to popularization as such. But the most dynamic conditioning factor was the zeal engendered by the reli-gion of science, as it has been called. The full formation of this new faith occurred rapidly in the late nineteenth century. Already well launched, as Lincoln C. Blake has pointed out, within a generation after the founding of the Johns Hopkins University graduate programs in 1876, the "scientific spirit" had seized the bulk of leading American scientific thinkers. They sought the truth themselves, and as "investigators" acted also as spiritual leaders, turning piety into "character" and "righteousness," which worked out in practical terms as "service"—service that included proselytizing the public as well as working as scientists. This vocabulary came of course from commonplace theological discourse of that time.[39]

For several decades in the nineteenth century, as will be discussed further in chapter 4, most Americans assumed that science reinforced their religion and the commonsense philosophy that went with it. Virtually all scientists and other well-educated people were at least nominally pious, and one of the major reasons that they gave for studying science was that it confirmed religious truths. The author of a children's geography and astronomy book published in 1818, for example, described the immensity of the universe and then noted "the greatness, the wisdom, and power of that Almighty Being who has created, preserves and governs this universe of worlds."[40] But about the time of the Civil War, these pious assumptions began to disappear from popularized science. In their place the religion of science flourished.

The religion of science consisted of an informal set of beliefs that filled followers with evangelical fervor. They thereupon attempted to convert both individuals and the public at large. Their enthusiasm and their approach were taken, as already noted, from Protestant evangelism. These enthusiasts had their martyrs to superstition—Copernicus, Galileo, Servetus, and, later on, the victims of antievolutionary churchmen. Moreover, the apostles had visible forces of evil with which to contend: superstition, ignorance, and, now, added in accordance with Anglo-American liberal political traditions, intolerance—since scientific findings presumably could stand up to any opinion. The goal of the evangelicals of the religion of science was to bring enlightenment by exposing everyone to the truth, that is, by popularizing science. They talked openly of "converting" people, especially after Darwinism came along. Given the religious upbringing of almost all of the American adherents, the religious parallels were not merely a metaphor but conveyed the style and manner of the evangelicals. Most of what did differ was merely the content.[41]

The religion of science was therefore, as A. Hunter Dupree points out, a Christian heresy. Such an interpretation recognizes both the Protestant background and the stream of naturalism that constituted a competitive explanatory, or religious, belief from the pre-Socratics to the Enlightenment. But in the nineteenth century the fundamentally negative element in naturalistic explanation became more prominent and characteristic.[42] In 1875, for instance, Howard N. Brown, a Unitarian minister, preached a sermon to his congregation at Brookline, Massachusetts, in which he underlined the negative animus of the followers of the religion of science. He knew, said Brown, that "the superstitions which the world has had most need to dread have sprung from too great assurance in what was thought to be known of God." But, he went on,

> there is a rapidly growing class both in point of numbers and influence which, in setting itself free from the superstitions of the past, is giving up all pretensions of either knowing or believing anything about God. . . . Among the young men who are being educated at our universities, Herbert Spencer, Mill, and that class of writers are in authority; . . . very generally, among cultivated people, the "positive" tendency of thought is uppermost.[43]

Of course many Americans retained some religious ideas, whether "modernism" or a late-nineteenth-century version of Deism. But the skeptics, after centuries underground, finally were having their day. Where once proscience theology had been an ally of science, now it, too, became an object of attack. In 1867, for example, Charles W. Eliot, who was then a young chemist, was delighted to find in a popularization by Herschel that "the inventive genius of the Creator never receives laudatory mention, the intentions of the Disposer of All are never appreciatively alluded to, and no surprise is ever expressed that God allows this thing or that thing to happen or exist. It is," Eliot went on, "a relief to find a new familiar treatise on scientific subjects which is accurate and logical, and free from the flippant semi-religious sentimentalism which mars so many of the popular books on such subjects." By 1901, Herbert Casson could write, "The best cure for mysticism is fresh air, exercise, bromide of potassium, comic opera and the study of popular scientific and economic books."[44]

The Program of the Religion of Science

As has been suggested, what the proscience forces opposed highlighted the positive elements that were implicit in their aspirations. Nineteenth-century figures did uphold Enlightenment values—faith in reason, suspicion of exploitation, and trust in civilization—that constituted the legacy of Voltaire's critique of superstition. But by the Victorian period, the superstition that science spokespersons opposed had been expanded by a further set of formulations with positive implications.

Victorian science advocates opposed mystery—superstition, of course, but also any supernatural explanation, especially when the explanation aroused fear and other undesirable emotions.[45] Not only reason, then, but demonstration took on the positive values. The paradigmatic victory against mystery was Benjamin Franklin's demonstration that lightning was electrical in nature and, therefore, rather than controlled by arbitrary and fearsome forces, was subject to the regularity of natural law. E. P. Evans in 1895, for example, referred to "the marvelous discoveries of modern science, whose achievements rival the annals of credulity in their appeals to the imagination, and render the visible and invisible forces of Nature, once a terror of man, now a tributary to his happiness."[46]

Scholasticism was a second ally of superstition, just as Bacon had suggested, for scholasticism stood not only for empty theory, contrary to fact, but for authority without an empirical basis. American thinkers in the nineteenth century openly invoked Baconianism, and well-read people recognized by that term the idea that facts gathered and arranged would lead to concrete and reliable generalizations, in contrast to both mystery and theory. John Wesley Powell, former head of the United States Geological Survey, wrote in 1896 that "the history of science is the history of the discovery of the simple and the true; in its progress illusions are dispelled and certitudes remain."[47] This empiricism was reflected in the twentieth-century term "unfounded beliefs," a category broader than superstition but including it.

Another negative term in the preachments of the science popularizers was "dogma." This term suggested two targets. The first was the rigid resistance of literal Biblicists to any change in their world view. The second was dogmatic persons' persecution of innovative thinkers. What the partisans of science advocated, then, in a positive way, was "open-mindedness," or at least tolerance—the Anglo-American virtue. Closely allied with dogma was conservatism in the realm of ideas; both stood in the way of progress. All that the scientists and their allies asked was a fair hearing; like all minority religious groups who for centuries had pleaded for toleration, they believed that if they could but present the truth, they would win.

Belief in progress had special relevance to superstition, particularly because on the popular level the way that protagonists of science measured progress was by the extent to which "science" had superseded credulity. The premier popularizer of science in the 1920s, Edwin E. Slosson, expressed in Voltairean terms the urgency of keeping up:

> Hunt out and destroy with great care every old rag of superstition, for these are liable at any time to start that spontaneous combustion of ideas we call fanaticism. . . . A little decaying superstition in the mind of a great man has been known to conflagrate a nation. . . . Go systematically through your intellectual equipment and see wherein it is deficient. Pick up each one of the sciences where you left off at school and bring it down to date. . . . This inspection of one's stock of ideas is necessary because they do not keep as if they were in cold storage.[48]

In their haste to adopt the new, evangelists in the religious wars of science encountered a particular difficulty: one of the major sources of outworn dogma and even superstition was yesterday's science, including such items as humoral physiology and alchemy. In 1883, the editor of *Science* complained that "camp-followers of the scientific army" traded upon the authority engendered by the wonders of science, which "accomplishes every day feats that witches, ghosts, and magicians performed only upon rare occasions. . . . It is curious to see how those, who, a generation or two ago, would have been the believers in witchcraft and all things 'supernatural,' are now turning to be caught in the toils of scientific charlantry [*sic*]." The solution that the editor offered for this deplorable corruption of popularization was more of the new "objective and experimental" teaching then coming in, in which students learned to judge—and doubt—for themselves. Half a century later, the same problem and the same solution surfaced at a meeting of adult education science specialists who advocated "the education of every individual in the essentials of natural science so that he may become his own critical authority. Lacking such education . . . , we are facing a new age of superstition and a new priesthood in which science is taking the place of the older dogmas."[49] Most people enlisted in the popular battles on behalf of scientific progress did not distinguish clearly between common misconceptions, outworn beliefs, and superstition, but they did know that the problem of error made it urgent that popularizers of science themselves know the latest findings.

Altogether this program, Enlightenment reason, altruism, and civilization, now supplemented by demonstration, appeal to facts, open-mindedness, and belief in progress, would have worked well for a skeptic in any age. But in the late nineteenth century most such skeptics also believed in the heretical and naturalistic religion of science. To spread the word of the religion of science in the Victorian era, from England came scientist-evangelists John Tyndall and Thomas Henry Huxley, not only by way of their writings but in person.[50] In addition, beginning in the 1850s, as large numbers of American physicians and scientists studied in Germany and were exposed there to classic materialism, reductionism, and positivism, these strains, too, showed up in all levels of proselytizing for the religion of science. In 1899, for instance, two Illinois educators quoted two German-language authors for the aim of science teaching in grades one to four: "The aim is to open up to a pupil an understanding of the present and to find thereby a frank and all-sided philosophical view of the world, founded upon reality and truth. Nature should not present to man the appearance of an inextricable chaos but that of a well-ordered mechanism, . . . ruled by unchangeable laws."[51] From every quarter, then, came similar messages, and the clumsily translated "all-sided philosophical view of the world" was a typical sign that on both shores of the Atlantic the aspirations of science advocates tended to go far beyond science. "The time has come," wrote an editor of the *Popular Science Monthly* in 1889, "when the claims of science to be the supreme mistress of thought and action can not be too boldly or earnestly advocated."[52]

Proscience advocates often differed among themselves, but their general program was clear. The major tenets of the religion of science, beyond the negatives, appeared consistently in the *Popular Science Monthly* and implicitly in other forums: scientists offered natural explanations of all natural events, and those included not only the universe but human beings and their thinking.[53] This general outlook persisted for generations as a recognizable creed—and also as a set of war aims while the universal application of a naturalistic, even reductionistic, approach invaded territories claimed by others.

The Scientific Method

Over the years, one other important element of the religion of science emerged, and it came from a negative element that turned positive. To correct credulity and demonstrate facts, typically in field or laboratory instruction, scientists and popularizers began with doubt. "Scientific training can hardly be regarded as completed until it has included the necessity of giving up cherished opinion," wrote geologist and geographer W. M. Davis in a popular article in 1922. Physicist John Trowbridge in 1879 had suggested the direction of this thinking: "Any plan of education which prevents a man or woman from becoming the dupe of those who pretend to use natural or supernatural forces is to be commended. One of the quickest ways of training the mind in the logical process which I have indicated is to undertake some simple investigation in physics."[54]

By thus emphasizing open-mindedness and then the method associated with naturalistic explanation, proponents found a distinctive element that helped identify science; namely, the essence of science was the method. By the twentieth century, this identifying abstraction was widely utilized, and many writers discussed the nature of ideal science (using "ideal" in a more or less Platonic sense). Moreover, emphasizing method was an immense help in popularizing, for it enabled members of the public to master indisputably genuine science without having to carry out difficult mathematical calculations or memorize formidable numbers of facts. Already in 1873 Youmans explicated the strategy:

> Science being considered as a kind of tough and forbidding knowledge belonging to laboratories, observatories, and apothecaries' shops, popular science was regarded as the same kind of knowledge loosely stated in common language. At the outset we rejected this view as narrow and false, holding that science, instead of pertaining to certain things, consists in a method of knowing, which applies to all things that can be known, and that popular science must be equally comprehensive.[55]

The mid-twentieth-century emphasis on scientific method (to be taken up in chapter 5) still echoed this view, that the subject matter of science was not as important as the method. Meantime, the method could be, and was, applied to any category of inquiry to which the imperialists of science wished to apply it. Altogether Jennie Mohr could summarize the aims of popularizers in the last days of the undiluted religion of science, the 1930s, as, (1) getting the reader to see the world as scientists saw it, an orderly and unified system, and (2) getting people to think as scientists did—the scientific way of thinking, as it came to be called.[56]

Because it came to embody an approach to knowledge and life, the struggle of the evangelists-cum-soldiers of science for the minds and loyalties of the people was a part of a more general cultural struggle. Intellectual historians have long since portrayed many facets of the contest: how the partisans of science defeated the classical curriculum in the colleges and how the emphasis upon innovation and method became the "revolt against formalism" as well as a part of the campaign against the "genteel tradition."[57] Science had always been part of liberal education, but in the late nineteenth century scientists hoped to have a larger part, and particularly to set the tone. William P. Atkinson of MIT in 1873 described the scientific liberal education of his day as a truly liberating process: "It will but cast old truths in new moulds, while it explodes old superstitions by adding new truths to the old ones." Atkinson had an explicit humanistic goal: to develop more regard for human life. Science led to this goal, he said, by defeating the fatalism of superstition. In this respect he anticipated the whole tendency of uplifting science popularization for a century (a tendency often conceived as part of the process of modernization). Insofar as people believed that they had more control over nature and their own lives, they embraced humane goals and the change that such goals required. The religionists of science would therefore grant nothing to opponents in level of idealism and concern for individuals.[58]

In practical terms, the goal of the proponents of science and culture was, in the words of Matthew D. Whalen and Mary F. Tobin, "the evolution, quite literally, of the moral, middle-class citizen within a progressively scientific civilization." Superstitious beliefs in children, wrote one proponent of science in 1934, correlated with not only fears and worries but "frequency of physical ailments, excessive attendance at movies, severity of discipline at home, and poor living conditions," which summarized in negative terms a range of values involved in civilization. Victorians who orated in favor of science utilized traditional lofty sentiments, but they did have a relatively consistent and definite program, easily recognizable in the early twentieth century, and they did not scruple, as David Starr Jordan, the ichthyologist and college president, on one occasion in the 1920s said, to guide both individual and social behavior—"to furnish a sound basis for the conduct of life."[59]

Men of Science

There was yet one more aspect to the forces popularizing science: the emergence in the late nineteenth century of the classic "man of science."[60]

It has already been observed that the personnel who did much of the popularizing were themselves practitioners of science on one level or another. Ideally, many people at that time believed, the most eminent investigators should also be those who were most prominent in popularizing.[61] What distinguished those who did take on responsibility for the fate of science in the public arena from colleagues who did not? The answer lies largely in the broad view that the men of science took of their enterprise, identifying science with both high culture and social improvement of all kinds. A writer, presumably Youmans, noted in the *Popular Science Monthly* in 1877 that many scientists, in contrast to men of science, were narrow and specialized, caught up in details of their study. "It is a great mistake," he noted, "to suppose that all the influences exerted on the mind by scientific study are necessarily of a widening or liberalizing character." And most regrettable, he continued, was the fact that excellent workers because of their narrowness were not contributing to popularizing.[62]

American men of science were, then, a special breed, more than just field or laboratory workers or thinkers. One mark of the man of science was that he took "more or less interest in all sciences," as one of them put it in 1916. However specialized, the man of science had, besides general breadth, an overarching identity that made him rise above parochial interests to embrace loyalty to science in general (an attribute, as will be noted in the last two chapters, that had largely died out among scientists by the mid-twentieth century). And clearly the intellectual justification for all scientists to stand together was the universality of the scientific method.[63]

A man of science thought of himself as a defender of traditional high culture, in part because of his high moral aspirations but also because the religion of science embraced all culture and life. When "science" (in, for example, the *Popular Science Monthly* and, later, the *Scientific Monthly*) included archeology, economics, history, linguistics, and politics, any cultured person might ideally be a man of science as well as a reader of popularized science, upholding a traditional view of culture while adding to it.[64]

The man of science, however, had one special attribute, and it grew out of his devotion to the scientific method: he had moral superiority. Over the decades, little changed. In 1896, the botanist John M. Coulter observed that the scientist brought observation and analysis, but so, too, did other disciplined thinkers. Likewise they all taught synthesis and even appreciation (the strong point of the then rival humanities). But what science alone stood for, Coulter said, was objectivity: eliminating the self. Many years later, just before World War II, the economist Wesley C. Mitchell made the same point. Scientists alone, of all social groups, said Mitchell, had succeeded "in emancipating themselves from the misconceptions and prejudices prevailing in their social groups." The moral superiority of the man of science therefore rested upon his denial of self— forswearing both subjective emotion and personal advantage. This was the end point in the negative battle against the irrationalism and cupidity of superstition.[65]

Finally, the responsibility of the man of science to popularize was explicit. He was expected to speak to the practical importance of science as well as to contribute to high culture and the liberal education of the public in general. An advertisement for the *Popular Science Monthly* in 1886 spelled out the program: "Leaving the dry and technical details of science, which are of chief concern to the specialists, to the journals devoted to them, the Monthly deals with those more general and practical subjects which are of the greatest interest and importance to the public at large. . . . Its leadership is recognized in the great work of liberalizing and educating the popular mind." Americans with these aspirations, then, were the chief popularizers in the nineteenth century and into the twentieth century, people who brought reason to all aspects of life and who later were part of the intelligentsia who tried to live the life of the mind.[66]

Men of science did have some successes against superstition and its allies, especially as secularization in general affected American life. But eventually, in the twentieth century, two elements changed: the personnel who carried out the popularization, on the one hand, and the institutions through which popularization proceeded, on the other. Whereas in the nineteenth century scientists tended to do their own popularizing, in the twentieth others gradually took over. And, simultaneously, as journalism changed and the public moved to electronic media, popularization, too, moved into a very different phase, in which popularizers faced a debasement of public taste and aspiration.

Popularization and Credulity

Popularization was not new in late nineteenth-century Anglo-American culture, although it was the 1840s before Americans started using the term "popularize" frequently. Already in 1830, for instance, Orville

Dewey, a Boston clergyman, could observe, "It is indeed one of the peculiar and great undertakings of the age, to communicate scientific knowledge to the whole intelligent portion of the mass of society." Citing recent publications from both sides of the Atlantic and also the growing lyceum lecture movement, Dewey concluded, "*Diffusion* is the watchword of the age." [67]

Even in the prehistory of popularization, the intimate connection between popularization and campaigns against superstition had already been established. [68] In order to popularize, someone had to know something that the populace (to use an appropriate, antiquated term) did not know. The earliest works typically involved an assumption that society is divided and that the ignorant and credulous lower orders could benefit from enlightenment by the privileged. But the relationship was ambiguous—for popularizing could also constitute the act of socializing the upper orders of society, the "intelligent portion," as Dewey put it. This basic ambiguity persisted through all efforts to popularize science and correct error.

The classic work of popularizing by correcting was Sir Thomas Browne's *Pseudodoxia Epidemica; or, Enquiries into Very Many Received Tenets and Commonly Presumed Truths* (1646). Browne, writing patronizingly in English instead of Latin, corrected ideas about any number of natural phenomena, from mistletoe to owls and ravens (the former had no "Magical vertues," and the latter were not omens). He took up, as he promised in the title, a large number of "popular errors" based on "misapprehension, fallacy, or false deduction, credulity, supinity, adherence unto antiquity, tradition and authority." [69]

This tradition of correcting erroneous thinking as the starting point for popularizing continued right into the nineteenth century. The major English-language book of popularization that was current when Americans were beginning to use the term, Scotsman Thomas Dick's *On the Improvement of Society by the Diffusion of Knowledge* (1833), started out immediately with a chapter, in the spirit of Browne and others, "On the Influence which a General Diffusion of Knowledge would have in Dissipating those *Superstitious Notions* and Vain Fears which have so long enslaved the Minds of Men." Astrology and witchcraft as well as ordinary omens earned Dick's scorn, and he had no patience for the vulgar folk who suffered "such absurd notions." Dick not only regretted the fear and cruelty that arose from superstitions but "the false ideas they inspire with regard to the nature of the Supreme Ruler of the universe, and of his arrangements in the government of the world." [70]

This tradition from the early nineteenth century that popularization involved the war against credulity continued right into the twentieth century, long after popularization was formally institutionalized in a more modern form. A century after Dick wrote, American sociologist Franklin H. Giddings took a stance similar to his and explicitly connected the struggle between science and superstition with the popularization of science. "It would be a deplorable case of wishful thinking," he wrote,

> to expect that the conflict between occultism and natural knowledge will be fought out on the uplands of scientific theory. It will drag on for generations in the fens of ignorance and moronism. . . . The first duty, therefore, of the intellectually honest and unafraid is to enlist for personal service and "for the war." It will be an unfortunate mistake to assume that successful hostilities can be carried forward by a paid army while gifted investigators devote themselves to their researches, in serene assurance that all goes well. [71]

As will appear below, Giddings's warning was all too prescient.

Popularization in the United States

As the diffusion of scientific knowledge in the United States turned into popularization early in the nineteenth century, educated Americans, at least, were exposed to increasing numbers of British as well as local efforts to spread knowledge about nature and natural law. By 1867, Eliot, quoted above, was observing, "These are the days of popular lectures and familiar treatises on scientific subjects." [72] Throughout the century, Americans continued to read many British in addition to U.S. books and magazines, and they followed and emulated popularizing activities in England such as lectures at the Royal Institution and the work of the British Association for the Advancement of Science.

The significant expansion of popularization and the rise of the term in the 1840s reflected the appearance in the United States of professional scientists, people whose knowledge and activities now clearly differentiated the group from their fellow citizens. People within the scientist group tended to speak the same language—at least enough to understand each other. Observers therefore spoke then and have spoken ever since of the need to simplify and interpret or translate for the masses outside of the expert group. Popularization, explained the editor of the *Popular Science News* in 1883, "means science put in language which can be comprehended; it means science adapted to every one's wants, to every one's necessities." As in Germany and England, then, the leading American scientists wrote textbooks for the young, and Americans joined some of the best English-speaking investigators such as Charles Lyell in making extensive speaking tours, pioneering the circuits soon followed by Tyndall and Huxley. Many of the professional scientists regretted the time lost in giving popular lectures and demonstrations—just as they resented drilling unprepared students. But a sense of duty and the customs of the day propelled them into the public arena.[73]

As professionalization increased in the decades before the Civil War, other terminology changed, also. "Science" tended to replace such expressions as "natural philosophy" and "natural history," and of course the language indicated shifts in attitude. The purpose of the coming "men of science" in reaching the public was not so much to show "wonders" as to keep the listeners or readers up with the latest developments.

In a modern form, then, popularizing started out as teaching what scientists knew. As scientific knowledge developed and especially as it became increasingly specialized and intellectually inaccessible to nonscientists, popularizers functioned to translate and interpret professional science for a lay audience. Both terms, "translate" and "interpret," were used, whether in the *Popular Science Monthly* in the nineteenth century or in *Science News-Letter* in the twentieth. Yet popularizers also were expected to summarize full-time scientists' work because ordinary people did not have time to learn all of the details. Obviously, in order for the major functions of modern popularizing, translation and condensation, to have functional value, the differentiation of the professional scientist from the public had to have occurred.[74]

Popularized science, as George Basalla has pointed out, is not the same as "pop" science. In the main, popularization was aimed at the educated classes. In Europe, the educated people tended to constitute an aristocratic patronage; but in the United States, where there was a large population of literate, upwardly mobile people, the dividing line in the nineteenth century was not a clear one. Superstition, of course, resided closer to the science information of what in a later day was the comic book and television element of the population, but at any time, American popularizers could aim low as well as high and still be popularizing. Nevertheless, they often manifested disdain at any time for mere entertainment. In 1882, for example, the editor of the *Popular Science Monthly* admitted that he published "a considerable proportion of articles so weighted with valuable thought as to require concentration of mind and often careful reperusal to grasp and assimilate their contents." Such material, he continued, "has provoked frequent protests on the part of our readers, who have complained that we deviate from the magazine-standard of easy reading, and are not true to our title, which promises a magazine adapted to the populace. Yes, but to the *improvement* of the populace!"[75]

Lines between pop science or "folk" science—as J. R. Ravetz calls it—on the one hand, and hard science, on the other, are not always easy to draw. Much folk science, however, consists of beliefs without regard to the way in which the beliefs were established and so has no special validity, any more than superstition; and, as will become clear, this phenomenon was not limited to preliterate or subliterate populations and peoples.[76] Moreover, in the United States, the highest-quality science, sometimes not even distorted by popularization, at times functioned to confirm traditional beliefs and attitudes—as in the early nineteenth century hard science reinforced the common belief in God and his beneficence and later in the century hard science confirmed folk atheism, that is, latter-day skepticism. Finally, to pursue this same stream, the difference was not just the change in science and popularization but in the composition of the population, including the "folk."

Institutions of Popularization

Beyond the professional scientists, then, the other requirements for popularization were an audience and, we can now add, institutions through which popularizers could reach the audience.[77] In the United States, middling sorts of people and upper classes patronized uplift and learning to an astonishing extent. Even before the railroad, wandering and resident speakers alike could attract listeners almost at will, as foreign observers remarked with surprise. The population at large seemed to those observers to be bent upon wholesale self-improvement and self-cultivation, and by the mid-nineteenth century, leading scientific lecturers could com-

mand audiences of many hundreds who would sit through protracted expositions of scientific material. Sometimes this lecturing was system-
atized, as in the lyceum and Chautauqua circuits. Sometimes it was
spontaneous or by special invitation. But the public lecture was a major
American ceremony of both substantive and symbolic significance.[78] The
enthusiasm for enlightenment represented by public speaking continued
unabated, from 1840, when a Boston mob broke a window in the Old
Corner Bookstore trying to get tickets to a series of Lowell lectures, right
down to the twentieth century.[79]

In addition to lectures, the written word helped slake the thirst for
knowledge by means of books, magazines, and newspapers—again into
the twentieth century.[80] During the 1840s, when popularizing was well
launched, the number of nonpolitical magazines increased from fewer
than 500 to over 600 and the number of newspapers from 138 daily and
1,266 weekly to 254 daily and 2,048 weekly. The amount spent on books
in that period increased from $2.85 million a year to a staggering $5.9
million, retailed through more than 2,000 booksellers (the federal government budget was only $25–40 million a year). The books tended to be
instructive and inspiring in nature, often directing readers what to do and
believe.[81]

The drive for self-improvement that fueled popularization reached a
high point in the 1920s, and the "general intelligent reader" who did serious reading played an important part in the culture well into the twentieth century. Increased literacy and greatly expanded education made
writers in good books and high-class magazines effective arbiters of society, widely imitated by other population elements who made more
modest popularization of science and health as well as literature and the
arts a flourishing activity. By the late twentieth century, however, cultural
changes had occurred. The increase in the number of books produced had
leveled off. Moreover, the readers of high-quality magazines, such as the
venerable *Harper's* and *Atlantic*, actually decreased in numbers. As the
population grew substantially, the proportion of Americans who were
"educated," that is, serious readers and thinkers for whom the best popularizers wrote and spoke, declined very substantially. Clearly, the balance
in the twentieth century slowly shifted, and there was in fact growing
concern that popularization should increasingly deal not only with the
elite but with the lower orders of society.

Even as some of the science for the cultured public died out, careful cultivation of journalists led to a substantial upgrading of popular science in the newspapers and magazines of the 1920s and 1930s. In 1936, an Associated Press science reporter pointed out that news about artificial fertilization of a rabbit egg made headlines all around the country, and the reporter used this as a demonstration that journalists were now able to communicate pure science stories in a way that would have been impossible a generation earlier. This improvement in newspapers and magazines persisted until the time that television had a substantial effect.[82]

In addition to general publications and national lecture circuits, during the nineteenth century Americans learned about and participated in science through myriad local groups, and many interest clubs persisted or left to the twentieth century other institutional legacies such as museums. But by then the amateur tended to be a consumer of popularization and relinquished participation (see chapters 4 and 5, below).

Finally, a major popularizing activity involved education of the young. Not only did scientists write (and later coauthor) textbooks, but they did what they could to influence teachers and curriculums at all levels. By the twentieth century, just as the number of students in school exploded, teachers themselves had become major sources as well as agents of popularization.

Other outstanding events in the history of popularization suggest some of the institutional determinants in the narrative to come. After Darwin's *Origin of Species* appeared in 1859, public interest in science became more intense, and in 1872 the first sustained, successful science magazine for the "general public," the *Popular Science Monthly*, began publication. Scandals over inaccurate and sensational (that is, misleading) "newspaper science" helped spark the founding of Science Service, a reliable news service, in 1921. The appearance of Science Service will be referred to repeatedly in the following chapters.[83] Also in the early twentieth century, forces within education, particularly progressive education, affected the teaching of science. The Great Depression of the 1930s, the atomic bombs of 1945, and Sputnik in 1957 all also had effects, including a major shift in the motive for popularizing, a shift from self-cultivation and general cultural uplift to the urgent need for an informed public to decide matters of science policy.

Along with events within the culture, audiences changed, as I have suggested. In 1874 the editor of the *Popular Science Monthly* said that his purposes were cultural—"to interest the non-scientific public, and to create a taste for scientific literature, and an appreciation of scientific knowledge in the reading community." By contrast, later popularizers had urgent business with all citizens. The American Association for the Advancement of Science, wrote an official spokesperson in 1981, had a special interest not just in "the selling, or 'popularizing,' of science"; rather, the group was moved by "a perception that the power of science is not neutral to the affairs of states or individuals, but is central to most of the critical choices and outcomes that will be resolved either by informal decision or by default, and that it takes a heap of understanding." Finally, transmutations in and additions to the media—the ingress of radio and television—and other social changes altered the institutions of popularizing. Not least of the other changes was the appearance, beginning in the 1920s, of a whole new group of major characters in the story, the science writers—journalists who specialized in stories about science and health.[84]

What was constant through all of these permutations over a century and a half was the basic concept of popularizing. One element that everyone understood was "simplification," particularly the practice of omitting both mathematics and memorization of detail. A second element alluded to above also was "translation"; a specialized scientist presumably thought on a level different from that of ordinary people, and a popularizer therefore had the function of explaining in ordinary, nontechnical terms and concepts the ideas in scientists' work. And, finally, popularization was "keeping up"—the idea that people should know the general events and findings from the cutting edge of learning and research. From time to time epidemics of "yearbooks" of scientific progress—the 1850s, the 1940s—provided transparent symbols of this impulse.[85]

Cultural Lag

Implicit in the idea of progressive updating is the notion of cultural lag. The latest developments in the laboratory or field usually did not reach the general public at once, and when they did reach "the public," often only a very small group of readers or listeners understood immediately the content and significance of the development, whether it was, say, the phagocyte, general relativity, or Gestalt learning. Only after a number of repetitions, with explanations, could consumers of popularization absorb the new development. In practice, in history, then, the actual process of popularization had a major additional dimension of complexity, particularly because some social groups did not absorb new knowledge and ideas until long after the cultural leaders did.

The cultural lag phenomenon meant that at any given time there was a whole series of different publics for any particular item of popularization—each of which publics was at a different stage of learning (i.e., a different stage of lagging behind). The object of the popularizers was not only to have everyone enlisted in the armies of science but to bring all of the publics abreast with the avant garde. But instead, reality—lag—always guaranteed highly variable levels of knowledge and comprehension. Popularizers often had, in effect, students from kindergarten to college (regardless of age) reading the same text. It is for this reason that the record of popularization is so complex. In part, the popularizers, to solve this problem, targeted different audiences, by age, by class, and so on, as has been noted. But the lag was temporal as well as social; a group did not miss enlightenment but simply came to it later. George Cotkin has shown, for example, how American socialists advocated scientific culture in popularizations for the common man a generation after Youmans and his contemporaries had initiated the same program for the better-educated classes.[86]

By the twentieth century, popularizers tended to develop a particular strategy. Catherine Covert has described the journalists' pattern of popularizing as proceeding as if in an upwardly tilted spiral. The writer would start at a low level with a general idea, giving a full explanation at the most basic level of presumed ignorance of the reader. Later the writer would assume that the reader knew the idea in question, and so the writer would feel free merely to allude to it in the course of a now more advanced exposition. Then the same writer would come back down and repeat the elementary explanation, for the benefit of those who had not yet picked it up. The next time the writer would assume knowledge—and subsequently in turn explain less and assume more until the idea had sufficient currency that little or no explanation was necessary, and finally the writer could assume that the concept or notion—missing link, germ, mutation, fission, complex—was a part of the vocabulary of ideas of the average reader.[87]

The progressive spiral model helps explain some of the otherwise confusing patterns of evidence in the vast literature of popularization. The model shows why simple and advanced subject matter and terminology existed side by side in a single organ of popularization as well as in the whole body of it, whether the Popular Science News of the 1880s or the *Scientific Monthly* of the 1920s or television presentations of the 1970s. The model suggests further one reason that popularizers and teachers frequently used a historical approach to explication: by following the sequence of discovery, they could cover both elementary and advanced material at the same time without offending the sophisticated or losing the naive. The model further suggests why popularizers often failed to convince parts of the public that science was understandable; because readers often came across advanced material before the more elementary material needed to understand the advanced material—even, for example, in the same book—many consumers simply gave up and considered science unfathomable. Finally, the disappearance of explanation and exposition of a particular item did not necessarily demonstrate that an idea was no longer of cultural importance—just that it was no longer necessary to talk about it. Around the beginning of the twentieth century, for instance, school textbooks in the health field no longer included extensive exhortations to bathe, since such advice had become unnecessary for middle-class students.[88]

In one way, Covert's spiral model helps simplify the task of tracing popularization. Because the high points of the spiral also suggest the low (or lagging) points of more elementary material appropriate for more naive audiences, concentrating on the most-advanced popularization permits a coherent line of advance to emerge—with the lag built in and assumed rather than distracting from an understandable sequence. The model also underlines how approximate were the boundaries of the eras in popularization.

The Bias of Basic Motives: Entertainment, Religion, and Health

The popularizers' public was never completely passive, and consumers therefore often modified or even frustrated the intentions of the most earnest producers of popularization. Many ordinary Americans not only did not have the background to appreciate science but were not entirely dedicated to self-improvement. From the beginning, then, some popularizers catered to the lowest tastes, popularizers who were not just essentially nostrum vendors or the authors of the notorious "newspaper science," but respectable figures who, for example, on the speakers' circuit did more amusing than educating. "Low public taste" of course existed, admitted Youmans shortly after launching his *Popular Science Monthly*, but he felt that there was no reason for the "degeneration" of uplift so that "the 'course of lectures' is transformed into a 'series of entertainments.'"[89] The same debate over popular taste continued in the twentieth century, first regarding yellow journalism and then the pervasive dominance of the entertainment standard in even the best television presentations. "Miracles" and "wonders" therefore allied with superstition in defeating the aims of many—but not all—American popularizers.

Even the best popularizers took account of the tastes of various parts of the population. In the laissez faire society of the United States, consumption of popularization was not required of anyone, outside of some school courses, and audiences would not listen or read or watch if the subject did not concern or entertain them. Entertainment did win and lose attention, but concern—the idea that some aspect of science was something about which they ought to know—was, after curiosity, the most enduring factor that made people want to learn about science.

The record of popularization shows that Americans whom popularizers could reach had, beyond intellectual curiosity, two fundamental personal concerns: religion, on one level or another, and health, in a broad sense, a sense in which awareness of self played a large part—so large that popular psychology was consistently the subject most attractive to audiences for popular science, whether in the time of phrenology and spiritualism in the nineteenth century or in the culture of narcissism more than a century later. Except for special motives in the age of atomic terror after 1945, only a very limited part of the population would consume popularizations of the physical sciences, and the appeal of biology, when it could be separated from health, varied with the intensity of religious concern. The three leading categories of successful volumes in the extraordinarily widely distributed Little Blue Books series of the 1920s, for example, were (1) sex and love, (2) self-improvement (often in the sense of social improvement, such as manners), and (3) skepticism and free thought (*The Life of the Infidel Ingersoll* sold more than twice *The Life of Jesus*).[90] It has never been a secret that sex was a major element in interest in popular health and psychology, and the element of skepticism in science popularizing has already been noted.

Where the health and psychology interest was more subtle in the earlier period of popularizing in the United States, the religious interest in science appeared most transparently precisely in the pre–Civil War period when speakers and writers about science argued that the Book of Nature, if read closely, furnished proof of God's existence, intentions, and will. In this sort of popularizing, intellectual wonder and religious awe were hard to separate. After that era, the theme of skepticism more often signaled religious interest in popularizing.

In all periods, then, patterns in the content of popularization to a substantial extent reflected consumer interests. The modern field of adult education provided an instructive test of the pressures on popularizers. In order to attract adult students, wrote an expert in the field in 1945, one should offer woodworking, clothes making, and personal psychology. But to kill the program off, he noted, schedule literature, history, and science.[91] When adult education programs were flourishing in the mid-twentieth century, not more than 4–6 percent of all adult—obviously voluntary—education could qualify as science, a proportion so low that science seldom came up in professional publications in the field of adult education. Such evidence confirms how great were the disadvantages under which science popularizers worked except where they could and did tie all of science to health and psychology.

Much of American popular science, therefore, rode on the audience's presumed interest in these two areas, plus of course religion versus skepticism. The health and psychology categories, moreover, often were confused with each other as well as with sex. At one point in the 1920s, the Science Service story that editors utilized most was "College Girls Have Best Physiques," which involved both psychology and health, not to mention sex. When psychological material increased in *Parents' Magazine* during the 1940s, medical content declined. And, to cite another example of blurred boundaries, for years in the mid-twentieth century, the editors of *Newsweek* could never decide whether psychology belonged under the heading of science or of health.[92]

As health and psychology intruded persistently into the popular level of all scientific exposition, neither popularizers nor members of the consuming public were able to maintain clear distinctions between health and psychology, on the one hand, and either purer sciences or the whole realm of science, on the other. It seemed entirely appropriate to all parties, for example, when a health and public health journal, the *Sanitarian*, merged into the *Popular Science Monthly* in 1904. The editor of the *American Naturalist* found as early as 1883 that he had to add "departments" for psychology and physiology. In the 1920s, despite the overwhelming representation of physical scientists on the board, Science Service from the beginning included at least 20 percent from the fields of health and medicine—not to mention psychology. In the first major survey of radio programs, in 1935, science did not even show up as a separate category, but psychology and health both rated above average. The *Science Yearbook of 1945* was at least 25 percent medical science, and in 1945–1946 the Sunday science reporting of the *New York Times* was evenly split between medicine and health. In the age of television, one survey from the 1960s classified about 75 percent of the television science content as medicine and psychology. And in the early 1980s, among journalists' calls to the Media Resource Service 24.5 percent were concerned with health and medicine, 14.8 percent with occupational and environmental health, and 9.4 percent with social science and psychology (in contrast to 3.1 percent with space and 6.0 percent with life sciences).[93]

In the popular field, then, the Comtean hierarchy of science was inverted consistently. Psychology and health were now at the top, in terms of avid interest and consequent effort; the questions of life followed, embodying health and religious concerns. At the other end, mathematics, the curse of popularizers, was reserved for the most limited, if most elite, audience. The search for patterns therefore follows this inversion of preponderances and goes first to the fields of health and psychology—and in fact patterns are more obvious there, as I have suggested.

In view of the discussion above, it ought also be observed that psychology and health were fields in which superstition has always flourished. Dick, in his 1833 classic, turned immediately from his introductory chapter on superstition to take up the subject of health. When Browne, two centuries earlier, claimed originality in his correcting vulgar errors, he excepted one single field that was a model even for him: for centuries others had written to explode the false ideas of the credulous in the field of health.[94] Both this venerable tradition of the negatives and the evidence of positive content lead now to the story of the popularization of health and then of psychology.

I have suggested that correction of error was fundamental in the process of popularization as it developed in the nineteenth century. People at that time and after advocated learning about science because science furthered thinking in terms of order, rationality, and naturalism, and superstition came to serve evangels of science in a negative way, to explain what science opposed and replaced. Superstition therefore constituted magical and unsystematic thinking in general, especially when based on some social authority. Men of science, as I shall show, were as ready to attack the authority of advertisers of patent tonics as they were to attack the folk belief in throwing spilled salt over the shoulder. Their successors were not as inspired.

Chapter 2
The Popularizing of Health

IN THE HISTORY of popularizing health, the themes of superstition and science appeared in the context of specific subject matter, and through the evolution of the changing patterns on which I focus there was nevertheless a powerful continuity in concern about hygiene. From the beginning of English settlement in North America, the inhabitants were well acquainted with attempts to preserve health that were known as domestic medicine; indeed, one of the classics, John Wesley's *Primitive Physick* (1747), was occasioned by Wesley's stay in the colonies. Colonial newspapers carried the usual recipes for cures that circulated among all literate people at least until the twentieth century, and ads for secret medical preparations supplemented the other reports of therapies that served as news items.[1] It is true that hygienic and preventive advice often accompanied domestic medicine in various kinds of publications, but only at the opening of the nineteenth century did new publications, out of both France and England, synthesize traditional teachings about personal health and create an identifiable modern hygiene tradition—although as late as 1834 the American physiologist Robley Dunglison still was regretting that "the study of the human frame—especially in its healthy relations—should not hitherto have been more an object of attention, as a branch of general learning."[2] But already by that time the popularization of health was in the first of the stages that provide a framework for understanding the public aspect of science as well as medicine.

In this chapter, then, I shall trace the stages through which health popularization went, pointing out that distinctive emphases in content changed as the format and agents of popularization also changed. Unlike the natural sciences, in which audiences ultimately tended to specialize so that a wide spectrum of popularizers developed, hygienic teachings tended to persist as a case of less complicated diffusion and translation from scientists to a less-segmented public. In this case, too, not only were superstitions conspicuous, but the role of commercial interest in perpetuating error and controlling behavior—the essence of functional superstition—was also relatively clear.

The Non-Natural Tradition and Nature

Early nineteenth-century writers on personal health drew for both debunking and positive content on traditional teachings, doctrines that were generally organized in terms of and recognized as the "non-naturals" (elements not in humans' original nature). In recent years several medical historians have called attention to the tradition of the non-naturals in popular writings about health in Western countries since Galen's time. Implicit in the historians' interest in the non-naturals was the striking and amusing fact that the specific content in the modern obsession with the health of body and mind closely resembled those ancient teachings about the non-natural elements essential to life. In the late twentieth century and in Roman times both, health writers believed that health was profoundly determined by those elements: air, food and drink, movement and rest, evacuation and retention, and harmonious "passions of the soul."[3] The continuities were perfectly explicit. In 1831, for example, William A. Alcott, one of the premier health popularizers of the United States, referred to "the '*non-naturals*,' to use the Physician's term," which factors, he noted, had "great effect upon the *mental temper* as well as the physical system."[4] By the 1980s only the term had disappeared from much of the health advice popularizers were still passing on.

Although the non-naturals persisted in health advice, the form of popularization of those ideas did change. The first conspicuous transformation occurred within the development of a health crusade early in the nineteenth century, when Alcott and his even better known contemporary, Sylvester Graham—now remembered for graham flour and graham crackers—enthusiastically urged health reform in a format that James C. Whorton has called "physical Arminianism." The religious terminology not only evokes the alliance between religion and the science of that time but reveals a wide recognition that the health reform movement represented one of the secularizing forces of the Jacksonian period. Graham, for example, did begin as a clergyman, and he made a success of himself as a temperance preacher. But he was able to lead a health crusade only when he addressed the inadequacies of the medical profession in confronting the threat of cholera in 1832 and when, in addition, he developed a scientific basis for his teachings out of the new physiology of the French physicians, Xavier Bichat and François J. V. Broussais.[5]

What Graham and others concluded, then, was that each individual could seek health—a health that was freedom from disease, the negative of illness and death—but a health that was also positive, a sense of physical well-being, the opposite of debility (and clearly a secular goal).[6] Already in the realm of curative medicine, botanic and other irregular physicians had engendered real enthusiasm among many Americans who were attracted by an often simplistic pathology and relatively mild treatments. When, in the pre–Civil War reform era, health crusaders went beyond therapeutics to hygiene and preventive medicine, they drew not only upon traditional advice but, like Graham, upon a new scientific rationale. Many Americans learned from this rationale to work with nature in the name of both health and social uplift. This point of view was expressed by Caleb Ticknor in 1836:

> A great majority of the cases of disease can be traced to an origin in some erroneous notions in regard to diet, dress, habits, or something else which greatly affects the human system. Our fellow-men are not altogether in fault, neither are they altogether excusable, for not acting more in obedience to reason and the requirements of nature. They are not well enough acquainted with the laws of their organization and the wants of the system to act, in all cases, in conformity thereto; yet, with the exercise of what knowledge they have, and the right use of reason, many of the miseries under which they now groan might be averted.

Ticknor therefore proposed to furnish this information which would both root out error and provide correct knowledge about the ways of nature. Worthington Hooker in his textbook in 1859 was even more direct; all workings of the body, he said, should be viewed as part of nature.[7]

The health reformers believed that nature was essentially beneficent, which was a contrast to some contemporary physicians who referred openly to "the nature-trusting heresy." Those who sought health therefore had only to obey "the laws of health" or "the laws of life," laws that had the status of the laws of nature. (No one was troubled that these laws so closely followed the traditional non-naturals.) Writing as late as 1872, in a book for the public, J. R. Black, a Baltimore physician, listed "ten laws of health": breathing pure air, taking wholesome food and drink, taking exercise, dressing sensibly, using the sexual function naturally, seeking a suitable climate, avoiding harmful occupations, keeping clean, seeking tranquility and adequate rest, and avoiding marriage with close relatives. These laws Black believed were demonstrable, just as were the laws of astronomy or chemistry.[8] And Black was merely typical. Such dedication to nature, and to the science by which one knew nature, continued to mark health popularization for a century and a half after the beginning of the health crusade.[9]

Despite the persistence of the non-naturals content in health advocacy, five epochs with distinctive emphases are discernible on the basis of health popularizers' objectives, assumptions, and personnel, and further patterns of popularization emerged around the epochs (bear in mind, of course, that the epochs were only approximate and contained many exceptions, both according to the Covert model and not). The first epoch was the early to middle nineteenth century, when reformers, moralizing, and an organic view of the body prevailed. Positivistic scientists and a mechanistic view of the body marked the second epoch, the late nineteenth century. The early twentieth century was the era of public health advocates and an atomistic view of the body ("dynamic materialism"). By the mid-twentieth century, journalistic specialists and a psychosomatic, holistic view of the body dominated popularization. The final epoch, after midcentury, was characterized by advocacy groups and an ecological and servomechanism model of the body.[10]

The First Part of the Nineteenth Century

Before the Civil War, in the first era, the means of diffusing popular knowledge centered on the book or pamphlet and the lecture even more than was the case in science in general. Early specialized magazines, such as the *Journal of Health* (1829–1833), did not survive, but the *Water-Cure Journal* (with broader content than the title might suggest), begun in 1845, developed a very large circulation (and lasted until a number of other health journals appeared late in the century). Health advocates in addition furthered their teachings effectively with an organizational device common in that day, namely, a network of local societies, members of which met in an annual convention. The *Water-Cure Journal* and other magazines also served to unite local groups and isolated individuals into a movement, at the least by conveying to them a sense that they were not alone in advocating health.[11]

Popularization of health was complicated in the nineteenth century because it often continued to appear as a part of medicine. At first, learning did not separate physicians from educated laypersons, and, in addition, any literate person could read "patent" medicine advertising. Even well into the century, discussion of strictly medical questions was not closed to the public. Indeed, the lively debates between the medical sectarians and the regular physicians were implicitly aimed at the educated public. Although these debates focused on therapeutics, preventive medicine and health—plus sanitation—also entered into the public purview.[12] At first, most health crusaders, like Graham, shared the antimedical prejudices of large parts of the population and often allied with sectarians who attacked the dosing and bleeding of regular medical practice. But the antimedical attitudes of health reformers tended to apply only to the therapeutics of the physicians, and the health crusaders in fact disseminated much information about anatomy and physiology as part of their attempts to develop a rational basis for healthy regimens.

As in the popularization of science in general, the campaign to educate, uplift, and convert the masses of Americans to health at first drew on ideas that were largely public already and required little if any translation and simplification. When Hattie Hopeful wrote about exercise in the health section of the *Lady's Home Magazine* in 1858, she explained that "exercise is a law of nature" as well as "God's law," and she argued empirically and naturalistically that both were true because "for want of daily, vigorous exercise, much bad matter is retained in the system, creating fevers and other diseases. . . . Exercise, when properly taken, increases and regulates the perspiration, imparts tone and power to the nerves, strength to the muscles, the brain, and consequently the intellectual powers, [and] promotes appetite and good digestion." Not much science was necessary to follow her connecting causes to effects. When Elizabeth Blackwell in 1852 talked on a slightly different level, mentioning circulation of the blood or exercise of the organs or even animal electricity, she assumed that educated readers could follow, although she graciously provided some minimal explanation of somatic workings to refresh the memory of the reader—and of course to undergird her injunctions to proper conduct.[13] Blackwell, however, unlike Hattie Hopeful, was already a transitional figure. As writers and speakers tried to keep up with the discoveries of physiologists and others who succeeded Graham's authorities, Bichat and Broussais, basic medical science discoveries (as opposed to therapeutics) eventually forced health advocates to translate and simplify. At that point, typically around midcentury, health tended to orient itself to science more than to medical practice.

But if the pioneer health reformers of the early nineteenth century were not functioning as translators and condensers in the standard sense, what was their relationship to the popularization of health? One answer lay in the fact that they did base their disseminating of knowledge upon the technical and popular science of that day. Their works therefore represented a substantial change from older writings, authors of which tended to appeal to the dogmatic authority of tradition or even the Bible—as did, for example, the author of a catechism of health published in New York in 1819.[14]

The health reformers of the pre–Civil War period were most distinctive, however, in that, like both Hopeful and Blackwell, they tended to speak in moral terms. In one of the very early health advice tracts, Benjamin Waterhouse of Harvard noted that "moral philosophers unite with physicians of the first rank in opinion, that all chronic disorders arise from either 1st. VEXATION OF MIND, or 2d. an INDOLENT AND SEDENTARY LIFE, or 3d. INTEMPERANCE." As Charles Rosenberg and Carroll Smith-Rosenberg, among others, have pointed out, the crusaders for fitness, as Whorton depicts them, wanted to convert each individual to health and, in the bargain, to uplift all of society. Thus in 1838, Elisha Bartlett, a physician of Lowell, Massachusetts, wrote a tract explicitly entitled *Obedience to the Laws of Health, A Moral Duty*. Catharine Beecher a few years later was typical in associating secular and spiritual by noting, "Our Creator has connected the reward of enjoyment with obedience to these rules, and the penalty of suffering with disobedience to them." Larkin B. Coles, a New England zealot, put hygienic rules on a par with the Ten Commandments. The Boston-based reform group the American Physiological Society included among their resolutions their explicit sentiments that "it is a duty morally binding upon man, to study the principles of health, and to understand and obey those laws which God has established for the perpetuation of his existence."[15]

The moralizing of the early health crusaders gave a tone to the popularization of health that never left it; clearly popularization was more than just conveying knowledge—in science also, as it turned out, as well as in health, popularization involved changing people's attitudes. And the attitudes affected not only looking after one's own health but also that of one's fellow human beings, and specifically those who died before their natural time or were unnecessarily weak or miserable. In this way, the goals of health went far beyond the individual. As Whorton points out in this regard, the vegetarians in convention in 1850 asserted that "a Vegetable Diet lies at the basis of all reform, whether Civil, Social, Moral, or Religious." Historians have correctly characterized all of this nineteenth-century popularization as "health reform" so as to place it in the context of general reform as well as secular evangelism.[16]

The fact that attitude change as well as knowledge was involved helps explain why the early health crusaders did not always have success in interesting the public in their teachings or their programs. When the organizers of the American Physiological Society tried to gain recognition in the 1830s by having the Massachusetts legislature incorporate it, newspaper writers and legislators ridiculed the "bran bread and sawdust pudding" diet they attributed to the reformers, and the legislators turned to other matters that did not involve what they considered to be mere personal customs. Yet by 1850 the same lawmaking body was passing legislation that required that "physiology and hygiene . . . be taught in all public schools," and in 1857 the legislature in New York tolerantly incorporated the Hygio-Therapeutic College of the hydrotherapist and leader of health reform, Russell Trall.[17]

Clearly, by the middle of the century, vast numbers of Americans had come to treat with respect the popularizers of health and their scientific and uplift programs. So the health writer in the *Lady's Home Magazine* in 1858 lamented that many Americans let themselves get run down: "When the sad consequences connected with this lack of health and vigor in the tenement provided by the Creator for the soul to live and work in are duly conceived of and considered, the vital importance of a Health Department in a Ladies' Magazine, and of all inquiries and efforts directed to the abatement of the evil and its many mournful consequences, will be readily perceptible."[18]

The Late Nineteenth Century

The second era of health popularization was that of the sanitarians and positivistic scientists of the late nineteenth century. The classical statement was that of John W. Draper, whose 1856 textbook for decades inspired many popularizers:

> Throughout the work Physiology is treated after the manner known in Natural Philosophy. It was chiefly, indeed, for the sake of aiding in the removal of the mysticism which has pervaded the science that the author was induced to print this book. Alone, of all the great departments of knowledge, Physiology still retains the metaphysical conceptions of the Middle Ages from which Astronomy and Chemistry have made themselves free.[19]

Gone, then, were the frequent appeals to moral sanctions and, often, to the Almighty in more general terms. Instead, leading physicians and scientists, now moved at least to some degree by the new religion of science, preached a heavily naturalistic gospel of health, targeting the educated public, school children, and even the masses.

Where the original health enthusiasts were often antimedical but still strongly based in nature and the natural laws of life, late nineteenth-century advocates of health were more often themselves physicians who, like Draper, combined the authority of medicine with that of science. For example, when Galen E. Bishop, a Missouri physician, in 1853 set out to popularize medicine, he did so for the dual purpose of advancing people's health and fighting quacks and nostrums. Bishop cited but one authority, medical science, to justify his focus on either hygiene or treatment, referring to "the firm basis upon which the science is based, and the perfection to which it has been carried, in the elucidation of the laws of life, and the phenomena and treatment of disease."[20] As later in the century physicians moved into the era of therapeutic nihilism when prevention rather than cure was the most effective means of attaining health, the goals of popular medicine and popular health tended to coincide.

In the new climate, the old health reform evolved in three directions. Particular concern for personal health turned into a new enthusiasm in which exercise was the path to well-being. The colleges erected gymnasia, and water treatments, both preventive and curative, were transformed into swimming for sport. The most colorful figure to appear in this metamorphosis of traditional health efforts was Bernarr Macfadden, who at the end of the century became the high priest of physical culture, as it came to be called, in which traditional health injunctions continued but always were subordinated to exercise. Macfadden's popular magazine, *Physical Culture*, launched in 1899, was selling 100,000 copies a month by 1901. Besides touting exercise, Macfadden was, like other standard health enthusiasts, making dietary pronouncements and denouncing such unnatural things as corsets and alcohol. Macfadden's pagan worship of the body, in which the gymnasium became a chapel and pushups substituted for prayer, was a conspicuous part of the American landscape in the 1890s and after and helped sensitize large numbers of people to the efforts of other popularizers.[21]

The second form that the late nineteenth-century health crusade took was more traditional but drew upon both evangelical religion and modern medicine: the chief figure was a man of great influence in turn-of-the-century America, John Harvey Kellogg. Kellogg was an eminent physician and Seventh-Day Adventist, and many famous Americans passed through his sanitarium at Battle Creek, Michigan. He published a journal and numerous books and articles in which he combined traditional fads, especially hydrotherapy and a Graham diet, with the most modern late nineteenth-century physiology.[22] The greatest influence of Kellogg and his imitators came only late in the period, however, for up until that time the dominant force in the public sphere was the sanitary movement, the third of the directions of late nineteenth-century health reform.

The sanitary movement eventually became the public health movement, and while it began with the idea that the environment to a substantial extent conditioned disease, it picked up momentum with the growing conviction that disease had to be prevented and, furthermore, that one's own health could depend upon the health of one's neighbors. The sanitary movement was particularly significant because it largely embodied rapidly developing sciences and provided an entry for scientists as well as physicians to take the initiative in health, simplifying and translating for both medical and lay audiences. Indeed, in the United States, scientists, not physicians, effectively introduced the public to the germ theory of disease, and in such journals as the *Sanitarian* (published in New York beginning in 1873), popular and technical material appeared side by side.[23]

Popularization of Darwinism reinforced the sanitarians' emphasis on environment by showing concretely, as a physician wrote in 1882, "that the organs must not only preserve equilibrium within the body, but that there must also be equilibrium between the body and its externals." Rapidly absorbing evolutionary ideas that man is an animal and his protoplasm no different from that of other organic beings, the life processes of which could potentially be explained in terms of physics and chemistry, men of science popularizing health made the authority of science an even more potent argument for following health advice than medical teachings had been. As Frank Overton, a textbook author, noted for his young readers in 1897, "It has been a great triumph for science to liberate men from the superstition that the chemical and physical laws of our bodies were governed by the arbitrary feelings of indwelling spirits, and so were different from the laws governing lifeless creatures." Clearly the reductionistic and mechanical, however complex, constituted a major prop in the campaign against mysticism and magic.[24]

Shifting the emphasis from body machinery—except as an adaptation to nature—and concentrating on the potentially dangerous environment helped popularizers effect change in both individual persons and whole communities. A popular health editor of the 1890s put it thus: "There is . . . an enormous amount of indifference and criminal ignorance to be combatted, whereby human life and happiness are indirectly sacrificed; and each individual whose intellect and conscience have been quickened has an immediate duty to perform . . . to the end that the area of knowledge may be enlarged and the comfort or safety of the greatest number ensured." The germ theory of disease in particular intensified social pressure for various kinds of cleanliness, both social and personal, until many good citizens rebelled. As one exasperated writer noted in 1898, "People are warned against so many fancied or remote or unimportant evils, for which there is no remedy short of a germ-proof room, that they are not disposed to listen when the case is really serious." He thought publicists would be better advised to denounce adulterated milk than the dangers of catching disease by kissing.[25]

All of this activity in popularizing various approaches to health advocacy in the late nineteenth century—hygiene, physical culture, and sanitation—appeared in the usual American formats of public lectures, books, newspapers, and magazines. Magazines in particular now assumed more importance and often contained popular articles by scientists and physicians. Editors of some of the general magazines carrying health stories, such as the *Popular Science Monthly*, aimed high. Others tended to target different parts of the middle classes; *Godey's Lady's Book*, for instance, initiated a rather elementary "Health Department" in 1868.[26] Moreover, especially near the end of the century, a number of specialty health periodicals appeared, suggesting that the demand for popular health material was very great indeed, beyond the capacity of general magazines to meet, as the success of Macfadden also demonstrated. In addition to Kellogg's *Good Health*, for example, there were, among others, such publications as *Health Culture* and the *Hygienic Gazette*. Many of these publications merged into each other or disappeared—but the rate of birth of such journals was striking.

It was at the end of the century, too, that the newspapers, which for decades had tended to mirror the magazines, degenerated into yellow journalism. Then and later, no area of life was more subject to irresponsible reporting than that of medicine and health. Among the seemingly infinite number of examples, one particularly outrageous item caught the eye of an indignant science editor in 1891: a journalist's report of an Omaha man who ran a fever of 171 degrees, well above the temperature, as the editor pointed out, at which albumin in the body would have coagulated. Respectable popularizers from this period on, then, found that they had not only overt superstitions to correct but widespread pseudo-scientific misinformation—far more than formerly, and misinformation that now was appearing outside of the advertising columns.[27] As noted above, people at the time lumped it all together as "error."

One important addition to popularization in the late nineteenth century was the successful program of members of the Women's Christian Temperance Union (WCTU) and their allies to bring health instruction into the schools. Unlike the first Massachusetts law of an earlier period, the new legislation was effective. By 1900, all states required instruction in hygiene and physiology in the schools. One major purpose of the instruction was to indoctrinate children against the consumption of alcohol. Albert Mordell later recalled from his school days in Philadelphia late in the century that "it seemed as if the reason for studying about the organs and skin was to learn the effects of alcohol and tobacco on them." But because, as Mordell observed, the dry propaganda was set in a context of physiology and hygiene, in fact children often learned a great deal about the machinery of the body, how to care for it, and why, albeit in tendentious presentations. In an 1889 text, for example, the authors used information about the working and resting of the heart to expose students to the concept of a normal person in good health as well as the specific strains that even a small quantity of alcohol would put upon the person's heart (250 extra strokes per hour, each one moving six ounces of blood). Regardless of bias, the quality of the American teaching materials was sufficient that they not only displaced imported books but were not infrequently copied—pirated—in England.[28]

As early as 1885, then, William Gilman Thompson, a medical reformer, could cite the progress under way:

> Popular medicine and hygiene are becoming everywhere the fashion. . . . In the most popular family magazines we read articles upon the "anatomy of the brain," or "how to trap a soil-pipe." We have a mother's magazine devoted to improvements in baby-feeding and the scientific development of the infant mind. . . . The importance of a universal knowledge of, and attention to, the laws of physiology and hygiene is becoming more and more appreciated, and the elements of these subjects are taught in the public and private schools.[29]

The Early Twentieth Century

By the time the twentieth century was beginning, the dual enthusiasm for public health and personal hygiene, especially physical culture, was conspicuous in both the highbrow and mass media. Soon, however, increasingly different emphases appeared. Health faddism of various kinds enjoyed a resurgence well beyond physical culture; the most notorious example was the food doctrine of Horace Fletcher, who advocated thorough chewing of food ("fletcherizing"). Moreover, costly public works showed that large and important parts of the population took their health beliefs most seriously, whether the germ theory of disease, which was reflected in an accelerated sewage disposal program, or the traditional belief in fresh air and exercise, which translated into the playground movement and continued gymnasium construction. Finally, changes in medicine, and most particularly the germ theory, the expansion of surgery, the x ray, and the prevention of tuberculosis, were popularized to the point that they became common knowledge for most Americans.[30]

The germ theory in particular affected not only the content but the whole configuration of health popularization. Along with new physiological discoveries, bacteriology transformed the certainty of many kinds of health knowledge and therefore the urgency of publicizing it. Within a few years after 1900, publicity destroyed a traditional institution, the public drinking cup, for example.[31] Above all, of course, the new certainty of pathology, whether of rickets or typhoid, meant that the possibilities for mysticism in health beliefs and especially superstitious attributes of cause had declined precipitously even as the authority of the spokespersons for scientific knowledge increased.

With the acceptance of the germ theory of disease, of notions of the efficacy of endocrine substances, and of other evidence that the body consisted of complex systems in balance or struggling to exist, the strictly mechanical model of the preceding era gave way to an atomistic model of the human body, a model that Garland Allen has called "dynamic materialism." A physician writing in *Good Housekeeping* in 1919, for example, described how "by proper feeding, sleeping, exercise in fresh air and bathing, so as to fortify the body against the inroads of marauding germs . . . [,] tissues and fluids shall be able to destroy whatever disease-producing microbes may gain entrance." The leukocyte concept was only the most obvious of the bacteriological-physiological ideas of independent atomic (in a generic sense) entities operating within the body, each with a function. The leukocytes were dramatic because they had free movement and a "devouring" function, but the idea that each body cell had "power" on its own accounted very satisfactorily for the complexities that scientists were discovering, and yet at the same time this atomic entity model continued to provide a reductionistic and antimystical basis for giving health advice.[32]

Innovations in the sciences of nutrition in this period helped to shift popularizers' attention away from the general environment that had engaged the sanitarians and toward the actions of the individual. It turned out in particular that Fletcher was only the early harbinger of popular interest in personal diet. Even in the field of public health, as an editorial writer in the *American Journal of Public Health* noted in 1921, "the center of gravity of the food problem . . . shifted from sanitation to nutrition."[33] The newly discovered vitamins, especially, lent themselves to extensive and urgent popularization, and diet continued thereafter the most conspicuous single element in most health popularization throughout the twentieth century.

All of the discoveries, in many fields, led to the early twentieth-century burst of enthusiasm on the part of those undertaking to convey health advice to the public. Where before, fear had been the most conspicuous motive in health education, recalled Iago Galdston of New York, now "health education was likely to be bound up with the Pollyanna spirit" with enthusiasms and joyous pageants and even a Foundation for Positive Health. "The more practical but less inspiring aspects of health were largely put into the background," Galdston continued. "Little was said about sanitation and pure water. There was little emphasis on vaccination and immunization. . . . In the 'well-baby' clinics there was strong emphasis on cretonne and lace curtains." Popularizers included not only physical culture advocates, educators, scientists, and an occasional physician but now an important new group: the public health workers who succeeded the sanitarians. Public health groups in 1915 formally launched what they called the Modern Health Crusade, emphasizing education more than the regulation that had been the traditional focus of public health. The new crusade was initiated by the antituberculosis organizations, leaders of which were experienced in propagandizing the public. They, together with other advocates of health, argued persuasively that prevention was cheaper (more efficient, in the parlance of the day) than cure. Life insurance companies joined the new public health, and by the 1920s Herbert Hoover himself played a critical role in the child health component of the movement. But the sparkplugs of the effort were salaried public health officials and counterpart elements in voluntary health groups. They used every form of communication that they could, starting with their own abundant special agency publications—typically pamphlets and leaflets—and moving on to publicity in newspapers and magazines.[34] In 1910, for example, Louisiana health authorities sent around the state a special train called "Gospel of Health on Wheels." It contained many educational exhibits about hygiene as well as more traditional public health. And as early as 1921, the U.S. Public Health Service went on the radio with health education. Eventually enthusiasts had to ask whether or not there was too much propaganda, but by then the momentum appeared to be beyond control.[35]

The modern crusade for health thus fed on itself and generated demand. Newspaper editors, especially in the 1920s, began to run health columns (usually written by physicians) that drew not only on the quest

for authoritative medical advice but on a new demand for health information. In 1923, the American Medical Association launched *Hygeia,* a
successful popular health journal. Clearly many Americans were taking
scientific health findings very seriously. Public-spirited leaders were
alarmed by the waste of human resources attributable to poor health and
then by the generally low level of physical fitness of World War I draftees,
and the leaders hoped to solve a national problem by persuading large
numbers of people to change their behavior. In the private, individual
sphere, many Americans came to associate their own feelings of well-
being with personal hygiene, and health popularizers—including, now
prominently, promoters of various commercial products—answered the
demand for knowledge about how to improve one's physical well-being.[36]

Part of the demand grew out of the efforts that health crusaders put
into mobilizing educators. Educators themselves, in the midst of adapt-
ing to increasing enrollments and rapid curricular change, still by 1920
had reaffirmed explicitly the obligation of schools to advance health by
teaching prevention. Such teaching went in two directions. One was to
discard the older physiology and hygiene materials, those which were
now satirized as vast amounts of anatomical data plus lurid descriptions
of the insides of drunkards' stomachs. Instead, educators tried to emphasize actual behavior. "The end to be aimed at," wrote one educator in
1919, "is not *information*, but *action*; not simply *knowledge* of what things
are desirable, but rather the *habitual practice* of the rules of healthy living."[37]

The other direction that health education for children took was to be
included within science teaching, rather than taught separately. Thus a
1927 study found that about 32 percent of the content of general science
textbooks and 50 percent of those in biology, the two most universal high
school science courses, consisted of essentially human health topics. Although, as will be observed in chapter 5, this strategy was a way of water-
ing down traditional science content, it also had the effect of trying to
keep health education in a context of nature and the natural.[38]

For some years, the new health education for the young showed up
chiefly in the form of the "health habits." With the health habits, educators attempted to emphasize attitudes and positive conditioning for actions, all appropriate to a child's age, as opposed to knowledge and fear
such as characterized the older hygiene-physiology tradition. In content,
the health habits grew in part out of the "Rules of the Health Game":

1 A full bath more than once a week
2 Brushing the teeth at least once every day
3 Sleeping long hours with windows open
4 Drinking as much milk as possible, but no coffee or tea
5 Eating some vegetables or fruit every day
6 Drinking at least four glasses of water a day
7 Playing part of every day out of doors
8 A bowel movement every morning

(A similar list for adults, "The Fifteen Rules of Hygiene," drawn up by Irving Fisher and Eugene Lyman Fisk in 1915, was widely influential; Fisher and Fisk advocated moderation in all of life, however, as much as breathing and evacuating.) [39]

At their apogee, the health habits were introduced in kindergarten and first grade—emphasizing cleanliness, diet, and sleep—as habits pure and simple. Only as children could understand the reasons behind the actions was the shift made from habits and skills to knowledge. The result was a lot of brushing of teeth and drinking of water, but the intellectual activities lent themselves to parody: children in dramas or parades or anything else that might get their attention as they dressed up as "Fresh Air" or "Leafy Vegetables." Behavior goals in fact often dominated in the classroom. As Benjamin Gruenberg observed at the beginning of the 1930s, health is a worthy goal indeed, "but . . . it becomes unnecessary so to emphasize the various health measures that the rituals and practices obscure their purpose." Others, too, were concerned about teaching health for the sake of health, blindly. "The child is to grow into a man or a woman," wrote the editor of *Nation's Health* in 1924, "and the real object of the school should be to furnish a sufficiently clear conception of the underlying principles of physiology, hygiene, and sanitation so that the child will be able not only to practise the routine of health habits imposed upon it at the moment but to meet situations as they arise in the future and to form its own health habits as an adolescent, an adult, a parent and a citizen." [40] In the face of such cautions, enthusiasts for health habits could and did reply that concrete results still were of primary importance.

The health crusade generated great enthusiasm regardless of whether children or adults were the objects of the crusaders. Anyone, without regard for philosophy, or even knowledge, could campaign for health habits. As a well-known public health official, Herman N. Bundesen, said in 1928: "My plea is that you live health, talk health, and think health. Sell it alike to young and old. Sell it by example and precept; by good health news published in the right way; through the press; by the motion picture, the radio, slogan and poster, or in any other way you will. But *sell* it. Science may outstrip public knowledge, but hygiene must remain to serve the public." And the new health educators had a paradigm that showed that mere ignorance—forget understanding—had bad effects, whereas disinterested instruction in fact solved many problems. The paradigm was sex education, and not enough could be said about the evil that could come of simply not having sound information in that department.[41]

Like the men of science of an earlier period, in one respect at least, the modern health crusaders opposed superstition and ignorance. "It is not enough," wrote two adult health educators in 1942, "to buy our boys and girls toothbrushes, to urge them to eat their spinach, to see that they get their vaccinations at the proper age. What about the 3 per cent who still say a cat will kill a baby by sucking its breath?" And the authors went on to cite other common beliefs such as the desirability and harmlessness of taking cathartic salts. "Until such superstitions can be uprooted from the folk culture passed from parent to child," they continued, "the health of our citizens must remain in constant danger of being undermined." The crusaders were particularly inspired by the campaign of the American Medical Association against quacks and proprietary medicine vendors and hoped to move large parts of the population away from emotionalism and subjectivity. Many early twentieth-century crusaders were, again, like their positivistic predecessors, willing to go far beyond mere health habits and to prescribe a whole attitude toward life. One pillar of public health, for example, regretted that extremists were writing about health, because their confusing assertions unfortunately could leave "the layman in serious doubt as to the best manner of life," a manner obviously known to the health forces.[42]

Despite the continuity of uplift and enlightenment from the late nineteenth century, the educators' emphasis on behavior was a sign, and a cause, of a subtle constriction in the meaning of popularizing. Some of the moral flavor in health advocacy was disappearing. Antialcohol propaganda seemed to many people no longer necessary. Advertisers more easily took on the coloration of health advocacy (a 1928 Macy's advertisement, for example, portrayed coats and raingear along with the family doctor as enhancers of health, and cigarette makers engendered much criticism by touting imagined health advantages of lighting up).[43]

Finally, and above all, the distance was growing between scientific medicine—practitioners and researchers—and the actual activity of popularizing health. D. B. Armstrong of Metropolitan Life, a particularly knowledgeable health educator, in 1935 voiced the viewpoint of the skeptic. "'Drink at least four glasses of water a day.' Sometimes this rule reads six, and sometimes eight glasses a day. This sounds like good advice, but have you ever attempted to verify it on a basis of scientific experiment?" he asked. Or, he asked, what evidence shows that fresh air prevents colds? "Then, exercise—" Armstrong continued. "'There is no better way to prolong life.' Of course, there is no better way to shorten life for some people. . . . 'Full bath more than once a week.' What health condition will that promote?" Armstrong admitted that frequent bathing would be esthetically advantageous but doubted that it would affect mortality statistics. But his call for enlightenment rather than injunction was seldom heeded.[44]

Critical Change in the 1930s

It was in the 1930s that a basic change in the popularization of health crystallized. Despite the prefiguring developments earlier in the century and despite continuities in many areas of popularizing, in approximately one decade two basic shifts occurred that separated the nineteenth and early twentieth centuries from the rest of the twentieth century. First, the types of people who carried out the popularization changed; that is, scientists and physicians distanced themselves from the public and tended to surrender popularization to journalists and educators. Second, the popularizers tended to shift from diffusing systematic knowledge to teaching about the products and consequences of medical science. Both of these changes had begun in the 1920s or earlier, as in the health habits campaign, but the not-entirely-coincidental combination of the two in full development made the 1930s a time of transformation (some of the underlying factors will be discussed in chapter 6). That something new was going on was suggested by the appearance of a fresh element in the media, the health pulp magazine and its congeners. Some of the magazines had the appeal of body concern (*Your Body*, 1934–1939; *Your Health*, 1939). Others emphasized the latest health news (*Health Digest*). And some exploited a sex motif (*Facts of Life*), embedded of course in a health context.

Lay participation in popularization of health was not new, whether in the antituberculosis campaigns earlier in the century or in the insurance-company-inspired Life Extension Institute (founded 1914). A few of the most enthusiastic crusaders of the new public health were laypersons, the most conspicuous of whom was Irving Fisher. Fisher was an economist at Yale who believed that he had won his own struggle against tuberculosis because he followed a strict regimen of personal hygiene. In 1908 he reported to the country on conserving "national vitality," that is, health, and he was the instigator and senior author of the inspirational and influential *How to Live: Rules for Healthful Living Based on Modern Science*, first published in 1915 and still being revised after World War II.[45]

Until the 1930s, however, representatives of scientific medicine tended to dominate popularization, and even Fisher had physician collaborators. Many medical figures continued to write for the public, but increasingly that new breed of journalist, the science writer, took over the field, especially the newspapers (where such writers represented an improvement over the traditional sensationalistic reporters). By the late 1940s, for example, only a quarter of the popularizers of medicine in major magazines were medical professionals. The rest were science writers or just generic journalists. By 1957 even the American Medical Association's popular journal, now called *Today's Health*, acquired a journalist editor, James M. Liston, who had been with *Better Homes and Gardens*.[46]

Moreover, medical and scientific professionals who did popularize in the 1920s and 1930s often did not write as professionals but instead took their format, standards, and message from the journalists. The best example was the distinguished medical scientist Paul de Kruif, who changed his role into that of a writer and whose sensational popularizations of various cures in the *Reader's Digest* in the 1930s and 1940s were a continual source of scandal.[47] The journalists in fact increasingly insisted on their own standards as they came to dominate popularization. The managing editor of the *Saturday Evening Post*, Robert Fuoss, complained, "It is . . . true that the doctors themselves make medical reporting very difficult. They seem to feel that they have a right of censorship which is enjoyed by no other group or profession. As a result, they frequently impose terms or conditions that are impossible to meet. In many cases they wish to take over the editorial functions along with their desire to promote scientific accuracy."[48] Clearly, as Fuoss indicated, it was the journalists who were going to have their way in the media.

The other group who tended to dominate health popularization, especially beginning in the 1930s, were the educators. They had started out working closely with physicians, and a whole program to succeed the older WCTU hygiene-physiology came out of a joint committee of the National Education Association (NEA) and the American Medical Association (AMA) in the early 1920s. But the joint child health group, the National Child Health Council, dissolved in 1935, leaving the field clear for the health educators, who organized themselves shortly thereafter. In part through their influence, health education in the midcentury period tended once again to become independent of general science and biology.[49]

This shift in personnel, from scientists and physicians to journalists and educators, continued over the years to reinforce the other major change in popularization that emerged in the 1930s, the displacement of emphasis from knowledge to product. Instead of science, nature, and uplift, popularizers more and more summarized the results of the biomedical sciences and explained how the reader or viewer could apply the latest findings—without particular attention to the rational or natural basis of the findings. Both educators and journalists—but especially journalists—carefully deferred to physicians in all matters of health. But it was the physician figure, not so much the research, to which they deferred. Much health popularization therefore became simply advice to consult one's personal physician; in practical terms, typical writers advocated an annual checkup for prevention, along with frequent visits to the doctor if any symptoms appeared (it was better to have the cold attended to before it turned into pneumonia)—as well as, finally, the practice of the now ubiquitous health habits, which still tended to be detached from scientific context. By 1934, one survey showed that little systematic teaching of physiology and hygiene had survived in American high schools.[50]

When Fisher and his physician collaborator, Eugene Lyman Fisk, set out in 1915 to enjoin Americans in general *How to Live*, their subtitle stated explicitly that they based their work upon "modern science," much of which was spelled out in appendices to the book. When the joint NEA-AMA committee drew up their health education program in the early 1920s, the committee had as goals inculcating healthy personal habits and attitudes and a desire to have a healthy environment, but they also made provision for basic knowledge of physiology and sanitation as well as moralism, including what the committee called a "health conscience." By the outbreak of World War II, however, educators could talk of habits without much context. Adult education, wrote Frank Ernest Hill, was largely "of the propaganda and habit forming type." The widely used standard booklet prepared for U.S. Army inductees represented the change well: authoritative practical advice on health and personal habits with a minimum of moralizing or knowledge about physiology and medicine—again the products of science without origins and context.[51]

The content of health popularization after the 1920s and into midcentury developed in a way that was remarkably compatible with educators' emphases upon the social environment. As one educator wrote in 1939, health instruction should have a context, but it was not to be moralism or science per se: "We do not want health facts taught in and of themselves, but rather an integration of all the pupil's interests, experiences, and environment in such a way that desirable health outcomes will result."[52] For decades afterward, such formulations meant social and personal, not natural and scientific.

As the mass media developed further with radio, more doubtful assertions about health assailed the attention of most Americans. "One has but to sit by the radio or read advertisements to appreciate the life destructive and youth-shortening enemies by which everybody is surrounded," noted J. Clarence Funk, a popularizer, wryly, and he mentioned "ailments that are both devitalizing and ostracising," such as halitosis, obesity, constipation, and eye strain that advertisers promised to correct. "Stating it baldly," he concluded, "great numbers of Americans [are] saturated with false or semi-authentic health facts." Authentic authorities of any kind were operating increasingly at a disadvantage.[53]

The Mid-Twentieth Century

The withdrawal of scientists and educators from popularization of health may have affected more than content. One of the notable aspects of popularization of health as such in the mid-twentieth-century decades was that it did not flourish. Some years passed before health education in the schools recovered from the educational budget cuts of the Great Depression. Publications, whether magazines indexed in the *Reader's Guide* or books and pamphlets of various kinds, tended to avoid health except for specifics of diet and other personal actions akin to the health habits. Gone were the extensive warnings about infectious disease that had graced the literature of the germ period. Even the vitamins, it turned out, had been oversold. Publications of public health offices at all levels less and less contained material for the general public and more and more spoke to the concerns of professionals and subprofessionals who were in the field trying to change behavior and administer laws. John Tebbel, in the preparation of his 1951 book popularizing up-to-date health advice, found very little good popular material available and had to draw therefore upon interviews with medical scientists.[54]

The non-natural elements that midcentury popularizers emphasized were nutrition (particularly in terms of body weight) and exercise. Americans increasingly were "running, stretching, starving." But instead of worrying about particular organs or diseases, the cultivators of health were concerned with their whole bodies, and, at least in the media, physical fitness came to enjoy a growing popularity, and not just because of patriotic concern about World War II draftees who had not measured up. Eventually one U.S. president, in 1956, called a "President's Conference on Fitness of American Youth," and another president, in 1961, sent a special message to the schools on the subject.[55]

Also around midcentury, American popular health came to contain a great deal of psychological explanation. Advocates were not emphasizing merely the tranquil passions of traditional health but the mutual involvement of psyche and soma, epitomized in psychosomatics, in which specific psychological elements joined the homeostasis of material particles and transformed the definition of health into a holistic human condition. As one educator put it in 1950, "Psychosomatics, with its emphasis on the singleness of mind and body, of physical and mental health, points up the long-recognized truth that the whole person is the proper subject of educational purpose." The extent to which such ideas were popularized was reflected in the request that psychoanalyst Franz Alexander received from a woman in Texas for "two bottles of your psychosomatic medicine." Altogether, popularized health material had shifted substantially to this holistic, cybernetic view of human beings, which for some time appeared also in a social context. On occasion, popular knowledge was sufficient that writers could focus on an organ, like the heart, rather than the whole person, but midcentury Americans, concentrating on the products and conclusions of medical science, stuck largely to diet, exercise, and mental health.[56]

In the health popularization that featured products and conclusions, the intrusion of the psychological was particularly appropriate in health education in the schools because the educators' goal continued to be that of learning how to change specific behaviors of Americans by motivating them and directing them. Health publicists focused on a general audience also were concerned that merely informing the public was not sufficient, because information alone was not necessarily effective when all they wanted was to change people's behavior. One such worker, Irwin M. Rosenstock, who headed what was actually called the U. S. Public Health Service Behavioral Studies Section, in 1960 noted that advertising techniques would not suffice, for health demanded not only action, but action by a large percentage of the population. Where an advertiser might make more than ample profits from a one percent share of the market, for instance, polio control, to take an extreme example, required action from 100 percent of the audience. Nevertheless, in the realm of personal health, the task of the educator could be much more like that of the advertiser, in which any changes in any person's health activity would be counted a gain. All of these concerns with behavior and motivation continued in later years.[57]

After Midcentury

After midcentury, in the final phase of popularization, masses of Americans took a special interest in health. They showed the interest by spending dramatically increased amounts on not only medical care but gymnasium and similar group memberships and paraphernalia. By the late 1970s, special-interest mass magazines joined older pulps that had come and gone in the limited circulation field. In addition to such magazines as *American Health* (founded 1982), which purveyed the standard commercial mix of advice along with news of newly discovered dangers and possible cures, both the Harvard Medical School, beginning in the mid-1970s, and the Mayo Clinic issued popular health newsletters. There was even a special cable television service carrying health news.[58]

Meanwhile, within the public health and educational systems, the health educators had been further developing a professional identity, with such organizational reinforcements as journals and associations, as well as establishing an independent niche in school curriculums. Health educators still believed that they had to provide not only the knowledge but also the motivation and practical skills that would make people of all ages effective in looking after their own health. Moreover, in the 1970s many educators and popularizers concluded that social as well as individual action might also be essential to health, but they conceived of actions more fundamental than quarantine regulation. The program that emerged was a remarkable combination of, as one health educator of that decade observed, "absence of serious environmental pollutants and extremes of poverty and wealth, regular physical and mental activity which does not abruptly come to an end at some arbitrary age limit, a fair degree of moderation and regularity in daily living patterns, a diet relatively low in calories, especially in animal fats, and a fairly stable family and community support system." [59]

Finally, although for some time public health officials had tried to emulate advertisers in order to get health messages across, after the midcentury period, the behavioral science approach to marketing provided an especially attractive model; and a special field, social marketing, including health, developed in the 1970s. Such interest intensified when social science evidence suggested that when health advocates were able to place their own content in the mass media they really could change some health behaviors effectively. [60]

One of the reasons that health advocates after midcentury took a very broad approach to health was the new awareness of the environment that has already been alluded to—an environment with which the holistic human being, as many thinking people conceptualized it then, interacted. In the 1940s, for example in the *Health Instruction Yearbook,* the environment had appeared specifically in connection with particular organs: feet and x rays, eyes and television, and, of course, teeth and fluorine. To immediately succeeding generations, "environment" embraced additional definite meanings, such as the cumulative effects of agricultural poisons. But the term also took on a more general meaning, one not just dealing with the effects of environmental factors on body organs but, in the traditional sense of the non-naturals, encouraging harmonious passions of the soul. [61]

In this new popularization, concern with infectious disease diminished even further. Although adjustment of the whole person to the natural and social world was seen as essential, and although there was even the brief concern about social action, the main thrust of popularizers continued to be toward getting individuals to control their own actions, whether ingesting, exercising, or carrying out other prescriptions from the nonnaturals. As the official Institute of Medicine report put it in 1982, "The heaviest burdens of illness in the United States today are related to aspects of individual behavior, especially long-term patterns of behavior often referred to as 'lifestyle'. . . . [Fully] 50 percent of mortality from the 10 leading causes of death," the authors continued, "can be traced to lifestyle." In addition to mobilizing people to change their lifestyles and thus reduce their physical deterioration, health educators were attempting to develop informed consumers who could use the health care system intelligently. Altogether, the popularizers' emphasis on individual behavior was striking.[62] Even in the 1980s, when there was a renaissance of interest in infectious diseases, the popular version of this interest took the form of concern about venereal diseases and easily translated into concern about self and personal actions rather than public health as such.

The bulk of the popularizers continued to be specialists in education or journalism, but a new and important element joined them in critical numbers by the 1970s: specialists in advocacy. Some advocated one emphasis in health, some another. Whole networks sprang up around so-called health food stores, for example. All such advocates believed in health for the sake of health in a context that led a number of writers to describe the advocates' romantic and obsessive preoccupations with the body and the person in terms of what Christopher Lasch has called *The Culture of Narcissism*. Another symptomatic group of health specialists stood for what observers called simply "the religion of running." Beyond the obvious self-centeredness of all of these enthusiasts, their emphasis upon an individual's taking responsibility for his or her own health took on an antimedical aspect reminiscent of the mid-nineteenth century as well as of the anti-institutional aspect remarked on in chapter 1. In the meantime, the mainstream health advocates continued to organize, not only in health departments but in the ever more powerful voluntary health groups; in 1971 there were, for example, 25,000 identifiable health educators.[63]

Health and Medicine

The phases in popularizing health, from moralism and scientism to arbitrary health habits and romantic self-centeredness, of course succeeded each other in a broader context of institutional change. Medicine, education, the media, and advertising particularly contributed to transforming the meaning of the popularization of health.

When the products of medical science—injunctions to behave in certain ways, and advice to see a doctor—became dominant in health popularization in the 1930s, an altered relationship appeared between health advocacy and popularized medicine, a relationship additionally underlined by the antimedical elements among health enthusiasts late in the century. Where for many decades the relationship between popularized health and popularized medical science had tended to converge, now once again in this confusing relationship they sometimes separated.

During the nineteenth century, following the laws of health meant coordinating with nature, not with physicians' various assertions about cures. Yet many physicians, as I have suggested, were also involved in popularizing health. When medicine became scientific in the modern sense late in the century, when cures went out and therapeutic nihilism and prevention came in, popularizers, as I noted above, could combine medicine and health. By the early twentieth century, sanitation and germ theory provided a basis for the new public health that depended upon educating people in preventive measures, both personal and public.

By the end of the 1930s, when infectious diseases became less consequential for Americans, health popularizers tended to shift to other types of problems, such as industrial hygiene, and particularly to degenerative diseases, which loomed larger as infectious diseases continued to diminish and the population grew older. C.-E.A. Winslow of Yale in 1942 saw how he and other public health workers would have to adapt to this elemental change in disease patterns:

> We can see without any question that the chief causes of death in the future will not be germ diseases and that the motive of protection against infection is not going to be a vital part of the picture. The chief causes of death are more and more going to lie in the individual and in his social environment, and our educational objectives will not

be anything as simple and obvious as the concept of distributing tuberculosis germs by spitting on the sidewalk.[64]

The shift to an emphasis on preserving oneself against heart disease,
cancer, and stroke did not occur without the complication of another
major shift that had been occurring in the role of medicine. As the effectiveness of medical intervention in specific cases of disease grew, starting
with the miracles of surgery around the turn of the century and culminat-
ing in the wonder drugs of the 1930s and 1940s, most Americans came to
believe that their health really could depend upon physicians. It was for
this reason that popularizing health came to involve popularizing medical
science and medical practice. As Daniel Fox emphasizes, new hopes for
scientific medicine already by the 1920s were causing Americans to identify health with curative health care. The growth of his confusion was a
major factor in the temporary decline in the classic popularization of preserving health, already noted, in the 1940s and 1950s—just when faith in
medicine increased. A widespread attempt to enlist the physician in prevention through patient education and the presumably informative annual checkup confounded the confusion between health and physicians'
institutions through most of the twentieth century. As early as 1928, for
instance, physician John B. Morrison pointed out that health education
could bring not only better health and the defeat of pernicious superstitions and cults but greater prestige for the physicians and a favorable climate for promedical legislation.[65]

In practice, one important way of popularizing the science of medicine—as it intertwined with health—was to glorify the heroes of medical
research, such as Louis Pasteur and Walter Reed or even more recent figures, such as Joseph Goldberger. The Metropolitan Life Insurance Company began as early as the 1920s to target schools with a widely read series of pamphlets called Health Heroes, in which children (and adults, as
it turned out) learned to connect the authority and products of scientific
medicine with heroes and the good, true, and progressive. Presumably,
however, some of the scientific content was also communicated. The
Health Heroes series was still going after World War II, and this general
approach, in which medical science justified the authority of the physician, was to be found in many media, including some famous motion picture dramas, for many decades. Because discoveries later were coming so
fast, the total effect of making researchers into heroes tended to leave

midcentury popularizers of medical science once again emphasizing authoritative cures.[66]

One particular effect of the explosion of the findings of medical scientists, it should therefore be emphasized, was to free popularizers from having to explain fully the health advice that they were purveying, for they could now appeal to the authority of scientists without establishing understanding in the particular audience. In his 1940 health textbook, Thurman B. Rice made the point explicitly:

> The body is so extraordinarily complex that the liberal arts student can gain no adequate notion of the real mechanism of his body in the time that he may reasonably be expected to spend in studying it. Nor is it necessary that he should. We learn to drive an automobile quite efficiently without taking a course in automotive engineering. We simply leave all that to the manufacturer and the mechanic, while we concentrate upon the problem of obeying instructions and using the car in a way that is conducive to the safety of the driver, the occupants, and the other fellow. For the purposes of hygiene we need a general understanding of the body but hardly need all the academic and technical details, which are after all the province of the technically trained physician or dentist.[67]

Special-Interest Groups

Physicians personally continued throughout the twentieth century to play an important part in popularizing, from the health columnists in the newspapers of the 1910s and after to television advisors of the 1980s.[68] But increasingly in the twentieth century, American society, including the field of health, developed special-interest groups to advocate various goals. Some groups represented commercial interests, and some were altruistic. Beyond physicians per se, a substantial number of these advocacy groups, as I have already suggested, were conspicuous in health popularization late in the century. They were also present and important earlier. Typically they focused on the schools, but usually they also mounted a parallel campaign to influence the public at large, especially as the press became susceptible to manipulation by means of the press release, not to mention advertising.

The precedent obviously was set by the efforts of nineteenth-century health reformers and then the WCTU to establish compulsory hygiene-physiology temperance teaching in the schools. By the time the WCTU courses were collapsing, a number of additional advocacy groups were ready to influence the new public health and the innovative school curriculum. The most conspicuous group was the antituberculosis association, which, at the least, caused a remarkable prominence of fresh air (not to mention outdoor living in general) to appear in health advice. Antivenereal disease forces also left their mark. At the same time, a number of life insurance groups developed formidable and sometimes inspired health education campaigns, including, as Bruce V. Lewenstein has pointed out, using insurance agents as active popularizers of health ideas. The insurance groups were biased of course toward preventing death rather than illness, much less fostering the positive elements traditional among health proponents. One of their great successes, for example, was making safety education a large part of health advocacy. The soap manufacturers, to cite another early twentieth-century example, through the Cleanliness Institute had a profound influence on school health education. They were joined in the 1920s by dairy interests, who made drinking milk sacrosanct in American schools. Many other groups made an impact on the schools and usually also on the general public. In the 1930s, 250 industrial corporations were supporting the American Hygiene Foundation, for instance. The American Heart Association was particularly successful in the 1950s, and planned parenthood advocates in the 1960s. The mental health forces had enviable successes after World War II, if not before, and by the late 1960s the anticancer groups were even affecting national politics.[69]

Over 100 private health organizations could be identified by 1933, and a quarter of a century later such organizations counted 15 million Americans among their volunteer supporters.[70] The problem with such groups was that with few ties to general medical and scientific knowledge, organizations could appear to the public to favor health but actually to have any goal. The best example of misleading appearance was the powerful National Health Federation, which in fact represented commercial interests that were exploitive as well as unscientific, to say the least (chiefly marketers of proprietary medicines and quackery).[71] In such an atmosphere, physicians could be reduced also to just another interest group, rather than concurrently represent traditional science and uplift. Even the best of the medical science institutions—those entirely philanthropic and divorced from physicians' political and economic campaigns—were forced into the public relations game. Not only did medical professionals have an obligation to report to their supporters and constituents, noted a Georgia journalist addressing a medical audience in 1953, but "the newspaper, radio-tv and magazine, as important social agencies, cannot ignore medical, scientific, and educational news. In the fulfillment of their obligation, journalists are entitled to the intelligent support of the medical world."[72] Under such pressures, it was no wonder that health workers turned to public relations and talked about their publicizing activities as marketing.

The Mass Media

Increasingly the institutions through which health popularization passed constrained its content. The major institutions were of course those involved in the shift of popularizing personnel in the 1930s, the schools and the mass media. The role of educational institutions as such was relatively clear, from replacing the WCTU hygiene courses with ones emphasizing general science and biology content to connecting health education to physical education and then to developing identifiable health education and health educators. The mass media, however, presented a different problem (not only discussed here but returned to in chapter 6). Unlike the schools, the media did not have any tradition of either moralizing or uplift, and yet they exercised a distinctive influence on the popularization of health.

The first popularizers, in the early nineteenth century, addressed a public made up of what Edward Hitchcock of Amherst referred to in 1830 as professionals and students—those for whom health was a special problem. Farmers after all did not need fresh air and exercise.[73] Professionals and students read books, pamphlets, magazines, and the personal journalism newspapers of the day—a situation that persisted, with the constant addition of an increasingly literate population, until, as I have suggested, the advent of yellow journalism. Indeed, except for explicit campaigns like those targeting workers or venereal disease and hookworm victims, health popularizers always tended to appeal to the upper classes. Clearly organic foods and jogging suits—the commercial face of more recent popularization—were not lower class. Yet as the population became more diverse, health workers often tried to aim at a variety of publics at once. Thus the readers of *Hygeia* for decades were berated for using patent medicines when in fact the teachers and other educated people who typically saw the magazine were not likely to be victimized by nostrums, quacks, and cures. But before very far into the twentieth century, all levels of the public were reached through essentially the mass media, as two 1941 observers suggested:

> Most so-called health education is acquired from publicity prepared for mass consumption: newspaper or magazine reports of medical news; "advice" of a physician-journalist; advertisements of pharmaceutical manufacturers; or pamphlets distributed by insurance companies. Innumerable posters, pamphlets, and leaflets of varying degrees of comprehensibility are forced upon the attention of the public. . . . Motion picture "trailers" and displays in the windows of public buildings or in health museums are among the visual media employed. On the radio the public hears popular or semipopular versions of the pursuit of the microbe.[74]

Popularizers in the age of mass media thus found themselves dealing with a set of institutions that originated in or took their tone from yellow journalism and continued to depend upon that kind of appeal so that neither truth nor balance could in the end be well served, whether newspaper, magazine, television, or whatever was involved. All continued the main bias of yellow journalism: sensationalism. Despite the best efforts of science writers, the indictment of sensationalizing health information was still valid almost a century after the birth of the yellow press. As late as 1976, for example, a former reporter, by then in medical school, criticized distorted writing about cancer; "Thus far," he observed, "science has been reported mostly as a curiosity. . . . Stories are meant to provide more emotion than information."[75]

Sensationalism in the health field showed up in two main practices. The first was that of emphasizing the prevalence and danger of certain pathological conditions in a way that went far beyond balance or sense. Cancer was a mid-twentieth-century concern, as was polio, and each was blown out of proportion. Other exaggerations ranged from food poisoning and tonsilitis earlier in the century to mental disease and heart trouble later— and finally acquired immune deficiency syndrome. Journalists using sentiment and scare brought them all to the attention of large parts of the public, sometimes very effectively. As one unwitting government official of the early 1950s is reported to have complained, "I can't imagine what's the matter with the girls in this office. They go about all day long pinching their breasts."[76]

Paradoxically, awareness of disease was often generated by the second sensationalistic practice: reporting cures. Editors of the twentieth century found that their readers were no different from victims of patent medicine vendors in any century: news of a cure was absolutely appealing. This was a clichéd approach in the early twentieth-century yellow journal, in the mid-twentieth-century *Reader's Digest* (the highest circulation magazine), and in the late twentieth-century supermarket rag: "Good News About . . ." or "New Hope for . . . ." Indeed, even the most ethical science writers had used the approach so often in medical stories that by midcentury they began to joke among themselves about it. David Dietz recalled that "if a biologist made an interesting discovery about the action of an enzyme in the living cell, the accepted lead for the story was, 'New hope for the conquest of cancer was seen today in the discovery,' etc. . . . The situation finally [became] so overdone that among ourselves we referred to this approach as the 'new hope school of science writing.'" Arousing false hopes was at best irresponsible, but it persisted, and sensational reporting of medical science was in part to blame for the antimedical movements of the late twentieth century when physicians and hospitals could not meet expectations raised by journalists. In 1983, for example, *Health* magazine announced the "Fourth Annual All-Breakthroughs Issue."[77]

With each addition to the media, health advocates themselves had new hope for popularization. Beginning in 1912, as many Americans were still seeing their first motion pictures, short feature films containing health instruction often introduced "the movies" to people who could look at images on a wall and learn, for example, how to brush their teeth. During World War I, the film was used very effectively for health propaganda for service personnel. But then Hollywood took over. As late as 1945 another round of army health indoctrination films led health officials again to develop new hope for the medium. But of course without captive audiences, which were found only in the schools and the armed forces, movies were a disappointment.[78] In the 1930s, the new picture magazines such as *Life* and *Look* were in fact sometimes effective, until television killed them off, but radio went commercial; not only was health popularization not especially appealing to radio audiences, but commercialization opened the door to the vendors of health and beauty aids, mostly of doubtful value, or worse, and the hucksters were quite successful indeed.[79]

If radio was a failure for health popularizers, television was a disaster. Indeed, scholarly researchers from time to time investigated and documented the dimensions of the disaster. Positive health information, such as that contained in public service announcements, appeared with rare exceptions at times when few people were watching or else was isolated on public television channels. One 1970 study showed that a full 5 percent of commercial television broadcasting carried misleading or inaccurate health information, chiefly in "entertainment" programs and in commercials. Another group of investigators, a decade later, concluded that television actively developed in viewers "poor nutritional knowledge and behavior, general complacency, and [unrealistically] high confidence in the medical community."[80]

Modern television displayed in its most naked form the commercial element that had traditionally had a special relationship to the popularization of health. Advertising in fact provided directly a substantial part of Americans' health information and advice in every period of history, from the nineteenth-century patent medicine almanacs (with their anatomical illustrations) and newspaper ads—sometimes constituting one-fourth or more of an ordinary newspaper—to the radio and television commercials with details of "pink toothbrush" (bleeding gums) and other horrors. Readers in 1840, for example, could learn much (for good or ill) from Dr. Evans' ad for medicines

> so compounded, that by strengthening and equalizing the action of
> the heart, liver, and other viscera, they dispel the bad acrid or mor-
> bid matter which renders the blood impure, out of the circulation,
> through the excretory ducts into the passage of the bowels, so that by
> the brisk or slight evacuations, which may be regulated by the doses,
> always remembering that while the evacuations from the bowels are
> kept up, the excretions from all the other vessels of the body will also
> be going on in the same proportion, by which means the blood in-
> variably becomes purified.

Sometimes advertisers took advantage of and reinforced other health popularizers, as in the cases of Dr. Evans, just quoted, or those who touted microbe cures in the late nineteenth century or fluorides for teeth in the mid-twentieth.[81]

Since such a very large part of the advertising was at best misleading, other popularizers for decades, as I have noted, denounced material that originated with people who were commercially interested. Therefore a large part of the efforts of health enthusiasts in the early twentieth century went into countering advertising, and by midcentury many social scientists were actually measuring the falsity of the commercial propaganda that reached its culmination in video. As the commissioner of the New York State Department of Health observed in 1960,

> Along with other mass media, television advertising is a ceaseless fount of health information. All day long the viewer is told how pills will end his nagging backache. He's offered tonics to pep up his tired blood. He learns what magic medicine is "strongest in the pain reliever doctors recommend most for arthritis." He can get a complete lecture on dental decay—and what product will end it—in 60 seconds. An end to sinus conditions, relief for sluggish intestines, a cure for skin blemishes, it's all there at the flick of a switch, a veritable flood of health knowledge. . . . But so much of it is so wrong, so spurious, so incomplete and so misleading. If the claims of medicine and toothpaste makers are to be the most persistent messages our people will get, then I for one am resigned to a low state of health knowledge.[82]

The nature of advertisers' misrepresentations has been detailed by Rita S. Rosenberg, using as a basis nutritional claims in advertising for the entire first half of the twentieth century. She found half-truth and suppression of relevant fact pervasive, as in the relatively benign nut marketers who touted the proteins in nuts but did not point out how they differed from other food proteins and were not as satisfactory from a dietary point of view. Rosenberg also found that advertisers effectively helped alert members of the public to various conventional health standards and concepts—calories, proteins, vitamins, minerals. Nevertheless, this educational effect was in turn but a response to previous successes of other popularizers. Members of the consuming public early in the century already were concerned that constipation was dangerous, and consumers therefore responded to bran cereal advertisers who praised "regularity." Later, those members of the public who knew vitamins were important were susceptible to the blandishments of advertisers of oranges. Yet if such ads reinforced contemporary health teachings, they always did so in a biased way. The bias was the same as that which commercial interest groups like the soap manufacturers introduced into the schools. Moreover, the bias was not filtered through responsible public groups or agencies. In this way around 1970 the three-pronged dental health program of brushing, seeing a dentist, and avoiding sweets in fact had its origins in toothpaste ads, and it neglected other elements, such as flossing, that experts at that time thought were important but that did not fit into the advertising.[83]

Advertising, moreover, had far-reaching effects on the popularizing of health itself. At best, advertisers corrupted the media. Even in the nineteenth century, the press so depended upon cure vendors that critics were largely ineffective. The press in the mid-twentieth century was similarly irresponsible in the case of the dangers of cigarette smoking, and even though the story was complex, only news magazines (according to one study) appeared free from quite realistic commercial concerns. As numerous health popularizers lamented over the years, the advertisers provided competition that was hard to meet, much less beat. By the 1970s, most people (88 percent in one poll) depended upon television commercials as the alternative to their physicians for health information.[84]

Flawed Missionaries of Health

The fact that the mass media were particularly susceptible to commercial influence underlines the importance of the shift in popularizing personnel in the 1930s era—and the more so since originally one of the major reasons for popularizing was to protect the public from commercial exploitation. Journalists and educators in fact were not able to maintain the standards of popularization that scientists and physicians had earlier tried to observe. And, more than scientists and reputable physicians, both educators and journalists were often not successful in maintaining perspective and, moreover, were themselves susceptible to influence by interested propagandists. The record of the performance of even the best of the journalists, the science writers, was lamentable in the health area. In a careful study of magazine reporting of health and medical stories of the 1940–1952 period, Carolyn Keith Cramp assembled a sorry record of

botched-up popularization that reflected on writers and also on editors—
the latter particularly for continuing to run articles written by unreliable
authors. Another of Cramp's findings was, again, the dramatic effects of
commercial promotion in conditioning the popularization of medical discoveries. Whether ammoniated toothpaste or chlorophyll tablets, items
available in trade generated grave problems in accuracy in ordinary popularizing stories.[85] Professional journalists clearly did not perform at a high
level as popularizers of health.

Twentieth-century educators often did do well in explicitly attempting
to undercut both superstition and advertising and develop in their students a scientific attitude along with healthy behavior. Educators who
saw their mission as essentially cultivating the intellect resisted introducing mere health training for the masses of students, but other educators,
aided by proponents of the new public health, relentlessly forced modern
health education on the schools. Problems did arise when health education fell into the hands of physical education instructors. "There is no
correlation between interest in physical activities and interest in science,"
noted James Frederick Rogers in 1933, "and it is little wonder that the
average teacher of physical education, excellent as he may be, is neither
adept nor interested in teaching hygiene."[86] But that era, as noted above,
passed.

Even in the hands of the best-intentioned educators, however, health
often lost something in the translation. As Rogers suggested, the crucial
element that went astray was science. A 1933 reviewer saw this problem,
for example, in a new textbook: "The lack of scientific background in the
text, the over-simplification of vocabulary, and the short sentences which
merely state facts—but rarely give explanations." Even the careful educators, then, tended to lose the science in mechanically translating and
condensing, and this problem was exacerbated as more child-centered
learning developed, as I have already suggested.[87]

Health in Isolation

The old positivistic tradition involved, besides opposition to superstition
and commercialism, an affirmative viewpoint, namely, that scientific
truths belonged in a systematic context. As the author of a popular
pre–World War II biology textbook wrote,

The study of biology thus helps us to know ourselves and to understand many of the requirements of safe and pleasant living, but it has still more to offer. With the other sciences, biology helps us to become intellectually free. It tends to rid our minds of superstitions and groundless fears and it shows us everywhere the universal working of cause and effect, the "uniformity of nature," by virtue of which we can rest secure in the certainty that what we discover today will be true tomorrow. . . . that nature is neither friendly nor hostile to us, but is in general beneficial or injurious according to our success in discovering natural principles or "laws" and acting in accordance with them.[88]

But even as he wrote, the changes in personnel in popularizing and changes in the media were altering the very meaning of the act of popularization.

Practitioners of journalism had long emphasized the products of science—discovery or cure, as opposed to scientific processes, much less the gospel of science. By midcentury, journalists were concentrating particularly on facts (in ways to be taken up in chapter 6), and this quest for objectivity in reporting helped shape the popularization of health. Earlier popularizers had not hidden their opinions, whether the moralism of early nineteenth-century health advocates or the harsh precepts of science of a later generation. As the quest for facts and objectivity grew in journalism, and as journalists more and more did the actual work of popularizing health, so increasingly the picture that both children and adults received was one of disembodied facts, disembodied even though discovered by scientists and clothed with the authority of science. It was in this way that health teachings became merely the reported products of science—vitamins are necessary for health in certain ways, or specified exercises develop certain sets of muscles—but hygiene no longer involved an explicit intellectual and perhaps social commitment or a way of looking at the world—only a way of looking at one's body, usually in a segmented fashion. In the mid-1950s, a science reporter reprimanded physicians who wanted to carry to the public more than the bare facts and products: "I think the doctors really have no kick coming about us reporters, because 98 per cent of the time I am writing about the wonderful discoveries and treatments they are making, and about 2 per cent of the time their foolish excursions into pontificating upon what is good for the public and things like that."[89]

As the change to products and facts was taking place, many commentators recognized the fact and deplored it. While knowledge expanded and people learned the "results of scientific investigation," complained a medical editor in 1920, "such information on these matters as is current among the general public is fragmentary, unrelated, and, for the most part, acquired through spectacular accounts of the Sunday newspaper." The editor went on to deplore "the tendency to mysticism in the absence of definite knowledge." A reviewer in 1933 criticized a textbook writer whose prose consisted primarily of "short sentences which merely state facts—but rarely give explanations." And a public health advocate from the interwar years warned, "It is desirable to form health habits which will be useful at the moment, but it is also important to give the child a sound knowledge of the principles of physiology and hygiene so that in the future it can modify its habits intelligently as the need may arise." The writer went on to say that children should learn to "think biologically" and not merely develop patterns of behavior advocated by the child health organization.[90]

The forces of change passed by such critics. By the mid-twentieth century, even scientists popularizing health, to say nothing of educators, conformed to the journalistic fragmentation as they tended to talk in terms of discrete actions—brushing the teeth, looking both ways before crossing the street—rather than in terms of a virtuous, clean way of living tied into a coherent rationale tending to physicalistic reductionism. As early as the 1930s, health educators were avoiding even science labels like the "physiology" of an earlier day and instead were talking about "healthful living."

By the 1970s, the health educators had moved even further from righteousness and scientism and now spoke of mere choices between styles of life. The authors of one book for health educators laid out as teaching goals not only developing desirable attitudes in the students but deferring to individual choice and background; these authors gave the subjective feelings of each child precedence over any set of teachings. In 1968 John S. Sinacore opened his college textbook *Health: A Quality of Life* by observing that "man's strongest desires are not for health, but for life and living," and in fact he emphasized sex and and mental health at the expense of instruction in hygiene. So far had health educators come that they actually tried to avoid teaching values in health courses; one 1973 set of precepts suggested the extreme to which the educators had moved from the uplifting and inspirational hygiene books of less than a century earlier: (1) teach individuals how to think without telling them what thoughts to have; (2) teach individuals to understand themselves in terms of their personal needs; (3) teach individuals to value without establishing a set of values for them."[91]

For the more general public, the important ancillary health "education" carried out by advertisers took the journalistic model of disjointed, isolated fact to extremes, so that a health worker in the 1960s was asked after a lecture on preserving nutrients in cooking, "Those vitamins you were talking about—are they the same as the stuff in the pills?" Contemporary observers in both the radio and television eras noted that repeated injunctions out of context were the basis for fundamental public ignorance. What difference did it make if a person learned from health advocates to sleep with the window open or if he or she learned from, say, 1930s advertising to reach for Feenamint "the minute dullness, laziness or headache show [sic] a condition that requires a laxative?"[92]

From one point of view, an overall context for health popularization in the twentieth century no longer made sense. The discovery of specific causes for infectious diseases—and specific cures—made following a general life strategy (a reasoned strategy, as opposed to a style) less urgent. The increasing prominence of degenerative diseases changed the priorities of health. Technical medicine, too, embodied and exemplified fragmentation, as I shall remark in chapter 6. Perhaps the life sciences were simply too complex to be used in health popularization in the recent period. All of these considerations in biomedicine complemented what was happening in journalism, in which discrete facts were welcome but not long, involved series or matrices.[93]

Change in the Meaning of Popularization

The problem was that the isolated-facts format was exactly the one that nineteenth-century popularizers had fought against, for it is the format of ignorance and superstition: singular beliefs repeated but never established or understood as part of a reasoned context. As long ago as 1939 a group of University of Missouri researchers saw the parallel. After reviewing assertions of advertisers, such as that a particular soap would make one beautiful or that a brand of face cream with vitamins in it would surely be effective, the researchers concluded: "Are these not just as much superstitions as the belief in lucky and unlucky numbers, the carrying of horse chestnuts for rheumatism or rubbing a rabbit's foot for luck?" [94]

As a scientific and rational faith tended to disappear from health popularization, leaving only "facts," the best that Americans could depend on from educators and journalists was a new set of competing superstitions, disjointed injunctions of scientific or whatever other origins. If the practice of chewing one's food according to Fletcher's ideas passed away, why accept jogging any more readily? Or why not? Under these circumstances, the non-naturals command respect. For many hundreds of years they embodied what was for their day a scientific viewpoint, and still generations later, in the 1980s, no one questioned their cogency.

But the context within which health knowledge of whatever antiquity was popularized had changed, as had its cultural function. [95] Health popularization was no longer a vehicle for extending advocacy of a robust scientism and uplift as well as a sound body. No one refounded the "League for Longer Life" that Harvey W. Wiley once promoted in the pages of *Good Housekeeping*. Each piece of health advice was reduced to just another among the many amoral, unconnected, often unreasoned assertions that passed for popular science in the late twentieth century.

Popular health advice nevertheless showed the concern of Americans of both the nineteenth and twentieth centuries for learning about ways that science impinged upon the self. But another area of learning, besides medicine, dealt with the self—namely, psychology. Since psychology for the public embodied both the popularizing of science and at the same time the most transparent concern with self that energized so much of the popularization of all learning, I turn from efforts to popularize health to the disseminating, translating, and condensing that constituted the popularization of psychology in all of its aspects—experimental, applied, and clinical. There, too, popularization went through stages and ended as a vehicle for fragments rather than viewpoint.

Chapter 3
The Popularizing of Psychology

ALTHOUGH popularizing of psychology went through stages very similar to those in the popularizing of health, the first stage was missing in the case of psychology. The reason was that for much of the nineteenth century it was not possible to popularize psychology. What psychology there was, was common property among educated people. Technical psychology would at most have been but a subfield within philosophy. It was not until specialized, distinctive, scientific psychology came along at the end of the century that psychology could be translated, condensed, and simplified for lay people. In 1838, for example, a savant of the day wrote on "The Power of Mind," by which he meant one's ability to control oneself and others—approximately what "psychology" meant to the public of a later day. The savant recognized at once the commonplace nature of his ideas: "What school-boy has not written something upon the power of mind?" he asked, "and what philosopher has ever fully analyzed it?"[1] In that day, any educated person could discuss the subject. Only beginning in the 1880s did a specialized experimental psychology begin to appear that was not already in the possession of the literate public, and therefore only then was there a psychology that could be popularized.

Psychological Subjects in the Diffusion Period

In the decades of mere diffusion, when identical information went to the public and experts indiscriminately, some of what would later be psychological subject matter attracted substantial attention in the usual newspapers, magazines, and lectures—and in the yellow press period just at the end of the century, even more so. Here, then, was the beginning of another narrative of popularization with internal determinants and momentum regardless of the general patterns that became discernible in it.

Americans particularly took up phrenology, which for many years functioned as a science of personality characteristics, the recognition of which supposedly could facilitate self-improvement. Many of the adepts of phrenology were offended when large numbers of Americans undertook to popularize the science and particularly to exploit it commercially. But even the itinerant phrenological practitioners and lecturers provided very large parts of the public with an introduction to the idea of character analysis and a naturalistic way of viewing human beings, including themselves. Despite the critics, the popularizers thought that they were contributing to the science of phrenology at the very same time that they were diffusing knowledge that was within the grasp of "any individual" American, as the leading publicists of phrenology put it in 1849; they did not differentiate technical from popular exposition.[2]

Another popular psychology that was available to anyone was mesmerism—at least until serious scientific studies at the end of the century turned it into hypnotism. The same reform groups that took up health and phrenology also tended to take up mesmerism, finding in it still other powers with which people allegedly could improve themselves. Then, after midcentury, spiritualism, which ranged from spirit rapping and ghost detecting to mental telepathy, received a great deal of popular attention. Like mesmerism, spiritualism suggested that the mind had special powers. Finally, members of the public at large knew about and discussed all of the various abnormal mental states. Physicians who specialized in mental illness indeed frequently voiced their frustration that they were unable to establish their expertise in the field; they found that every lawyer and also every person on the street thought that he or she knew about insanity and mental aberrations of all kinds. As expertise in such areas grew, popularization came only slowly, and to a grudging public.[3]

This popular, or even, to some extent, folk, psychology was applied psychology. It had meaning in terms of everyday problems, especially those which "every school-boy" knew: controlling oneself and others. Even abnormal phenomena appeared in practical as well as sensational guises, chiefly relating to the question of individual differences. In each of the varieties of popular applied psychology, the belief or hope was that phrenology or mesmerism or spiritualism or insanity revealed a natural force that science somehow should or did comprehend (which was of course a comment on the growing prestige, if not understanding, of science). Moreover, this popular lore involved a phenomenon parallel to that of the laws of health—somehow there were other natural forces with which it would behoove one to live in harmony. Indeed, tranquility of the passions, as in the non-naturals, was often an explicit goal of the pre-psychological writers and speakers. In short, popular psychological interests tended to involve prescriptions of correct attitudes and behaviors as one learned to use new powers. Some of the spiritualism evolved into mind cure and the New Thought inspirational movement of spiritual perfection—which a later generation sometimes still confused with psychology. But the scientific aspirations of other proponents tended to carry them into psychology proper, but only after a distinguishable science by that name had developed.[4]

As in health popularization, when phrenology and other popular applied psychology appeared in publications and lectures, frequently the usual enthusiastic organizations materialized to reinforce and spread the ideas. Sometimes the best journals published accounts by the best proponents, and sometimes ignorant practitioners and lecturers made wild claims, claims that of course showed up in the newspapers. A writer in the *Southern Literary Messenger* in 1838, for example, denounced "the blundering ignorance and quackery of many of [phrenology's] professors" who "imposed upon the public [a] false representation of character deduced from a superficial view of the external organs; whereas the chief excellence of the science consists in its beautiful classification of mental phenomena." And when the yellow press came in to exploit the worst aspects of popular applied psychology, the professional psychologists showed up just in time to try to rescue the public. With the new experimental psychology, wrote John Bigham of De Pauw University in 1896, "the popular interest in mental phenomena, shown by the prevalence of public hypnotic exhibitions, spiritualistic séances, faith healing, and similar perversions of true science can now be gratified in a way that is wholesome yet thoroughly scientific and naturally attractive to the keen American mind."[5]

Professional scientific psychology developed directly out of academic philosophy and only later absorbed the applied, popular strain. The immediate ancestor of modern popularization of psychology was therefore popularization of philosophy in the nineteenth century. Philosophical psychology—as opposed to experimental psychology—was, in that period, usually an integral part of the required instruction in moral philosophy, and in this context psychology was tied closely to ethics and metaphysics, at the least. This psychology was the science of the soul, which meant ambiguously both moral agent and personality (and, later, mind, or willing consciousness). Psychology in this tradition was already involved, then, in prescribing how people should live. But the method by which philosophers proceeded was largely limited to commonsense observation and logic, plus the concepts of the faculties through which, traditionally, a person exercised perception, feeling, and will. The ultimate appeal in establishing "laws of the mind, or mental facts," in such a psychology, was the person's "own mind and the minds of the people with whom he comes in contact," as an old-fashioned textbook writer put it in 1890. Such a formulation meant that anyone could establish the laws of psychology; there was, once again, no effective distance between the expert and the public. Occasionally a philosopher would advocate popularizing this kind of philosophy through precollege instruction. Why should the pupil, asked Joseph Haven of Amherst in 1857, "learn everything except the one thing, which, of all, it would seem he ought to know, that is, *himself?*" But for younger students and the educated public in general, popularization was not a serious issue.[6]

Unlike popularization in the health field, then, popularization of psychology did not usually involve the schools but only the print and lecture media and the college textbooks. Indeed, one of the major aims of the pioneers of the new discipline was to establish an identity and to get psychology established on its own in the curriculums of the colleges, the original entry point of the new discipline.

The Advent of Experimental Psychology

What in practice established the discipline of psychology was the introduction of instruments and the use of experiments. Psychologists borrowed heavily from physiology for their apparatus and from other parts of post-Darwinian zoology, neurology, and physics for their science. With this armamentarium, and the rise of the elective system, lecture and laboratory instruction in psychology rapidly began to establish itself in the colleges in the late nineteenth century, although still usually within

the philosophy department. Only later did separate departments of psychology become common. But just the courses brought the beginnings
of an audience, and this was the base for most of the psychologists who
initially undertook other popularizing activities. One of their rationales
in fact was that they had to win over the educated public in order to gain a
place in the college curriculum, just as Joseph Jastrow observed as early as
1896: "Nowadays, when each branch of study must make good its claim
to a place on the curriculum, it is more than ever necessary to acquaint
the cultured and powerful public with the general problems and broad
outlines of your science." [7]

The psychologists who popularized turned out to be a special breed—
special particularly in their dedication to expanding the public who
learned about their science. An element of self-interest was involved; yet
the zeal of the campaigners for their subject matter showed that larger
issues were involved. It is easy, for example, to compare the routine,
tepid popularizations of the older philosophical psychology—the tone of
which was, yes, of course everyone should know how the mind works—
with the ardor with which proponents of experimental psychology tried
to sell what they called in the 1890s "the new psychology." John Dewey,
for instance, writing as early as 1884, in the *Andover Review*, claimed that
"a revolution in psychology" had occurred. Superficially, great differences between the old and the new were hard to find. E. W. Scripture's
1895 *Thinking, Feeling, Doing* provides a good example. It was the first
major popularization as such, and it sold an amazing twenty thousand
copies within the first five years and was, in addition, plagiarized by a
textbook writer. Yet even the title of the book reflected the traditional tri-
partite philosophical psychology. What nevertheless was fresh was the in-
strumentation that permitted measurement of what now had become not
abstract "laws of the mind" but "psychological facts," which "new" psychologists treated on a par with material facts. "The new psychology is
entitled to its special adjective," wrote Scripture, "because it employs a
method new in the history of psychology, although not new in the history of science." [8]

Americans who read Scripture's book were answering to an interest
other than fascination with photos of mechanisms that measured human
reaction times or color vision. What the psychologists had to offer was
demystification of the most holy mystery, the person's thoughts and feelings, as psychologists translated them into naturalistic phenomena. The

most potent concrete information, in popularization at least, was explanations of illusions. Thus G. Stanley Hall of Clark University, in a heavily illustrated article in *Harper's* in 1901, noted how measuring the speed of reactions "lay[s] bare even the structure of the soul, and show[s] the thoughts we think oftenest." Hall went on to other experiments and concluded that "imagination, sentiment, reason, volition, and all the rest are taken into the laboratory, and its instruments and methods have taught us a sharpness and refinement of introspection and self-knowledge which makes these methods almost comparable with a microscope for the soul." And right from the beginning, eager psychologists who ran short on demonstrated facts pointed out that theirs was a young science and that in the future they would explain the mysteries that they had not yet plumbed. As John M. O'Donnell points out, psychological laboratories in the colleges in this period served not so much to train laboratory workers as to induct them into the culture of science.[9]

What the psychologists who popularized were doing, then, was acting out the role of the man of science. Indeed, the psychologists tended toward the extreme in that role. It was no secret that for thinking people the great issues of the nineteenth century were, is there a God? an individual soul? or any reality other than the material? The psychologists were not only on the firing line in addressing the issue of materialism, but many psychologists represented the naturalistic (implicitly reductionistic) side strongly. Even the nonreductionists invariably started their textbooks with an account of nervous system functions, and demystification proceeded from there. People at the time were aware of the direction that psychologist men of science were going. Isaac Cook, of Nebraska Wesleyan University, for example, in 1895 portrayed psychology and metaphysics "in unnatural war, like a child entering suit to overthrow its mother. In some recent presentations of the claims of the new psychology, as well as of other sciences, there is this species of antagonism, with a spirit of matricide as unwise as it is unnatural, ungrateful, and unscientific." As early as 1888 J. H. Hyslop, then at Lake Forest College, noted that "a proper examination of the new departure, as represented by a large number of its advocates, will reveal a more or less disguised form of 'psychology without a soul.'" It was no wonder that another contemporary could note, "Few physiologists, mixing in general society, can have failed to notice how common it is to hear their psychological brethren (if referred to at all) stigmatized as atheists." The direction of the efforts of psychologists was well known, and even in this early period, then, they had a public relations problem with some parts of the public who opposed reductionism in the mental sphere.[10]

Establishing the Presence of Psychology

The science of psychology therefore developed against a background of popular interest in controlling oneself and others (applied psychology), on the one hand, and, on the other, of the extreme of the nineteenth-century tendency to antimystical reductionism and even materialism. Even though popularizers tried to maintain the philosophical legacy and to emphasize not iconoclasm but the neutral objectivity of the experiments, clearly at the time people recognized that psychologists' interest in control and application and their bias toward mechanistic, if not materialistic, reductionism away from mysticism animated the popularizers. And one further factor, which marked almost all discussions, came into play: because it was so difficult to attain scientific objectivity when dealing with human beings, and because psychology was the "youngest" of the sciences, psychologists had to try much harder than other scientists to be "scientific." One aspect of this superscientific stance was of course the obligation to attack mysticism and superstition; and in fact popularizers of psychology, like popularizers of health, soon made antisuperstition campaigning a special feature of their popularizations.

But in the late nineteenth century, popularization had as yet evolved only incompletely. The work of William James—particularly as embodied in his great synthetic contribution published in 1890, *The Principles of Psychology*—illustrates the problem. Parts of that book were actually popular essays published in *Scribner's* and the *Popular Science Monthly*. Insofar as they constituted textbook material, publication in a high-class popular magazine was not inappropriate. But other chapters of the same book functioned as advanced treatises that other psychologists used in research.[11] This confusion of technical and popular, however, did not persist for many years; even though leaders in the new science like James were most often among the popularizers, they addressed different audiences at different times, as would any man of science.

Psychology at the Opening of
the Twentieth Century

By the opening of the twentieth century, differentiation was well under way, and the psychologists knew what their program had to be. Initially, the popularization proceeded through conventional channels, and the aim was to establish psychology and advocate the gospel of science. But later in the twentieth century, popularized psychology changed in two aspects. First, the strategies through which popular audiences were supposed to use psychology to fulfill their aspirations, to control self and others, altered fundamentally. The content, technique, and purpose of popularized psychology all became very different. And the other change was in the amount of public interest that psychology generated, from relatively little to a great deal. At the beginning of the century, James Rowland Angell of the University of Chicago wrote, "In the mind of the average man there are probably few things so supremely unimportant for the welfare of society as psychology." [12] Obviously he and his colleagues wanted to do better, and, eventually, they did.

If most members of the public in 1900 had heard of psychology, they tended to persist in using familiar images to conceptualize the discipline and its practitioners. Initially, and typically, the psychologist might be stereotyped as an absent-minded professor, preoccupied with abstruse matters. [13] And, given the philosophical ancestry of psychology, that image was not inappropriate. Or psychology appeared as simply common sense, the wisdom of a person of perception; such a view was of course a holdover from the time in the nineteenth century when in fact no difference existed.

Psychologists in the turn-of-the-century years also drew on existing images when they undertook to inform the public about what they were doing, and they pictured the discipline as legatee of the scientific tradition. Lay people responded by using psychology as a code word for the mysterious—the psychologist had (or claimed to have) knowledge that common folk did not possess. Psychologists, by identifying themselves as researchers who were privy to the laws of nature, were ironically bringing on themselves not only the prestige that they coveted as scientists but an association with the mysteries they were trying to dispel. As a group, psychologists continued therefore to attack occultism and superstition, to the point that they were subject to what Warner Fite of Princeton in 1918 called "the scientific prepossession." [14] Yet for years, many members of the public did not heed psychologists' protests that real psychology did not countenance telepathy and spiritualism and faith healing, rail against them as the popularizers would.

Regular academic psychologists of course tried in popular writing to convey the enthusiasm they felt for their work and yet to establish an acceptable public image. One persistent popularizer, Jastrow, of the University of Wisconsin, spelled the major problem out clearly. "The popular misconception," he wrote, that associated psychology with both mysticism and attacks on religion "is nothing short of a calamity; and it is so not mainly because it imposes upon the psychologist the discipline of suffering fools gladly, but because it deprives him of a ready and comprehensive communion with his professional colleagues and the wider colleagueship of earnest and sturdy students." [15]

Trying to Reach the Public

The one subject with which psychologists could attract the attention of at least parts of the public for that which was solidly scientific and even philosophical was the mind-body problem, the fear and wish that subjective thinking and feeling have physical—or at least physiological—determinants. Whether a somewhat sensationalized account of technological devices that could objectify emotional responses, an announcement that physiology could explain and correct bad habits (in one case simply a discussion of the synapse), or a more or less technical consideration of the fate of free will in interactionism and parallelism, under the title "Is Man an Automaton?"—reductionism did excite many Americans' interest in free will and control. [16]

In general, however, such popular attention as existed was drawn in more sensational directions. Any number of mental self-help books, for example, filled library and bookstore shelves. [17] An excellent example of subject matter catering to public interest was provided by the editor of a journal for lay persons, *Practical Psychology*, which appeared briefly in the opening years of the century (1900–1902). He featured such subjects as mental healing, suggestion, hypnotism or magnetism, self-improvement, extrasensory perception, and spiritualism. His version of reductionism was a lively interest in the newly discovered wireless, which at the time was widely believed—though certainly not by professional psychologists—to confirm the probability of the existence of telepathy.

Most of the leaders of psychology who wanted to address a general audience—beyond the students whom they reached with lectures and textbooks—turned to the better magazines and to books, although they of course, like other scientists, made public and semipublic addresses whenever possible. The number of magazine articles that they placed rose sharply during the first quarter of the twentieth century, and at least some newspaper coverage (often written by psychologists) reflected the public interest that educated Americans gauged by conspicuousness in the press.[18]

Professional leaders who popularized tried very hard to describe the technical problems that interested them (chiefly in the realm, in those years, of perception and thinking), but they also tried to meet the public interest in livelier topics. A good example was E. B. Titchener, who came from England to Cornell in 1892 and within a few years was following the American pattern of writing for well-educated popular audiences. Although he emphasized an experimentalist's interest in mind, sensation, and neurophysiology, he catered to public taste by mentioning work in optical illusions, attention, feelings and emotion, and in animal psychology. Moreover, he did not forbear discussing social, educational, and mob psychology as well as telepathy (he denied that it was parallel to Roentgen and radio waves).[19] The leading publicist ultimately, however, was Hugo Münsterberg, a German faculty member at Harvard. Like Titchener, Münsterberg resorted to practical matters like industrial efficiency and court testimony to attract attention to psychology, but in addition he often used sensationalistic tactics and exaggerated claims that, while often effective in gaining journalistic exposure, offended a number of his colleagues.[20]

Before World War I, then, many psychologists continued to believe that as psychologists they should obtain public recognition and, presumably, support. Yet their claims that their work had important practical consequences were either programmatic, like the behaviorists' assertions that they could predict and control behavior, or were superficial attempts at applied psychology that were vulnerable to observations like those of an anonymous reviewer of one of Münsterberg's books: "How Dr. Münsterberg can have the face to ply the American public with these shallow, platitudinous half-truths as the fruit of a profound study of 'the psychology of feeling,' we are unable to conceive."[21]

Attention and Controversy in the 1920s

World War I transformed the place of psychology in American culture. Both the mental hygiene crusade and mental testing came out of the war effort as important movements that, with appropriate publicity, were applied to civilian life. Moreover, psychology gained a place as a science in the National Research Council, and when Science Service began in the 1920s to issue authoritative news releases on all scientific subjects, psychology (as opposed, for example, to sociology) benefitted, and for decades thereafter the findings of established psychologists were widely and effectively publicized as science.[22]

All contemporary observers commented on the fact that during the 1920s the media—magazines, books, newspapers—called attention to psychology, and surveys show as well that particularly in the early and mid 1920s this production of popularization reached a peak—what satirist Stephen Leacock described as an "outbreak of psychology." A substantial amount of the publicity originated with the psychologist men of science, but many other writers and speakers and even practitioners took advantage of the public interest. Since not only the public but the psychologists themselves were willing to include as psychology anything remotely having to do with human behavior, popularizers could hardly keep up with demand. More than ever, public interest, often channeled through editors, seemed to control popularization.[23]

In the media version of psychology, mental testing was the psychologists' own, but mental hygiene was largely, and confusingly, in the realm of medicine, although psychologists, to say nothing of social workers, were also part of the mental hygiene team. Moreover, the content that was usually associated with the mental hygiene movement was now called "the new psychology"—ignoring the "new psychology" label of the 1890s. Between the new psychology and applied psychology, which in fact tended to merge into each other, the discipline flourished and received vast amounts of attention in the media of that day. Psychologists were even receiving the flattery of having various greedy people take the title of "psychologist" in order to make money by preying on members of the public who had come to value psychology.[24]

The entire entity, "psychology," therefore expanded greatly, especially in "applied" areas. In so commonplace a guide as the *Reader's Guide to Periodical Literature*, for example, the topic became almost hopelessly divided into specific headings in this period, again chiefly because of applied psychology activities. As early as 1920 a number of leading psychologists formed the Psychological Corporation to try to set standards for commercial applied psychology.[25] And the media publicity went further, so that the psychologist developed a new public image, becoming a pundit, an expert on all of human behavior, the kind of authority whom journalists could cite or who could serve as a straight man in formal jokes.[26]

Yet what attracted most journalistic attention, and presumably the public's, in technical psychology were the controversies among exponents of various schools of technical psychology in the 1920s and 1930s. Combative statements made good copy. In particular, John B. Watson, advocate of behaviorism, goaded any number of opponents into public denunciation. Psychoanalysts and other proponents of the new psychology were not far behind, and even the Gestaltists were notably aggressive in their crusade to win converts. For the educated public, the debates, with figures of speech that suggested warfare—*Behaviorism, A Battle Line*, was one collection—dramatized the content and implications of psychological teachings.[27]

During the 1920s, then, psychology prospered in many ways. Academic psychologists had many students. Applied psychologists found demand for their services in education, mental hygiene, business, and industry. Psychology interacted with other forces, too, that were affecting the media, and these cultural forces showed up in the two types of appeal that psychology had. One was social awareness, which led writers to suggest that science of that day contained the potential to reform society or at the least to explain and control group behavior. The second force appeared in attempts to use psychology for personal purposes—an extension of the traditional spiritualism–New Thought stream in which the word "psychology" substituted for other descriptions of the power of positive thinking.[28] In fact, a large proportion of what was labeled psychology for the masses derived directly from the how-to-become-a-success literature, ironically dragging in antiscientific features such as faith healing and nature cure as well as hypnotism and telepathy. One journal, for example, took the title *Psychology—Health! Happiness! Success!*[29]

Even in the highbrow versions of popular psychology–success literature in the 1920s there was a subtle change in focus. Where once success had involved, as one careful observer noted, "honor, dependability, courtesy, etc.," now with the language of inferiority complex, neurosis, conditioning, and the like, psychology came to signify manipulating other people: "One should be polite because politeness will get one a job." The new psychology part of this success literature not only purported to reveal the hidden self—the power of "the real me"—but taught students (and at other times such people as advertisers) how to appeal to humans' instincts and weaknesses in ways that would benefit themselves. Above all, one was supposed to develop one's personality so as to triumph in business and social relationships. The ultimate in this type of success literature was Dale Carnegie's bestseller, *How to Win Friends and Influence People*.[30] Professionals of course looked upon such uses of the term "psychology" as misuses, however common in the press and elsewhere.

In one area during the 1920s the psychologists were still the controlling and driving force in popularization, although, as will become apparent in a later chapter, they were operating in harmony with other scientists. This area was the traditional fight against superstition and occultism, and it occupied a large part of the conscious efforts of psychologists as well as a conspicuous part of the public press. Part of the campaign was aimed at spiritualism, telepathy, and the mystical and superstitious in general. But, inevitably, part of the campaign also targeted folk beliefs and false ideas propagated by defective popularization. Colleagues did studies revealing not only that students were influenced by superstitions, such as that the number thirteen is bad luck, but that they subscribed to folk and popular notions, such as the ideas that fat people are always good natured or that any physical or mental disease can be produced by thinking about it too much. In the classroom and the media, then, psychologists undertook to expose not only fraud but "unscientific thinking" and so to help confirm that psychologists excelled in scientific thinking.[31]

Change in the 1930s

In the 1930s, many psychologists continued to popularize in much the same way as in the 1920s, but, as in health popularization, an ever larger proportion of popular writers on psychological subjects were writers and journalists or, sometimes, mere amateur psychologists. Both psychologists and journalists—but especially the latter—exploited the usual media-conditioned opportunities such as, for example, the human interest element in the account of a Yale psychologist and his wife who reared a chimpanzee alongside a human baby. When regular academic psychologists did popularize academic psychology, it was, again with increasing frequency, not a result of missionary zeal so much as a response to a publisher or adult education agency. The academicians still had students, of course, but the Great Depression that began about 1929 seemed to blight the quantity and perhaps the intensity of popularizing activities. Psychologists did appear occasionally in the new medium, radio, as for example on "The University of the Air" or "Science Service Radio Talks." Their efforts in that medium, however, were almost always very restrained, a pale reflection of the most unexciting classroom teaching (and not comparable with the presentations of the health popularizers).[32]

Nevertheless there were still in popular psychology some fireworks left over from the 1920s. The behaviorists, especially, wrote with zeal, and controversy continued to please the journalists. As all science came under attack in the better magazines—and presumably elsewhere—in those years, so psychology, too, was assailed for being, among other things, successful. Reductionistic, behavioristic psychology blighted humanism, complained one writer; it undermined ethics, reason, religion, and philosophy, complained another. Such complaints suggested that psychology held a prominent place among cultural influences, but the resurgence of those traditional attacks also signaled that new issues, beyond superstition and occultism, would be coming into the popularization of scientific psychology.[33]

Hard times, everyone believed, were inhibiting the progress of psychologists in instructing the public. As late as 1939, when members of the newly founded Society for the Psychological Study of Social Issues tried to take their insights directly to the masses in an exhibit at the New York World's Fair, the effort was not successful. But rather than just hard times, other factors were operating contemporaneously: the withdrawal of psychologists from the public arena because they were increasingly caught up with new developments in their science, and the ingress of more technical material in psychology that was hard to translate for the public, such as statistics and apparently abstruse theory.[34]

The most important changes of the Depression era, however, showed up in the vulgarized psychology journals. As psychology became harder to market, sex became even more prominent than in the educated Americans' new psychology literature of the 1920s, as if in the economically hard times the meaning of success tended to change from material and social success to sexual conquest. In general, sexual material titillating to people of that day was frequently smuggled to the public under the heading of psychology.[35] The very first article in the new *Popular Psychology Guide* of 1937, for example, was "I Married a Sadist." The whole tendency was neatly summed up in the title changes of one magazine, which went from an inspirationalist periodical called *Successful Living* to the magazine *Current Psychology and Psychoanalysis* and finally, in October 1937, became *Current Psychology in Pictures*—many of which pictures were of the unclad female variety.

Another important change was the introduction of the psychologist as psychotherapist, a role in which the psychologist was indistinguishable from the M.D. psychotherapist. *Psychology* magazine, which had temporarily dropped *Health! Happiness! Success!* from the title, in October 1933, began to carry a new feature, "In the Psychologist's Office," which consisted of case histories recounted by a clinician. This feature had been preceded by letters to the editor detailing personal life experiences. In the 1920s such an emphasis on the personal narrative had produced *True Story* and other confessional magazines and many more sophisticated counterparts—one notable version of which was the clinical case history with an essentially narcissistic appeal.[36] It is entirely possible that 1930s editors did not know the difference between a psychologist and a psychiatrist. But the point is that even in relatively uninformed publicity, a new identity for psychologists was emerging exactly when more general popularizing was at a reduced level. This identity was symbolizing not just the ideas of the 1920s new psychology, but a concrete social figure, in contrast to, for example, the absent-minded professor stereotype. When popularization expanded, during and after World War II, the clinician identity of course became much more widely and vividly established, and at that point the popularization of psychology began to share more characteristics with the popularization of health as well as of science.

Mostly the popularizations and textbooks of psychology in the 1930s followed the familiar pattern of emphasizing the results of experiments on sensation and thinking, although discussions of behavioral, and particularly animal, experiments were becoming more prominent, along with the new psychology, which sometimes included the customary abnormal psychology along with Freud, depending on the author. The negative element, too, continued strong. Edgar James Swift of Washington University, for example, apologized in a popular book for emphasizing the "foibles of the many rather than the achievements of the few"; he did so, he said, because he wanted to replace superstition and error with knowledge. "Psychology is not a patented process for making one healthy, wealthy, and wise," he wrote, "but it does reveal the curious ways in which the mind works, and it also throws a spotlight into the blind alleys of credulity which thoughtful people wish to avoid."[37] But the days of such standard formulations in popularization were coming to an end.

World War II and "The Age of Psychology"

As early as 1939–1940, memories of the successes of American psychologists in World War I and the subsequent expansion of applied psychology inspired leaders of the profession to try again to use a military emergency to advance the interests of their discipline. Reinforced by unanticipated circumstances, particularly the dramatic rise of psychiatry, they eventually succeeded. By the late 1940s, both the demand for psychological services and the numbers of psychologists answering the demand began a dramatic expansion, developing a momentum that continued into the late twentieth century. As early as 1946, two officers of the American Psychological Association (APA) noted, "Psychology has been badly oversold; we cannot deliver the required number of qualified personnel. . . . It seems as if the ivory tower ha[s] literally been blown out from under psychology." The change in demand, of course, was in part related to publicity in the highbrow and mass media as well as the "selling" of psychology to authorities in the armed services—which was in effect a particular, targeted popularization.[38]

The numbers of psychologists did increase dramatically, at such a rate that within a few years it was possible to project this growth so as to predict that in the year A.D. 2100 everyone in the world would be a member of the American Psychological Association. In 1951, the APA executive secretary observed that "the age of psychological man is upon us." With all of the growth came other changes, too. The average psychologist became younger, better educated, and more clinical. Although the APA had reintegrated applied psychologists—who had been organized outside of the APA for a few years—into the organization in 1942, still the additional numbers of psychologists became so great that within a few years they spoke about the "fissioning" of the profession and discipline into endless specialties and subspecialties and other groupings. By the 1950s, leaders could anticipate the wealth, leisure, automation, health concerns, education demands, industrial and scientific development, and demographic changes that would undergird a continuing demand for psychologists of all kinds, a demand that was to some extent independent of deliberate popularization. One of the leaders in clinical psychology, Roy Schafer, characterized activity in the field as "boom-town excitement." [39]

The nature of the demand for psychologists reflected a complex public image. Students, wrote Franklin Fearing in 1947, take psychology courses "because they believe that in the study of psychology they will find something slightly glamourous, slightly dangerous but very exciting and mysterious, *and* practical. Successful businessmen 'use' psychology, you know. It is hard to analyze this curious compound of superstition, awe, glamour, and hardheaded practicality." A decade later, a survey of students showed that after actually taking a course they found most interesting the topics "Frustration and Stress," "Personal Adjustment Problems in Group Living," "Emotions: Inner Springs of Action," "Psychology and Social Problems," and "Motivation." The study of perception, by contrast, interested students little. [40]

Like students, midcentury journalists were attracted by aspects of psychology that were useful and somewhat sensational. By and large, journalists believed that their publics wanted to hear about mental hygiene, child guidance, sex, and applications of psychology to current concerns, such as brainwashing. Among the headlines that were assigned to journalists' stories out of one 1950s convention, for example, were "What Makes Us Love as We Do," "Criminals Aren't Family Men," "Psychology Analyzes Causes of Infatuation," "Overrating Seen Likely for Tranquilizing Drugs," "Subliminal Ads Should Cause Little Concern," and "War Prevention—Can Science Help?" [41]

The general popularization of psychology, in magazines and books, had fallen to a very low ebb during World War II. Publicity for psychology did increase, however, particularly in the services, where both psychotherapy and psychological testing were widely used and came into the common experience of many Americans. Since for psychology, just eliciting awareness was at least a beginning of popularization, proponents were jubilant as well as gratified by the midcentury explosion of attention in the media. In 1957, the public relations person for the American Psychological Association observed that "magazine and television interest in psychology and psychiatry seems to grow exponentially." He might also have mentioned the movies, which drew on both popularization and literature; authors, in any event, used popular notions about psychology and disseminated them.[42]

Both public and professionals saw that the expansion of psychology was taking place within what was broadly designated as applied psychology. Already in the 1940s, large firms were alerted to the advantages of hiring psychologists who were shifting from psychometry to clinical work. Likewise, after World War II the government generated demand for psychological services, operating, as one bemused observer noted, "under the oddly mated slogans of 'total human welfare' and 'total military efficiency.'" A representative and very widely circulated *Public Affairs Pamphlet*, "Psychologists in Action," issued in 1955, was devoted almost exclusively to applied and clinical aspects of the discipline.[43]

The fact of the postwar explosive increase of clinical psychology is well known. The increase followed and answered public demand, as is evident, for example, in the one area in which journalists' writings about psychology were entirely out of line with psychologists' own publications: popular publications showed a disproportionate bulge in the area of abnormal psychology.[44] What happened, in short, was that "psychology" became a word to cover the public interest in defining problems and coping with them. As early as 1948, Frederic Wertham, writing in the *New Republic*, diagnosed what was happening: "The tremendous amount of popular reading in psychopathology is an important social phenomenon," he observed. "Focusing the minds of people on their own individual problems and seeking solutions only there, is . . . an evasion of the adult problems of social life, from responsibility to reminiscence, from the immediate to the remote, from social action to individual therapy. It is," he concluded, "a cult of contentment." Wertham was seeing the genesis of the later culture of narcissism, one important aspect of which was still psychological professionals' helping to free people of their personal problems.[45]

The popular image of the psychologist was changing, and the new one was generally indistinguishable from that of the psychiatrist. The first halting steps of the 1930s ended in an almost complete transformation in the 1950s. As early as 1948, one survey of attitudes toward psychologists confirmed that members of the public believed that "psychologists deal with mental problems, both intellectual and personal," and respondents not only knew little of other fields of psychology but could not differentiate between a psychologist and a psychiatrist. In 1959, an acute observer, Elton B. McNeil, noted that the psychologists' "quest for professional identity had yielded only a distorted mirror-image of psychiatry." One yield, however, was to attract a whole new crop of pseudopsychologists who for some time could practice legally as "psychologists" in most states. One of the major aims of midcentury popularizers therefore became to warn the public against the "psycho-quacks" (and incidentally to campaign for licensing laws for practicing psychologists).[46]

Insofar as the public did differentiate the clinical psychologist or psychologist of any other kind, that public image continued to be favorable (although not as favorable as the image of the physician, of course). Beyond psychotherapy, what McNeil characterized as "the Sunday-supplement popularity of the mysteries of the mind" as well as the attractions of applied psychology—all of which tended to constitute products of the science of psychology, not the science itself—continued to receive publicity. The most notable help with the image came with the appearance of Joyce Brothers, a very bright psychologist who appeared on a television quiz show and then stayed in the mass media solving people's personal problems and saying wise things. Another very important piece of public education came through a series of well-informed articles, "The Age of Psychology," in the most influential publication of that time, *Life* magazine, with a subhead noting that "the science of human behavior permeates our whole way of life—at work, in love, in sickness and in health." Although in that series psychology had only equal billing with psychiatry—regardless of the use of "psychology" in the title—the writer, Ernest Havemann, explained the differences clearly.[47]

Midcentury: The Products of Psychology

In the midcentury period, the emphasis of popularizers on the findings or products of psychology increased still more, even though many older themes persisted. The use of psychology to cover interest in sex continued, at least on the most popular level—in the August 1943 issue of *Popular Psychology Guide*, for example, eleven out of eighteen articles fell into the sex category. Yet, as in the earlier work of Science Service, the reporting of the better journalists (not the pulp writers) reflected with surprising accuracy subject matter distributions in scientific publications listed in Psychological Abstracts (as opposed to distortions in the interest of sensationalism).[48] What did emerge strongly, however, was the idea that psychology was a tool for manipulating other people. This conception evolved with an emphasis much different not only from the older self-improvement but also from the more recent simple personal advantage of "personality" and appealing to people's instincts. By the 1950s, psychological warfare, brain washing, and subliminal suggestion in advertising were attracting a great deal of notice and comment. Most literate people had heard about what Vance Packard had described in his extremely successful 1957 book, *The Hidden Persuaders*. All of this practical application of psychology represented social, as opposed to personal, manipulation. The latter was of course far from dead and seemed to make psychology on either level at least a little dishonest. One teacher suggested that his students expected to be taught "how to fool an employer" and other aspects of what he referred to as "slycology." But on either the personal or the social level, psychology seemed to popular writers to be potent. Even within the profession, there was continuous debate—including a well-known confrontation between Carl Rogers and B. F. Skinner—about how manipulative benign psychologists should be.[49]

A whole series of concerns, both negative and positive, were impinging on psychology at midcentury. As the American Psychological Association grew and increasingly developed a professional function—not unlike that of the American Medical Association, as some purist members noted—officials and committees repeatedly voiced the belief that the APA should employ the same public relations methods that other organizations were using. The psychologists had two goals: (1) to get the public to distinguish the psychologists from the psychiatrists and (2) to develop favorable attitudes toward psychologists and their work, the stipulation being that the goals be pursued in a dignified way. Robert Tyson of Hunter College summed up the problem in 1949, the year that the APA did hire a public relations consultant:

> The profession suffers from chronic ambivalence on the question of informing the public. On the one hand, a fixed apprehension, namely that non-technical, interesting material for popular consumption is not entirely respectable, leads to academic aloofness. With reliable psychology inhibited, the quack steps in to fill the need, and in true-

neurotic fashion the psychologists are dismayed by a situation caused by their own conflict.

In the 1950s, the ambivalence persisted, but in fact official publicity activities accelerated, although of course public relations did not necessarily involve conveying knowledge beyond what was necessary to identify psychologists and their work. But there soon were workshops on public relations on the state level also; and both national and state efforts persisted even in the face of universal belief that the most effective public relations activities were those carried out locally by myriads of individual psychologists.[50]

Part of the public relations work of the psychologists grew out of genuine concern about what people at the time noted as hostility to intellectuals in general and the social sciences in particular, which in psychology showed up vividly in attacks on mental testing and manipulative techniques. Like other segments of American society at that time, psychological professionals had become extremely sensitive to bad publicity. But as the 1950s drew to a close, a new element appeared in the public face of psychology. Psychologists were increasingly talking in terms of official recognition and even, rather frankly, the use of power—particularly their own power—in American society. The phrase "public affairs" occasionally replaced "public relations."[51] But at that time it was only a hint of what was coming in the 1960s.

Meanwhile another context shifted. By midcentury, the very nature of publicizing psychology had changed significantly. Some of the old persisted, but long, systematic articles in essentially high-culture magazines like *Harper's* and the *Atlantic* almost disappeared. Instead the style of journalism predominated, just as in the health field, and it was in this context that the results rather than the process of doing psychology were emphasized. Moreover, those results were presented in short, interesting snippets unrelated to one another but widely distributed. Particularly common were watered-down psychological tests. In "How Do You Feel about Your Boss?" for example, one could in 1953 diagnose oneself as "an individualist," "a willing worker," or "a success in today's business world." Psychology, in short, was no longer high culture but was all news, even though some of it was not simplistic, involving, for example, detailed descriptions of complex mental and physiological processes. Thoughtful pieces, however, were more and more restricted to professional or very highbrow outlets. Even the semiofficial popularizations of Science Service at no time confronted basic problems at length.[52]

Popularity, Products, and Power

In the decades after midcentury, the specialization of the profession and of popularization intensified. The great breakthrough in public relations was a prime-time television show about a clinical psychologist in private practice ("The Bob Newhart Show," 1972–1978).[53] But in many ways ideas that came from psychology became more and more a part of all aspects of American life, and observers had the impression that in the 1970s, after the relatively social 1960s, psychology tended to enjoy a renaissance of attractiveness for college students and an even more vigorous interest among reporters for the mass media. In 1969, for example, *Time* magazine initiated a department called "Behavior." Throughout these years commentators still talked about "The Age of Psychology" as well as the culture of narcissism, and popularizing psychology therefore involved many kinds of workers operating at many levels. "A year's subscription to a typical women's magazine is akin to an encyclopedia of applied psychology," complained two academic psychologists in 1974; "it is impossible today to escape from being bombarded by psychological terms, psychological concepts, psychological advice, and psychological information."[54]

The major development in deliberate popularization, however, was the appearance in 1967 of a glossy magazine, *Psychology Today*. The event was significant because the magazine within a few years had a circulation of over one million. And when an imitative competitor, *Popular Psychology*, sprang up, the publisher of that magazine noted candidly, "We entered a market discovered (if not created) by *Psychology Today*."[55] That the market for *Psychology Today* may have existed already was suggested by the fact that much of the content in the magazine was drawn from or reflected recently published books on a level higher than the usual sensational psychology of pulp magazines.

The editors of *Psychology Today* carried relatively authoritative popularization that often was written by respectable academicians and was therefore of much higher quality than that in earlier magazines or in other media dependent upon journalists. Although traditional subjects such as uplift, healing, abnormalities, and sex—especially sex—did show up in *Psychology Today*, for years quality did not suffer greatly.[56] Individual psychologists, as well as allied pundits such as Erik Erikson and Paul Goodman, were featured, giving a number of leading professionals an opportunity to address—at least through an interview—a very wide audience indeed, and even, as was common in that period, to appear as gurus of a sort.

The initial pitch of the publishers was to self-interest, or popular narcissism. "No other scientific subject affects everyone as frequently and as deeply as does psychology," wrote the editor, Nicolas H. Charney, in 1968. "However," he continued,

> newspaper and magazine articles on topics in psychology like racial prejudice, psychedelic drugs, mental illness, brainwashing, extrasensory perception, and intelligence testing are often superficial or just plain wrong. . . . At last, the information gap has been closed by *Psychology Today* magazine. . . . Psychology can insure our personal integrity and freedom if we understand its discoveries and use them wisely.

The articles, he promised, would "concern you *personally*."[57] In fact over the years the editors focused not only on schools of psychotherapy, each in turn, but on every new fad that hit the mass media. In the 1970s, sociology, anthropology, and social psychology became very conspicuous in the magazine, and whereas brain studies showed up at appropriate times, still the rigorous laboratory and rat studies of an earlier day became relatively rare.

Psychology Today was not unrepresentative of the public aspect of psychology in general in the decades after midcentury. Psychologists were markedly sensitive to cultural and mass media influences. At appropriate times, so-called community and environmental and ecological psychology appeared, neatly labeled, in both professional and popular publications. The romantic movements of the 1960s and after were reflected in psychologists' newly discovered concerns with parapsychology and what came to be called humanistic psychology.[58] From their concern with heredity and the aged and women to their social reformism, articulate psychologists made psychology appear, both within the profession and in public, to be at least up-to-date and even trendy.

Psychology was, in fact, changing, and even the "service provider" emphasis of the 1970s, which grew out of clinical psychology, was in the 1980s turning into attempts to find applications for psychology that were compatible with the resurgence of business and defense interests. Between the growing size of the enterprise, the frequent adaptations to a changing society, the general transformations of American culture, and actual subject matter innovations in scientific, clinical, and applied psychology, many observers felt that psychology was in a fundamental reorientation in those decades after midcentury.[59]

So popularization, too, was changing. Psychologists thought even more frequently in terms of conventional contemporary public relations, and they continued to develop organizational means with which to deal with the media. The American Psychological Association finally established a Public Information Office in 1974 to cope with the flood of inquiries that writers and even television producers were directing to the national organization. Whether through local institutions, such as universities, hospitals, or corporations, or through professional organizations, public relations had become the standard mode through which psychologists popularized what they were doing.[60] Implicitly, of course, public relations focused on a person or on a specific, limited product.

But psychologists also continued more and more after midcentury to attempt to exert power directly, beyond cultivating general image and public relations. Exerting power meant primarily influencing legislation (particularly social legislation), public and charitable appropriations, and governmental administration—all of which meant that psychologists had to operate as another effective interest group in American society. As the APA executive officer observed in 1967, "Psychology is swept up in the affairs of men in ways and to an extent undreamed of a decade or two ago." Of course psychologists still had their own approaches, however attuned they were to the larger world; thus in 1969 a committee of the APA used the metaphor of receptor, decision making, and effector mechanisms to report on ways in which the organization might influence public policy.[61]

Psychologists' aspirations to gain power and change policy reflected more than just interest group maneuvering. Many wanted to make the world a better place in which to live. Meliorism and closely associated mass media faddishness showed up in *Psychology Today* and its congeners as well as in the professional publications of the APA. As Leona E. Tyler observed in her APA presidential address in 1973, psychology had attracted many recruits, including clinical and applied workers, who believed that they should and would improve the the world, and they increasingly set the tone for the whole profession. Moreover, they moved into the community and brought psychology to many people in many different settings, in ways not altogether different, in effect, from the efforts of itinerant phrenologists of a century and a quarter earlier. Altogether, however, neither the practitioners nor the leaders of organized psychology were ever able to discriminate between representing the interests of a profession and popularizing ideas.[62]

Regardless of whether in the community or in Washington, psychologists were still mostly selling the products of psychology, rather than the doing of psychology. In 1972, for example, Eli A. Rubenstein expressed his delight with the impact of a report on television violence. "To the best of my knowledge," he said, "this is the first time a major social science research program report has been publicly accepted by the 'target audience,'" who were of course policymakers in business and government.[63] And psychology—or science or health and hygiene—as product was transparently dependent upon the authority of the producers. It was ironic that a group who had wanted recognition as scientists ended up as authorities with a public that did not have the critical abilities really to appreciate the basis of the authority. Furthermore, as innumerable psychologist practitioners complained, as the "psycho-quacks" continued to dispense their bogus products, they appealed to the authority of psychology.

Fragmentation

Beyond the issues of products and authorities, the public relations approach to popularizing psychology reinforced another trend, that of fragmenting the popularizations so that each result, typically a handout to the press, was not connected to psychology as a whole or to anything else other than the originating authority. The specialization within a large discipline augmented this sense of fragmentation in psychology, and the consistent journalistic emphasis on controversy, splits, and schools also contributed. Finally, the controversies generated when various psychologists cited selected research results to uphold social points of view compounded the impression that psychology was a science that consisted of unconnected conclusions. So far, at least, the psychologists had not established an authority comparable to that of exponents of medicine and health.

Yet over the years it was clear that popularized psychology as well as pop psychology continued to maintain an identity. The best evidence appears in the textbooks that psychologists wrote for their students. Three books, for example, in their very titles represented different preoccupations at different times over eight twentieth-century decades: George Malcolm Stratton, *Experimental Psychology and Its Bearing upon Culture* (1903); E. G. Boring et al., *Psychology for the Fighting Man* (1943); and Nathaniel Ehrlich, *Psychology and Contemporary Affairs* (1972). In terms of topics treated, these books show a basic similarity. It is true that sensory perception was relatively neglected in the 1970s, esthetics in the wartime 1940s, and ethnicity in the 1900s. Yet in one way or another, abnormal psychology, memory and learning, social influences on behavior, and many other standard topics were covered in all three volumes, suggesting that psychology, at least as psychologists presented it to the student public, had a persistent identity in terms of subject matter, even though the different authors clearly had different goals for their expositions. The diverse aims did contribute to the problem of identifying psychology, but so also did the shifts in audience that popularizers were addressing.

Turn-of-the-century popularizing had as a target primarily the well-educated readers of the cultured, genteel tradition and those Americans improving themselves in imitation of that model. They all read magazines and books more or less seriously, as well as newspapers, which when not to some extent sensationalizing, carried material that aped that of the well-bred and literary people. Initially popularizers aimed at this audience and to a substantial extent the intelligentsia of the midcentury decades. Many of those readers would have been familiar with, for example, James Harvey Robinson's classic *The Mind in the Making* (1923). Contributing to high culture was an important element in the aspirations of the psychologists writing for the public, and they hoped that all of high culture would trickle down to the masses. By the later part of the twentieth century, whereas products were welcome, science and encompassing theory often were not. Douglas G. Mook of the University of Virginia, for example, complained in 1983, "Students, like laypersons (and not a few social scientists for that matter), come to us quite prepared to point out the remoteness of our experimental chambers, our preoccupation with rats and college sophomores, and the comic-opera 'reactivity' of our shock generators, electrode paste, and judgments of lengths of line segments on white paper." [64]

Fragmentation was particularly characteristic of psychology in the mass media, where, as in popularized health, journalists set the tone as well as the format. In the days when research with rats made for intellectually interesting contributions, a reporter from New England covering the American Psychological Association meetings threw into the wastebasket abstracts of the animal researchers' work, exclaiming, "People in Boston don't care to read about rats at breakfast." When such reporters did not, or could not, see a wider significance of the findings, no story existed, and when scientists turned to application or otherwise followed the lead of journalists, their own agenda in popularization diminished. Joyce Brothers, for example, came to be treated as just another newspaper columnist. Good journalists were of course aware of the problem, whether or not they were able to do anything about it. "*We* are missing the big stories for daily preoccupation with trivia," noted the science editor of a Minneapolis paper in 1965. [65]

Psychologists as Standard-Bearers of Science

Throughout the twentieth century, the psychologists who popularized without totally surrendering to journalists' standards and fragmentation generally had two aims, one negative and one positive. The negative was the familiar campaign against mysticism of every kind. "The psychology of the past," wrote Knight Dunlap in 1920, "has fought a good fight against mysticism: it is demanded of us that we fight a better fight. . . . No one can accept the fundamental hypotheses of scientific psychology and be in the least mystical." [66]

It was in the role of "keeper of the gate" against "philosophical mysticism," as Dunlap put it, that psychology became the advocate of science, and it was in this service that psychologists developed their "scientific prepossession." Because they were less certain of themselves and lower in the Comtean hierarchy of sciences, psychologists, as has often been observed, were more self-consciously scientific than colleagues in other disciplines, and this advocacy of science was, then, their positive contribution. Their veneration of scientific method led psychologists not only to seek objectivity in dealing with their subject matter but to look increasingly at the externals of human beings (as opposed to the internal workings of the mind) and their place in biology.[67] Reductionism was always inherent in this approach to psychology, and, in terms of popularizing, fascinating to many parts of the public—not least, of course, to the skeptics.

If the message often was lost in the flood of applied psychology in the mass media, psychologists nevertheless persisted in one area in their identity as defenders of the scientific outlook, an identity distinctively more self-conscious and deliberate than other scientists' and, indeed, a hallmark of the psychologist. The evidence is in textbooks of general psychology. As will be noted below, textbooks in various natural sciences varied in the extent to which they contained explicit discussions of the scientific method and scientific procedures. Textbooks of psychology did not vary. The authors expected readers to learn and understand what it meant to address a problem or a series of events—and, implicitly or explicitly, life—in a scientific manner. Even an iconoclastic 1975 textbook, *Psychology: A New Perspective*, included the usual discussion of what it meant to address human phenomena from a scientific standpoint.[68]

This tendency, to try to make students conscious of the difficulties of investigating humans objectively, showed up alike in textbooks of the earliest period and in those of the 1980s. Edward John Hamilton's philosophical textbook *The Human Mind*, published in 1882, for example, began with a section on method. Moreover, the authors of psychology texts were unusually explicit in stating that psychology was important because learning to study man scientifically would counteract false beliefs. A person with an "unguided interest" in psychology, wrote F. C. Dockeray in 1932, can become "a victim of fakers who have mixed a few facts with a mass of convincing language which the uninitiated accepts as truth. This frequently leads him to believe that psychology is simple and easily understood without study, and that scientific data . . . are relatively unimportant." In 1966, Howard H. Kendler, in his textbook, asserted that learning the scientific approach to psychology would remove the student from among "those who are willing—almost eager—to accept superficial answers to complex questions," especially those answers doled by "self-styled psychological experts"—not only "naive psychological advice" but "harmful," even "dangerous . . . misconceptions about psychology."[69] Psychologists, in short, like popularizers of health, connected the scientific approach with protecting the public from exploitation.

Whatever the dilution of psychological research in the mass media, teaching psychologists deliberately undertook as their mission inculcating objectivity and the scientific method. If many came to think that the mission could be fulfilled through products and applications, still the pristine dedication showed through in the textbooks. In later years the touchstone was the idea of a controlled experiment. As the texts showed, if American students who flooded psychology classes in the mid- and late twentieth century learned the scientific skepticism which that one idea, the controlled experiment, could convey, they often learned it in a class in psychology, for that was where they were explicitly exposed to the strategy.[70] And in the better journalistic popularizations of that period, too, the two textbook aspects of scientific psychology were not infrequently present: accounts of controls in experimental results, even when the experiments were reported without context, and attacks on the unreliable foundations of vulgarized or exploitive popular psychology. A writer in *Look* magazine in 1950 quoted Samuel Stouffer, speaking from his lab at Harvard: "Here we turn our backs on the arbitrary, unproved statement."[71]

The psychologists did feel that out of their hardheaded work they had something positive to offer, beyond their symbolizing in the larger culture the quest for objectivity. In the depths of the Great Depression of the 1930s, Edward S. Robinson of Yale, for example, chided his colleagues for not speaking up about the possibilities of psychology. Psychologists, he said, were not mere technicians, they more than anyone had worked out "a fundamental and scientific perspective of human nature" and had acquired an approach to problems that involved not only methods but values. Robinson's was an unusually candid statement of what psychology stood for in those decades: the faith that disciplined scientific knowledge, even about homo sapiens, provided both intellectual satisfaction and solutions to human problems. Popularization, in short, involved a generally agreed-on point of view, one that provided a frame of reference within which facts about humankind made sense. In 1952, in their textbook section explaining and extolling the scientific study of behavior and experience, Ross Stagner and T. F. Karwoski spoke explicitly and frankly about "the psychological frame of reference."[72] It was easily recognizable in other writers, too, who may not have labeled it as such.

The Weakening of the Sense of Mission

In the last part of the twentieth century, however, much of popularized psychology proceeded largely without the earlier deep concern for a wider framework that made sense of the wonders and peculiarities of humans in a changing world. Where once there had been an audience for psychology as high culture, specialization—particularly in the form of fragmentation—and vulgarization undermined the community of intellectuals, and, as was noted in discussion of the health field, self-improvement took on decidedly uncultural connotations.

One reason that the traditional negative program of psychology was attenuated was that it had been successful to the point that part of the motive for popularizing scientific psychology no longer operated. As noted in chapter 1, by midcentury, serious writers were not very often defending mysticism, or else "soft-minded" thinkers had retreated behind such unassailable positions as an ironical view of life. Moreover, the specific campaigns of an earlier day were effective in changing the public's ideas about psychological matters. Whereas in 1925 significant numbers of college freshmen agreed with such statements as "Adults sometimes become feeble-minded from overstudy," in 1964 another survey showed that such foolish beliefs had almost completely disappeared. Psychology as the correction of error therefore no longer had so urgent an appeal, although of course traces still appeared, and a few psychologists still urgently took on the mission of unmasking overtly mystical fraud.[73] None of the psychologists seemed to see that superstition had taken on a new form.

Another reason that popularization changed was that psychology itself split in the 1920s over the issue of method, and psychologists argued over the question of what it meant to be scientific. Because of this split, the positivist point of view became ever less viable—nor could lay people then easily discern anything consistent or valuable in psychology other than what could be applied. The combative language that made such a good story for a reporter was fatal to the mission of psychology as keeper of the gate of science. As noted above, the popularizations reflected genuine divisions within psychology, not so much over subject matter as over what psychological science was. In 1969 philosopher Sigmund Koch was asserting for a popular audience that psychology could not be "a coherent science" since it was crowded with pieces of "pseudo-knowledge" largely "unrelated to each other."[74]

By the 1960s and 1970s, the large volume of popularized psychology showed patterns but embraced no great themes. As exemplified in *Psychology Today*, the only general viewpoint, aside from a modish anti-institutional liberalism, involved, as in hygiene, a life style, not an intellectual stance. Indeed, in *Psychology Today* as in other types of contemporary journalism, the content of the articles showed substantial compatibility with surrounding advertising materials and went through a period a later APA official characterized as the era of "the shlock or 'hot-tub' approaches." [75]

By that time, psychologists could once again have pursued an aggressive campaign for the scientific prepossession and against mysticism, for there was an abundance of targets not only in American culture but in psychology itself. With the romantic movement of the 1960s and 1970s came a resurgence even among the better-educated groups of the nonempirical and frankly irrational. So-called humanistic psychologists, for example, based a large part of their appeal not only on subjectivity but on a consistent point of view, a point of view that had not been evident in the mainstream of science for generations. But instead of regrouping for the grand battle, most psychologists insofar as they spoke to the public joined the enemy, or at least collaborated in the name of eclecticism. The humanists, for their part, explicitly attacked reductionism. By the mid-1970s not only had journalists given them much exposure in the press, but even the editors of *Psychology Today* were publishing papers debunking science and objectivity.

Although trendy and fragmented journalism as the model for popularization fitted well into the bureaucratically segmented and episodic nature of American life in the midcentury period and after, yet some psychologists still spoke of psychology as high culture and wished the discipline—now increasingly a profession—would stand for knowledge rather than power. [76] Nor was such an aspiration merely a longing for the good old days when a psychologist was a cultured intellectual and before the wars of the schools of psychology interacted with the yellow journalism mode. Popularization had important consequences for psychology, just as it did, as will appear below, for all of science.

Popularization was increasingly important not only in recruiting young psychologists but in helping all psychologists conceptualize psychology. [77] Popular works on the new psychology, for example, were influential in opening up new areas of study within the discipline because psychologists such as the influential Robert S. Woodworth of Columbia were part of the intellectual community and read those popularizations. Between public expectations and such impacts on working psychologists, patterns of popularization had momentous consequences because they did help both public and professionals make sense of psychology and through it of their own places in an age of rapid change. In this final sense, then, too, popularization of psychology serves as a paradigm for all of the sciences.

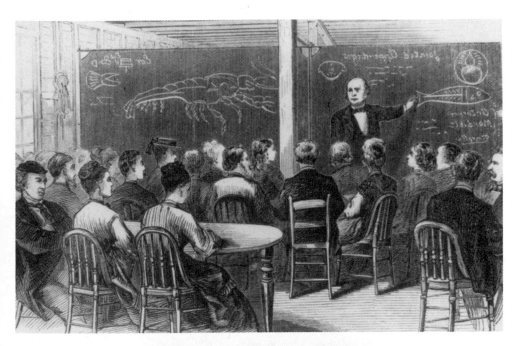

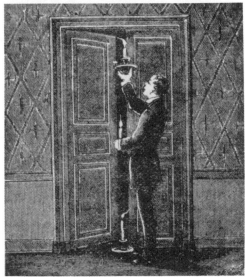

2. Louis Agassiz (1807–1873) lecturing to ladies and gentlemen at the Anderson School of Natural History. *Leslie's Illustrated Newspaper*, 1873. Courtesy of the Carnegie Library of Pittsburgh.

3. A simple physics experiment, demonstrating the cause of wind by showing air movement. *Popular Science News*, 1886. Courtesy of the Library of Congress.

4. Use of photography to show illusion and explain it: an illustration from *La Nature,* reprinted in *Popular Science News* in 1892 for the purpose of demystification.

5. Newspaper science, from a somewhat battered library copy of the *New York Evening Journal,* 1898.

6. Nature study students learning gardening, early twentieth century, New York. *Cornell Nature Study Leaflets,* 1904.

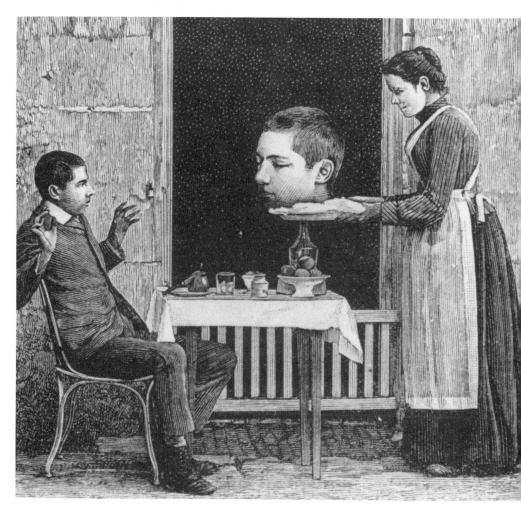

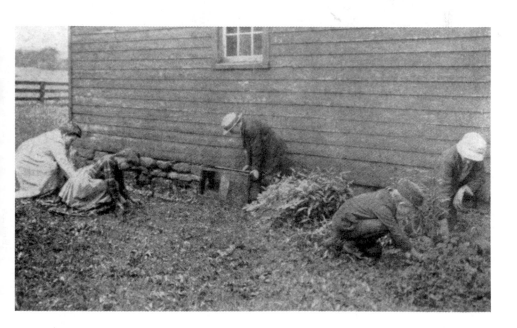

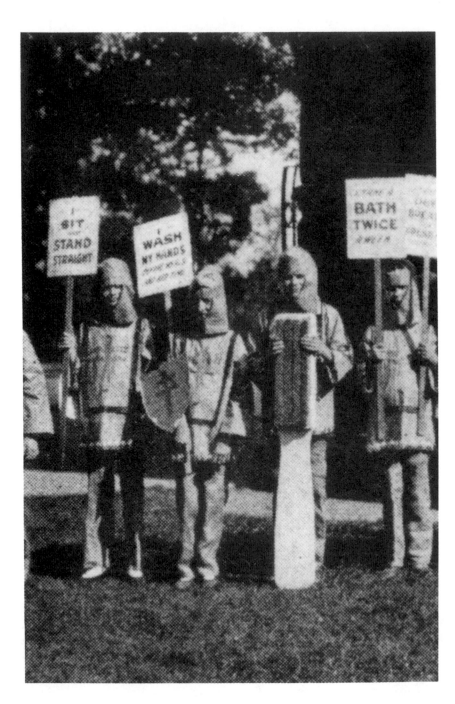

7. Learning health habits. "The awe-inspiring formality of the old school medical inspection has given way to a fascinating game of health impressed on the child mind by pageantry and parade." *Nation's Health,* 1922. By permission of the *American Journal of Public Health*.

8. Edwin E. Slosson (1865–1929), founding director of Science Service, as a young chemist teaching at the University of Wyoming. Courtesy of American Heritage Center, University of Wyoming.

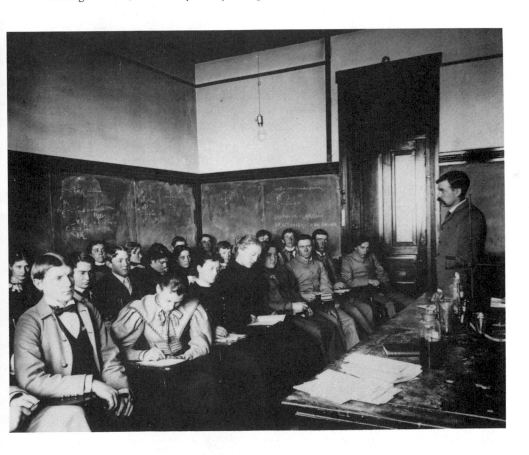

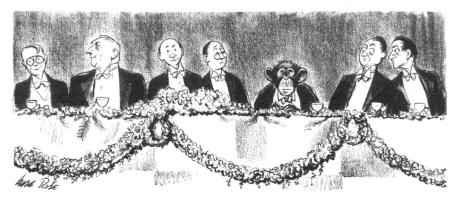

"I'm not sure,
but I think he's from the Yale Psychological School."

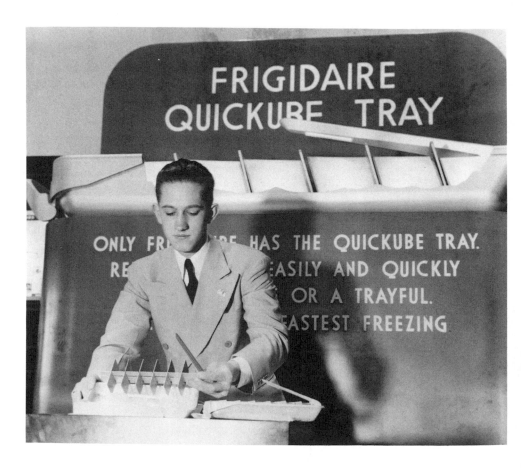

9. Popular satire of experimental animal psychology. *New Yorker,* 1934. Drawing by Carl Rose; © 1934, 1962, the *New Yorker Magazine,* Inc., by permission of the *New Yorker.*

10. Teaching physics with a brand name; commercial influence on science display at the New York World's Fair, 1939. Courtesy of the Smithsonian Institution, Science Service Collection, Archives Center, National Museum of American History.

11. Watson Davis (1896–1967), director of Science Service, on the radio, mid-twentieth century. Courtesy of the Smithsonian Institution Archives, Science Service Papers.

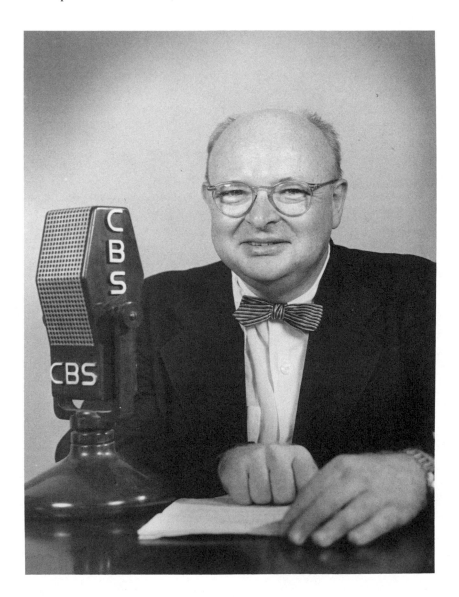

12. Scientist briefing a group of science writers, Minneapolis, 1952. Journalists included in the front row are Thomas Henry, *Washington Star;* William Manchester, *Baltimore Sun;* Arthur J. Snider, *Chicago Daily News;* Marguerite Clark, *Newsweek;* and in the second row are Wadsworth Likely, Science Service; William White, *Look;* Earl Ubell, *New York Herald Tribune;* Alton Blakeslee, Associated Press; and Victor Cohn, *Minneapolis Tribune.* Courtesy of American Cancer Society.

13. Ad for *Psychology Today,* appealing to reader self-interest, 1968. Reprinted from *Psychology Today* magazine, © 1968, American Psychological Association.

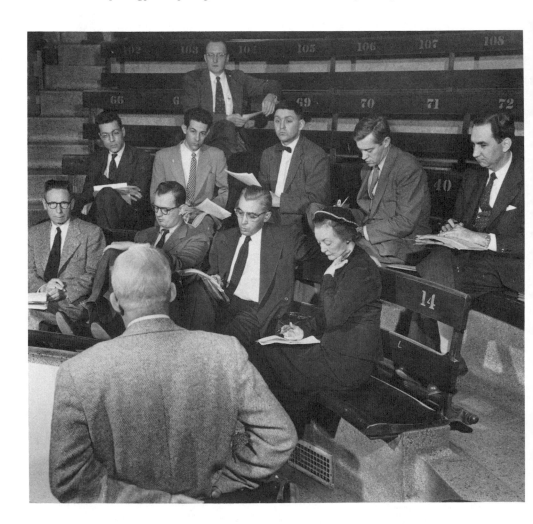

Do you want to know
what Psychology Today readers
are really like?

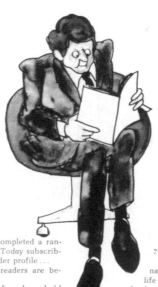

Survey Tabulating Services just completed a random sample survey of *Psychology Today* subscribers. STS computers drew this reader profile ...

You're young — 70% of our readers are between the ages of 18 and 44.

You're well educated — 87% of our household heads have attended college ... 73% graduated ... 46% hold advanced degrees.

You're prosperous — 46% of household incomes are $15,000 plus ... 73%, $10,000 and over.

Here are some more nice things about you.

You're highly literate — 78% bought a hard cover book in the last 3 months ... 31% bought five or more.

You swing a little — 82% entertain at home ... 85% use alcoholic beverages at home.

You buy now, pay later — 72% hold credit cards.

At the same time, you're financially responsible — 90% own life insurance ... 28% own mutual funds ... 45% own corporate stock.

In short, you are generally younger, brighter, more prosperous and classier than the readers of any other class consumer magazine.

We thank you for being what you are—and for spending an average of 2½ hours of your time with every issue of

psychology today
Del Mar, California 92014

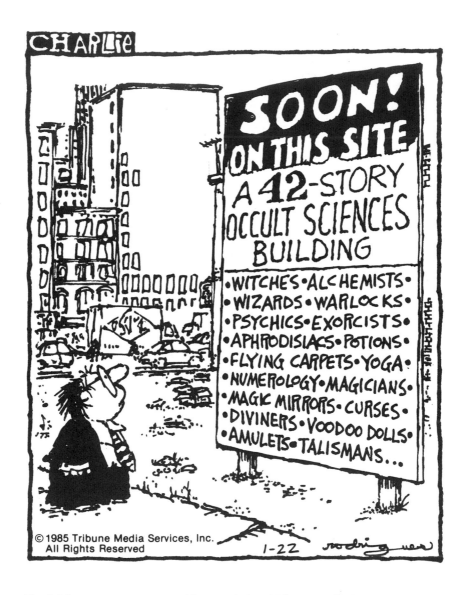

14. Truthful satire, 1985. Reprinted by permission: Tribune Media Services.

Chapter 4

Popularizing the Natural Sciences in the Nineteenth Century

THE WAYS in which Americans popularized health and psychology revealed the pattern that popularizers of the natural sciences generally followed. Health and to some extent psychology tended to be derivative, and they did not represent physics, chemistry, biology, and other "hard" sciences directly. Rather, the course of popularization in health and psychology was more linear and involved fewer complications than was true in the more basic sciences. With the physical and biological sciences, however, the issue of science was necessarily explicit. Moreover, without the distraction of personal interest in health and psychology, the importance of curiosity and the full momentum of popularization as a social phenomenon emerge clearly.

Popularization of mainstream science paralleled that of health and psychology in that the phenomena of the religion of science and the men of science, not to mention the ultimate fragmenting, all showed up, and in the same major time frames. The patterns in popularizing the natural sciences fell into four main phases: two in the nineteenth century and two in the twentieth.

A period of natural theology and increase in the number of full-time scientists covered roughly the first half of the nineteenth century, perhaps until the Civil War, and was succeeded for the last decades of the century by the period of positivism or scientism (the term here used in the general sense, not in the sense of Whalen's popular scientism). Tension and transition marked the first half of the twentieth century, a phase during which the religion and ideology of positivistic science peaked and at the same time popularization slipped out of the hands of scientists. Then during the decades after 1945, the media changed the context of popularized science, which no longer nourished the religion of science. Like all historical divisions, these eras were not clean-cut but instead represented dominant trends—complicated, we can now add, as were health and psychology, in Covert's model of the constant mix of levels of popularization (see chapter 1).

This chapter therefore deals with the rise and flowering of popularization and the religion of science—how transmission of science shifted from diffusion into the institutional form that was familiar for a century as popularization. The chapter also forms an account of the rise of the enthusiasm that sustained the men of science and their vision and of the way in which their vision and popularizing fitted into American culture. It was this enthusiasm, particularly, of the nineteenth century, that was ultimately derailed in the twentieth century.

American Science at the Opening of the Nineteenth Century

At the century's opening, surprisingly little remained of the Enlightenment enthusiasm for science that had sparkled among the educated elite of the Revolutionary generation in America. Despite the growth of population, interest in science languished, especially in contrast to political and literary activity. Some spontaneous interest in natural philosophy and natural history persisted, but the essential local leadership did not replace itself. Of the 1,338 books printed in the United States and listed in a bookseller's catalog in 1804, "not more than twenty," according to John C. Greene, "can be considered works of science," and those were mostly textbooks.[1] No magazine was devoted to science, although the few general magazines took note of scientific items such as the uncovering of Peale's mastodon. In New York City, John Griscom gave a course of lectures on chemistry, and here and there a few other popular lecture series also drew crowds from time to time. Science organizations, which functioned to encourage both amateur and professional (of course usually indistinguishable at the time), were with few exceptions relics of a period of earlier enthusiasm. The only notable institutional innovation of the period was Peale's Museum, which, although it led a tenuous existence, for years enabled the general public for a small fee to view the wonders of nature exhibited not randomly but in a systematic and orderly way, with domestic and exotic natural history specimens and even a menagerie, all set in a context of high culture. Despite the ephemeral nature of many scientific efforts and institutions, as Greene shows, the impulse to learn and to carry out scientific activity kept springing up here and there in the United States with remarkable persistence. Moreover, scientific workers tended from early in the century to separate themselves, or at least their scientific activity, from the work of technological and agricultural organizations.[2]

Two factors overwhelmingly determined the nature of such popular science as existed in America at the end of the eighteenth century. The first was the continued hegemony in the United States of English writers, publications, and thinkers. Moreover, this colonial relationship in the realm of intellect continued throughout the nineteenth century; when it was occasionally modified, the modification often consisted of the substitution of French and, later, German influences for British. Residents of the New World had habitually, if reluctantly, looked to the Old World for civilization and learning. American readers read the English reviews, and American publishers reprinted (usually pirated) English books. American magazine editors for decades borrowed openly from English magazines, or writers in American periodicals summarized European articles and books. As late as the 1880s and 1890s, for example, the *Popular Science Monthly* consisted to a very substantial extent of articles written by English and Continental authors.[3]

The second factor that placed science in American culture in 1800 was the lack of full-time scientists. In 1802, there were in the United States but 21 people who earned their livings as scientists. As George Daniels, especially, has shown, the absence of a critical mass of scientific workers was a factor that did change, particularly in the economic expansion after 1815 and the subsequent cultural ferment of the Jacksonian period.[4] As was observed in chapter 1, it was only when this full-time group differentiated itself from generally well educated people who were not scientists that the term "popularization" came to have meaning and substance.

As institutions of science developed in the pre–Civil War decades, so, too, did institutions that embodied the popularization of science: books, magazines, schools and colleges, public lectures, museums, almanacs, newspapers, and amateur science organizations. The material expansion of those decades and the rapid growth of population together provided the basis for the agencies of popularization to expand and evolve. By midcentury a basic pattern of popularizing media was well developed and changed only slightly as increasing educational levels expanded the mix and emphases of the various agencies of enlightenment toward the end of the century.[5] In all of this growth, as both high and popular culture flourished and spread, science by any measure became an increasingly significant element in American culture.

Books and Magazines

At the beginning of the nineteenth century and for many years, textbooks constituted the major class of books that embodied scientific subject matter.[6] Textbooks both reflected and shaped science teaching and therefore belong properly to the subject of science education. Yet they also represented one of the major means by which a reading public could learn about scientific matters. Textbook writers were well aware of the dual audience of school pupils and independent adults who might buy and use their books; frequently books were explicit in this appeal, such as Mrs. Almira H. Lincoln's *Lectures on Botany* (1835), which was designated "for the use of seminaries and private students," or another, the author of which expressed the hope that the book (in this case, *Peterson's Familiar Science*) would "prove an interesting and useful companion to both old and young, either in the family circle, or in the school-room." Moreover, many text authors, particularly in the field of natural philosophy (physics), modified their presentations to minimize the mathematics required so as to broaden their appeal.[7]

Even before the appearance of a large number of books aimed explicitly at a popular audience, the constant proliferation of textbooks already provided a fundamental agency of popularization. In the 1840s, the editors of the *Scientific American*, for example, a magazine designed primarily for upwardly mobile artisans and mechanics, stopped trying to carry extensive expositions of basic science and recommended that mechanics instead use basic textbooks then on the market to learn the science that they needed to know.[8]

The nineteenth century, however, was the century of the magazine, on both sides of the Atlantic. The magazine was a particularly important popularizing vehicle for both general and specialized readers, as has already been noted especially in the area of health. As the editor of the *American Journal of Microscopy and Popular Science* explained in 1875, many amateurs had both instruments and good books available to them:

> But it is well known that a regular visitor in the shape of a journal is calculated to sustain a much deeper and more lively interest than can possibly be excited by any book. Just as the living teacher has more power to interest and instruct than any printed page whatever, so a journal has more power than a text-book; it has a closer and more immediate influence, and seems to be more nearly like a personal friend. In addition to this, a book is, in a measure, fixed and stereotyped, while the periodical is progressive—reflecting the latest news and giving information of the most recent discoveries. Therefore books can never entirely fill the place of periodicals; and we believe that there is a sufficient number of persons interested in the microscope to sustain a periodical devoted entirely to that subject.[9]

Despite the late-nineteenth-century tone, this description of the special function of the magazine was valid for all of that century and at least part of the next.

Early in the nineteenth century, a substantial number of new general periodicals, such as the *North American Review* (1815), appeared. Such journals carried many notices of scientific events and writings, typically, for decades, in the form of review articles. In some of these early journals, the contents included a substantial proportion of scientific and technical material. The *American Monthly Magazine and Critical Review* (1817–1819), for example, contained a regular section edited by the eccentric naturalist Constantine Rafinesque, as well as other special articles on science. The *American Quarterly Review*, to cite another example, for several volumes after its beginning, in 1827, included a very substantial amount of material about science and the arts (technology). Even before the term "popularization" became current, then, the general magazine reader was subjected to the "diffusion of knowledge," including particularly natural history and natural philosophy.

So vigorous was the interest in science in the post-Napoleonic era that a few brave editors attempted to capture a popular science audience with specialized magazines. The *American Journal of Science and the Arts*, started by Benjamin Silliman of Yale in 1818, was aimed at the growing number of very active or completely full-time scientists but cautiously included a pitch to the more general public, or at least to only weakly interested amateur scientists.[10] *Silliman's Journal*, as it was known, managed to survive, however, because it functioned as a professional journal rather than a popular magazine. Other exclusively scientific ventures that were dedicated frankly to the public did not fare as well. The *Scientific Journal*, for example, also founded in 1818, featuring elementary mathematical problems and chemical experiments that one could do at home, did not last the year out. In 1823, a more ambitious work appeared, the *Boston Journal of Philosophy and the Arts, Exhibiting a View of the Progress of Discovery in Natural Philosophy, Mechanics, Chemistry, Geology, and Mineralogy; Natural History, Comparative Anatomy, and Physiology; Geography, Statistics, and the Fine and Useful Arts*. The title alone suggested that well-educated people should take an interest in both science and applied science. Moreover, the editor's preface spelled out additionally just what popularization meant then: "The scientific labours of European philosophers . . . are spread over so wide a surface, are scattered among so great a number of Journals and volumes of Transactions, and the valuable are so connected and mingled with the worthless, that it is very difficult for individuals in America, except under uncommon advantages, to get a complete view of science and the arts."[11] The *Boston Journal*, with its "complete view," perished for lack of patronage after three volumes, and although a number of other popular science magazines appeared from time to time, it was 1872 before the *Popular Science Monthly* showed that Americans could sustain such a venture. Meanwhile general magazines continued to include scientific and medical articles and reviews as part of the information that any cultured person should absorb.[12]

Educational Institutions

Another institution for the cultured, the college, radically expanded the place of scientific teaching in the required curriculums. The change occurred most rapidly in the 1820s, but continuing expansion contributed substantially to the growth of full-time scientists, as college after college acquired additional teachers and expensive "philosophical apparatus" in an effort to modernize. Eventually Harvard and Yale and other institutions added special scientific courses of study parallel to the classical arts curriculum, in a last attempt to stave off what became in the late nineteenth century the elective system.[13]

One of the reasons that college-level instruction could expand was that the preparatory academies and other secondary schools likewise were upgrading instruction in science, to the point that college students came better prepared to take up natural sciences. Although school science patterns varied greatly, nonetheless schools as well as colleges noticeably developed momentum in extending the science content of the curriculum, especially in the 1820s. Since much of the function of secondary education for many decades was to prepare students for college, the trends naturally paralleled those of the colleges. Some secondary academies, however, like those institutions that evolved into Norwich University (founded 1820) and Rensselaer Polytechnic Institute (founded 1825), went much further and had essentially a science curriculum; some other academies, perhaps most, of course had little or no science. After the 1820s, science instruction persistently claimed a place in secondary education, and by 1850 a modern pattern of instruction was coming into place, including the substitution of "physics" for "natural philosophy." The momentum that had developed carried well past the Civil War. Two late nineteenth-century surveys showed that natural science—and particularly physics and, to a large extent, chemistry, both often now with laboratories—was by that time offered in virtually all U.S. high schools, even though, as Sidney Rosen remarks, schools invariably located laboratories in the basement, along with the coal bin.[14]

Although most science instruction was confined to colleges and high schools, the common schools in many places also developed some science instruction. The major impediment to introducing science was the fact that the teachers were largely ignorant of the subject themselves. As both secondary and college curriculums came to include more science, teachers and administrators at all levels found it easier to expand instruction in those subjects. In 1857, Massachusetts set one standard by requiring that high schools in towns of four thousand or more population offer natural philosophy (physics), chemistry, and botany. Although rural school children obviously received less, and the law was not rigorously enforced, the ideal was at least a sign of aspiration. In 1861 the Chicago graded curriculum provided a substantial amount of science instruction even on the grammar school level and served as another model for educators.[15]

One way of getting around ill-prepared teachers was to employ text-books, and in fact most instruction for decades in both elementary and secondary schools tended to be based upon the rote learning of textbook materials. Memorization of textbook terms, in particular, became noto-rious throughout the nineteenth century as constituting instruction in science, as was suggested by a satirical set of "Nursery Rhymes for Little Scientists" that appeared in an education journal; one of them was "For the Young Geologist":

> Trilobite, graptolite,
>   Nautilus pie,
> Seas were calcareous,
>   Oceans were dry.
> Eocene, miocene,
>   Pliocene, tuff,
> Lias and trias,
>   And that is enough.[16]

One common form of textbook in the early nineteenth century, espe-cially in the common schools, was the science catechism, in which rhe-torical questions presumably aroused the children's curiosity as well as set the stage for learning that could be tested (recited upon). *A Catechism of Botany*, for example, published in New York in 1829, included the follow-ing exchange:

Q. What are the different parts of a plant?
A. The perfect plant consists of the root, the trunk or stem, the stalks, the leaves, the flower, and the fruit.
Q. What are the functions of the root?
A. The root serves to fix the plant, and to imbibe nourishment from the earth for its support.

Not all of the catechisms were as informative and clear as this one. Jane Kilby Welch's *Botanical Catechism* of 1819 consisted almost entirely of definitions of terms ("Q. If a plant in the twentieth class, has the stamens united by their filaments in the staminate flowers, to what order does it belong? *A.* Monadelphia, the sixteenth order.")[17]

Another question-and-answer form also appeared in many children's books on science, that of the dialogue. Typically the dialogue took place between a young person—with whom the child could identify—and an older person, and in the course of the conversation the younger, amid many exclamations of wonder and gratification, learned science as, it was hoped, did the reader. In an 1833 children's magazine published in Charleston, for example, the young aspirant says, "We are greatly obliged to you, brother John, for giving us such pleasing information; Botany is a beautiful amusement and not such a dry study as I thought it was: I do not wonder you are so fond of it." [18]

The dialogue format tended to inculcate appreciation as well as learning. The primary purpose of catechistic training, by contrast, was to impart factual information that would also be useful. As William Mavor, the English catechism author, observed in 1820 in a book widely used in the United States, "Names and distinctions must be acquired before any further program [i.e., progress] can be made in the study." Beginning in the midcentury period, another approach to learning facts appeared in the "object lesson" method for elementary school students. Under the influence of new, and especially Pestalozzian, educational theories, teachers (who now obviously needed to have some knowledge) were to start with familiar objects in the child's environment and draw lessons from them. The method eventually died out because the subject matter was not organized, but for about three decades after 1850, many American school children learned to use their senses and then memorize explanations— right or wrong—in object lessons: that ice floats, that flint is very hard, that the presence of mountains affects the wind. As in mathematics, so in science: one should learn the objects first, explained one proponent. "Lessons on plants, animals, minerals, qualities of objects and manufactures will, in like manner, lead directly to Botany, Zoology, Mineralogy, and some of the truths of Physics and Chemistry. Lessons in size and position of objects introduce Geography." In both catechisms and object lessons, not only some regular knowledge of science informed the answers to the lessons, but also moral and sometimes religious justification, for they offered flexible modes for drawing lessons. The method was in fact not inherently defective, but in practice teachers often did not make sense of the material. Nevertheless, when well taught, as in the pioneering "Oswego system" in New York, the method helped elementary school pupils learn to observe and even, in the upper grades, to generalize, so that, for example, observing a number of animals or plants led to learning classification. [19]

By the midcentury decades, American as well as English school text-books of a systematic kind were becoming increasingly available as science teaching spread. Often science content in school curriculums appeared in but two types of courses. One was physical geography, which included astronomy and meteorology and to some extent natural history (and paralleled the preoccupation of American scientists with what has been designated geophysics). The other was one already noted, physiology and hygiene. Both geography and physiology-hygiene emphasized facts, usefulness, and morals. But increasingly children and, where appropriate by the use of textbooks, interested adults were in one form or another studying natural history (botany, zoology, geology, and mineralogy), chemistry, and physics.[20] Always, of course, man's relation to nature appeared in a pious and moralistic context, and especially in books for younger readers authors did not raise difficult questions that might have undermined Biblical literalism. Yet as the Civil War approached, more and more Americans were gaining educational background sufficient to appreciate at least some science in a cultural or avocational role.

Popularizing Institutions for Adults

One avenue for enhancing one's appreciation was the public lecture. As I suggested in chapter 1, lecturers offered their services to the ladies and gentlemen of communities in all parts of the country. The lecturers represented an extremely wide variety of ability and learning. Some gave merely amusing nitrous oxide ("exhilarating gas" as it was known then) demonstrations or appeared for just one evening, but other lecturers over many weeks gave the equivalent of full college courses. Amos Eaton, a good scientist who was very successful with chemistry presentations in New England and New York in the years around 1820, offered this advice:

> In commencing an itinerating course, let the Clergymen, Doctors,
> Lawyers, and other principal men in the village or district, send
> printed cards (prepared by the lecturer) inviting the citizens to attend
> a gratuitous lecture. At the first lecture . . . the plan and object of the
> proposed course should be illustrated by striking experiments. But
> never introduce those blazing, puppet-show-like experiments, com-

mon with quacks and imposters. . . . Itinerating lectures on Chemistry, Natural Philosophy (including astronomy), Geology and Botany, are of great use to small villages and country districts where permanent courses cannot be supported.[21]

The American lecture and its audience came increasingly to represent a fundamental public institution. The lyceum system dominated public lecturing by the 1820s, and after railroad lines expanded dramatically in the 1840s, national speakers preempted lecturing everywhere. Within these flourishing public lectures, scientific subjects always played a conspicuous role. The Lowell lectures in Boston, for example, which constituted a version of the lyceum, included initially a large proportion of science subjects. Indeed, between 1839 and 1847 all of the science series were repeated, in contrast to only two of those on nonscience topics. Similar patterns appeared all over among lecture series, whether in lyceums or not, and regardless of the quality of presentation. A "Professor" Sanders, for instance, in 1847 lectured in Norfolk, Virginia, on chemistry, demonstrating with his apparatus, according to the local newspaper, "many surprising facts in practical and experimental philosophy never attempted before." Sanders was followed the same year by the well-known Dr. Boynton, whose area was electricity and magnetism and whose demonstrations included stringing a short telegraph line over which members of the audience could send messages from one part of the lecture hall to another. Beyond and parallel to the standard lectures, a series of workingmen's or mechanics' institutes also developed, which included a special emphasis on the connection between science and practical matters. For decades, there was no part of the population that was not targeted for science instruction and entertainment in the lecture hall. The best lecturers, who often led members of the audience into lifelong interest in science, performed memorably, as did Benjamin Silliman:

> During the lecture hour there was no lull or intermission; all was rapid movement, a constant appeal to the delighted senses. Here were broad irradiations of emerald phosphorescence, there the vivid spangles of burning iron, or the blinding effulgence of the compound blow-pipe, or the galvanic deflagrator. . . . As forms of matter once regarded simple were torn into their elements, or these again compounded in manifold ways, a very kaleidoscope of changes came

into view, of which the greatest was the transformation of the whole seeming phantasy into science, through the lucid rationale of the gifted lecturer.[22]

Closely connected with the lectures were the museums. Typically a museum collection was an amalgamation of private "cabinets of curiosities" such as cultured people had assembled for their own wonder and amusement throughout the Enlightenment and after. They often included stuffed animals, dried plants, and rocks and minerals. As groups of amateurs gathered in various urban centers around the country, they often established, in conjunction with their societies, such museums, which were, naturally, highly variable in quality. Since typically the museums were private or institutional, as agencies of popularization they were therefore limited in their effects.[23]

With the rise of Peale's Museum, another pattern was available, however, that flourished in later decades: commercial museums. Part of the remnants of the Peale collections, for example, passed into the hands of one of the most spectacular showmen of the century, P. T. Barnum. He had purchased Scudder's American Museum in 1841, before he added the Peale material. For decades, Barnum brought natural history to all parts of the country, most vividly through the menagerie, and through donations of material, he was a patron of the collections at the Smithsonian and other large academic museums that developed late in the century. Barnum's museums and traveling shows gave rise to a number of imitators, and the sight of all of the exotic animals, ancient Egyptian relics, and Siamese twins stimulated popular interest in natural history for generations.[24]

Although the magazines, colleges, and especially the lectures and museums could, and often did, include many citizens who were not in any way elite, by and large, as I suggested in chapter 1, it continued to be those who were already well educated who benefitted from the "diffusion of knowledge." "Every man of liberal education," wrote Granville Sharp Pattison in his *Syllabus of a Popular Course of Lectures* in 1819, "knows something of Botany, Mineralogy, &c."[25] From the eighteenth century on, however, two particular institutions, almanacs and newspapers, provided for scientific enlightenment not only of the well read but also, to some extent, of the masses, including those with only some common school education, that is, the vast bulk of Americans.

The almanac, which had once served as a major means of diffusion, especially regarding astronomy in general and the Newtonian mechanical universe in particular, in the nineteenth century tended to become commercialized and specialized. These later almanacs continued to include recipes for both cooking and doctoring, and weather predictions were fundamental to the existence of the publications. But the kinds of information available in almanacs was no longer scientific in any substantial quantity. Whereas Espy's theory of storms, for example, received a substantial exposition in the *American Almanac* for 1843, most of the rest of the volume was filled with official facts, such as the officers of government and population statistics, and it did not serve to popularize natural science—despite the subtitle, *Repository of Useful Knowledge*. Editors of other almanacs did continue to include amusing stories, child-rearing advice, and moral injunctions, but increasingly patent medicine ads substituted for the odd scientific facts. In an 1887 commercial almanac for farmers, for example, one could read, "The most perfect, and at the same time the most wonderful of the land animals, is the mastodon. Its dimensions were truly gigantic, sometimes measuring twelve feet in height by twenty-five in length." This particular science example, however, came not from the editorial content but from an advertisement. In one important way the nineteenth-century almanacs did differ from earlier ones: editors less and less repeated superstitions, which they had done so often in earlier decades. Thus in 1832 one compiler commented: "The moon's supposed influence on the human body is entirely omitted, as one of those uncertainties which is incapable of demonstration, and which furnishes a play to the imagination, in which there is no rational dependence." At least in a negative way, then, the newer almanacs appeared to foster common folks' receptivity to science.[26]

While almanacs declined in effectiveness as agents spreading scientific knowledge, the newspapers expanded, especially as technological changes reduced the price of dailies and weeklies. Colonial papers had carried a great deal of information about health and medicine both in sustained stories and in short extracts such as appeared also in the almanacs. Natural history, particularly, and such items as the 1769 transit of Venus received some attention, but still not in proportion to original work that was proliferating in the sciences at that time.[27] By the post-Napoleonic years, the pattern of science in the newspaper had become well established. Sometimes editors published magazine types of articles, including the publication of public lectures. Sometimes newsworthy material appeared as news, including, for example, accounts of explorers and inventors. Finally, science showed up in "fillers" of miscellaneous but (it was hoped) curious information, the presumption being that the information was true, even when it included laconic reports of supposed medical cures. Much of the material printed consisted of knowledge of that day, but a great deal reflected credulousness, and people already began to connect unreliable stories with the rise of the "penny press" of the 1830s and after. In 1835 the *New York Sun* published an account of the discovery of furry, winged men and women on the moon. These batlike creatures had been sighted through a telescope on the Cape of Good Hope, according to the reporter. This notorious hoax, and others like it, made popular newspapers particularly problematic agents of popularized science.[28]

Like the editors of magazines, editors of newspapers often reprinted material from almost any source, starting with other newspapers and local lectures. Major midcentury lectures, for example, often appeared in the *New York Tribune* and then were cribbed by editors all over the country. When T. H. Huxley traveled in the United States, innumerable editors provided him an audience through reprinted lectures far beyond the throngs who actually heard him speak. Editors also sometimes ransacked even highly technical publications that involved on occasion esoteric vocabulary from geology, astronomy, or some other discipline. In 1824, for example, the editor of the *Providence Gazette* lifted an item on geography directly from the *American Journal of Science*. Most of the newspaper material, however, was at the elementary level, if not the credulous level of the penny press. A writer in the *Constitutionalist & Republic* of Augusta, for example, in 1855 reported the possibility that the moon is inhabited, reasoning that atmosphere probably exists on the side that terrestrial observers never see. In general, material on natural history tended to consist of curious facts, such as a toad with five feet, or accounts of natural phenomena such as petrification. Chemistry stories typically appeared in connection with practical applications—what a substance or process would do for agriculture or manufacturing. Only physics and astronomy occasioned any general theories. As the school textbook writers did, newspaper editors emphasized the factual, but they also commented freely, and often skeptically, on reports of scientific matters, such as, for example, the 1854 report of a sea serpent.[29]

The chief subject areas that appeared in the usual newspapers—medicine aside—were astronomy and meteorology, as might be expected of people who were still in many respects directly dependent upon nature. As Donald Zochert points out, science was of general interest, and local readers felt as qualified as the editors to report scientific events and ideas as well as to argue about the feasibility of inventions or the likelihood of both scientific and pseudoscientific events as both skepticism and the thirst for knowledge flourished. The basis for popular interest in science was not different from that on which Americans were pursuing other popularizations: items that were curious in themselves; those that (again as in the textbooks) were awe inspiring—a large fish, an aurora, a great steam engine; and those that were practical. Most notable of all, of course, was the substantial incidence of science material of any kind, especially in an age in which newspapers were organs of personal opinion that concerned mostly politics.[30]

The Appeal of Popularized Science

The varying levels of science exposition in the newspapers suggest how diverse was the audience for such material. Readers of course represented different levels of education. But editors, like educators, clearly believed that science was part of the general high culture for which everyone should strive And, moreover, notices in the papers of lectures and of the activities of amateur groups also revealed that the editors were well aware of a special constituency, the scientific amateurs and enthusiasts who, representing cultural aspiration, received disproportionate publicity in the press.

Amateur groups, which conspicuously embodied the special constituency, thrived in every part of the country, even, occasionally, on the frontier. At first, at the beginning of the century, no difference other than source of livelihood separated the amateur from the full-time worker. Then over the decades, both level of understanding and self-identification removed professionals from amateurs. Yet until almost the end of the century, in group after group, the two elements frequently worked together, particularly in natural history.[31] Sometimes a local scientific society or academy continued to be dominated by amateurs; at other times, the group and its assets and publications were captured by professionals. Where the two elements came together in the social relationship of a scientific organization, the mutual reinforcement helped create and sustain a demand for high-grade popular science, and this effect was not lost altogether if the professionals departed. The groups provided not only mutual encouragement but institutions through which lay enthusiasm for science could spread directly. Amateurs acted both as interpreters to each other and as consumers of popularized science. Everyone knew that the conviviality of amateur groups brought in additional participants at the same time that it reinforced existing interest. Where people—including newspaper editors—believed that learned societies were a badge of civilization, local pride as well as belief in culture encouraged natural history societies or academies of science. Typically the earlier local societies developed around "cabinets." At some colleges, similar interest groups sprang up, emphasizing natural history with the goal of supplementing curriculums deficient in such subjects. Occasional later groups, more national in scope, such as the microscopists, developed around technologies as well as either topical or generalized interest in science.[32]

All of the institutions of popularization showed that a wide variety of motives for learning about science existed among members of the American public. From the beginning, there was of course the usual quota of hardheaded citizens who opposed credulousness—exemplified in David Reese's ruthless exposé of the "humbugs of New York" (phrenologists and medical sectarians). On a more humble level, other skeptics relished exposing the fallacies of so-called common sense. "Tom Telescope," for example, in an 1803 Philadelphia book, pointed out to his fictive auditors that a body in motion will continue forever unless disturbed by an outside force:

> This seemed so absurd to Master Wilson, that he burst into a loud laugh. What! says he, shall any body tell me that my hoop or my top will run for ever, when I know by daily experience, that they drop of themselves without being touched by any body? At this our little Philosopher was angry, and having requested silence; Don't expose your ignorance, Tom Wilson, for the sake of a laugh, says he; if you intend to go through my course of Philosophy, and make yourself acquainted with the nature of things, you must prepare to hear what is more extraordinary than this. When you say that nothing touched the top of the hoop, you forget the friction or rubbing against the ground they run upon, and the resistance they meet with from the air in their course which is very considerable, though it has escaped your notice.[33]

Science also had very concrete positive appeals. Amateurs in astronomy, botany, zoology, and geology had hopes of making discoveries and adding to knowledge as scientists, and many other consumers of popularization used science as a hobby in one way or another. Many mechanics hoped to use scientific learning as an equalizer as they applied their knowledge to become upwardly mobile; in 1847 Robert Macfarlane, editor of the *Scientific American*, told an audience of such mechanics: "A more general knowledge of the sciences governing our respective occupations, would in a great measure give us that advantage over the merely booklearned, which they have [had] too long over us."[34] Other Americans connected science with another kind of upward mobility, for, like the editors, they viewed science as part of high culture. Lectures, particularly, were extremely fashionable among social leaders in different cities at different times. Moreover, even after scientists developed professional self-consciousness, they continued to mix socially and intellectually with many nonscientists; Agassiz and Holmes and many others through personal acquaintance affected literature and philosophy and other areas of thought throughout the century.[35]

Finally, the function of science as entertainment was transparent, from Franklin's early electrical experiments on. In 1816, for example, a writer in the *National Register* suggested how amusing it was to attach different metals to parts of a newly killed bird and watch it move and flap its wings. John W. Webster of Harvard (hanged for murder in 1850) used entertainment to get students' attention in ways Eaton (quoted at the beginning of the previous section) would not have approved of. According to one account, Webster "gave the class two or three chemical lectures, which were brought to a sudden end by his show experiment called *the volcano*—a large heap of sugar and potassium chlorate piled on a slab of soapstone. After he had lighted it with a drop of sulfuric acid, he saved himself by dodging out of the room, and in a very few seconds all the members of the class found themselves obliged to jump out of the window."[36] Spectacular and moving presentations were successful with the public, whether solid displays or mere show; they all made science appear attractive.

Testimony from and about the public also shows that from the beginning of the nineteenth century on, excitement about progress fascinated many literate Americans. They made no distinction between the discovery of a new comet and the development of a new machine—they wanted to learn about what was new, and presumably better. They hoped, too, to share in this progress. As historians long ago made clear, middle-class Americans in the pre–Civil War decades had a mania for self-improvement, a cultivation of the mind and spirit for which science was exquisitely suited and which served as a somewhat secular version of virtue and godliness.

Yet, as Margaret Rossiter points out, the extraordinary level at which Americans patronized popular science was far from exclusively caused by trying to improve themselves. The interest in novelty or progress also was merely an added dimension to efforts to popularize science. Science had a basic, inherent appeal. There was available an abundance of high-level popularization that Americans patronized in significant numbers—attractive popularization that mobilized interest, curiosity, and wonder, with Silliman and Agassiz on the lecture circuit, dozens of first-rate scientists working with amateurs, and elegant English as well as American writings and compilations of progress.[37]

Institutional activity permits some attempt to gauge quantitative changes in the intensity of all of this popularizing in the nineteenth century. From comments already made about schools and colleges, magazines, and lyceums, it is clear that during the 1820s popularizing activity grew remarkably. By the 1830s, much of this interest had tended to focus on the practical applications of science, especially in the wake of the introduction of the steam railway. Then beginning around 1850 another surge in interest in science as such appeared; not one, but two yearbooks appeared—the first in 1850, the second in 1852—to chronicle the progress of science and technology. The plateau of popularization that they symbolized may have continued to the next peak of interest, the years around 1870; the record is not clear. What is clear is that by midcentury the institutions of popularization, complete with school curriculums, were in existence in a pattern that would change relatively little for decades.[38]

Pious Science

Audiences of the ante-bellum period expected that popularization would be tendentious, that the popularizer would include a point or moral in his or her exposition. Most of them emphasized the traditional view that learning about science was pious and practical. But, in addition, popular science also carried the message that the world was orderly and therefore predictable and controllable—a message that, as James Turner, especially, has pointed out, was welcome to theologians and meshed with piety.[39]

Pious science took the form, usually, of natural theology; indeed, in many colleges, natural theology was the title given much or all of the formal science teaching, and certainly most commonly that outside of the physical sciences. It was, of course, in the area of natural history that the complexities of design showed the need for a Great Designer. Complexities typically were exemplified by the eye—but any other discoveries that suggested the complexity of biological organization served the same purpose. Such were the wonders of anatomy and physiology, wrote lecturer Pattison in 1819, that he could show that the being "who created a worm, required to be the Creator of a Universe."[40]

But natural theology went beyond merely proving that there is a God. In combination with Scottish commonsense philosophy, natural theology served virtually all American intellectuals as a point of departure and furnished an approach to the content and method of science—typically the Baconian method, which people at that time understood to consist of gathering large numbers of facts to show the workings of God and the world. As the Unitarian Orville Dewey asserted in 1830, "It is not enough to say, in the general, that God is wise, good, and merciful. . . . We want statements, specifications, facts, details, that will illustrate the wonderful perfection of the infinite Creator."[41]

Science, according to popular writers, was peculiarly valuable because one could learn about God from "those boundless regions where the perfection of his conceptions has never been marred by sin." Astronomy, wrote an anonymous reviewer in 1828, "is the highest triumph of human intellect, and is calculated to give us the most exalted idea of the intelligence and penetration of man; while on the other hand, this intelligence and penetration sink into insignificance, when compared with the wisdom and power of the great framer of the celestial machinery." The better theologians also saw that scientific investigation provided evidence not only of God's design and his care in creating the world, but of the perfection that the universe embodied. The theologians had ample support from such scientists as Edward Hitchcock of Amherst, who often preached on the subject of the ways in which science contained "the most beautiful exhibitions of the divine wisdom and benevolence." "What admirable skill and benevolence does the doctrine of definite proportions and atomic constitution in chemical compounds present!" he exclaimed. "Here we see nature incessantly performing processes, on which organic life and comfort depend, with a practical mathematics as perfect as the theory." Hitchcock had no difficulty in finding much other evidence "recently discovered" that in his eyes affirmed God's workmanship and the greatness of his plan alike.[42]

With such support, religious leaders could place themselves on the side of the openness of investigation, for all new facts would confirm the kind of God and universe that their theologies posited. Indeed, wrote one reverent essayist in 1823, the materialists were the ones who were dogmatic and bigoted, and he went on, therefore, to speak scornfully of "the *superstition* of 'materialism.'" Another commentator of that same era asserted that he had "no fears that science and learning can, on the whole, or in the end, be converted into weapons of hostility against Christian faith; for thus far, the more searching they have become, the more have the fears of the timid believer subsided, and the conviction of the ingenuous inquirer been strengthened."[43]

Benjamin Silliman, Jr., in 1852 summarized the set of beliefs that underlay most educated Americans' approach to science in the pre–Civil War years, combining Baconianism and commonsense philosophy with enthusiasm for encouraging people to learn about science. "Our knowledge of nature begins with experience," he wrote, and so knowledge began with observation. But, he went on, "our knowledge would . . . be very limited, without a constant effort to extend our experience by experiment," an extension, he pointed out, that advanced modern people far beyond the ancients, who did not know the relationship between cause and effect. When, then, Silliman spoke of "facts," he meant not just simple observations but the relationships between phenomena. And "facts in nature," he concluded, "are the expression of the Divine will in the government of the physical world." Silliman was therefore content to study the "laws of nature" because he knew that they were but "laws and forces which proceed directly from the mind of God."[44]

Useful and Naturalistic Science

Textbooks, essays, orations—all actively and explicitly affirmed the compatibility of the hardheaded knowledge of nature with theism and theology. But as often as popularizers affirmed the truths of natural theology, they also argued that science was useful. "Useful knowledge," the customary phrase, totally confused pure and applied science, the distinction between them being, as has been remarked, virtually unknown in the first half of the nineteenth century. Americans grouped invention and technology with any other science under the heading of science, or progress, or both. In 1849, for example, in the *Literary Union, A Journal of Progress, In Literature and Education, Religion and Politics, Science and Agriculture*, published in Syracuse, of the items labeled "science," over half were technology and another one-eighth medicine. Or, for another example, by midcentury the *Scientific American* was virtually all technology. In emphasizing the usefulness of science, writers sometimes had problems with the higher mathematics and descriptive botany, which could not be connected easily to surveying or housekeeping. But the evidence of practicality was overwhelming: the titles of magazines that tied science to the useful arts, the transparent economic interest in the investigations of geologists, the need of farmers for meteorological information, and innumerable additional testimonies spelled out how ante-bellum Americans believed that science was and should be useful. Of course most popularizers continued to distinguish science as discipline, and textbook writers, for example, often did not bother to mention applications.[45]

Beyond mere economic development, which was desirable enough, science had additional social utility in the eyes of popularizers. Learning about nature was inspirational and recreational in a constructive way. Science served other ends, such as encouraging ambition and helping develop democratic social changes, because science, as an essential part of culture, furthered civilized as well as productive behavior on the part of the masses. Of course full-time scientists used all of these arguments to suggest, with both sincerity and self-interest, that scientific activities should be supported, and such contentions overlapped other varieties of popularization. One of Barnum's advertising brochures for his menagerie and museum in 1866 brought together the whole range of arguments for everyone's learning about science:

> There is no study that is more important to the youth of a rising generation or to adult age, than that of Natural History. It teaches man his superiority over the brute creation, and creates in his bosom a knowledge of the wisdom and goodness and omnipresence of a supreme and All-wise Creator. . . . Hence, it became necessary that

man should study the history of animated nature, make himself master of a science on which his own happiness depended, and which, when developed, could not fail to advance the great causes of civilization and learning.

Knowledge, as such popularizers argued, then, was to bring happiness and social benefits alike in material, religious, and cultural terms.[46]

Popularization increasingly tended to convey a sense of human power, power connected to the natural sciences and the idea of progress; this sense of power was involved in the force that later became known as modernization. The sense of power came from the idea that the world was orderly, and it was a sense more precise and vivid than that in classic formulations connecting knowledge and power. As late nineteenth-century thinkers made explicit, if the world was orderly, it was predictable and therefore subject to control. By learning about the regularities of nature, then, human beings could to some extent control their fates—whether through harnessing steam or following the laws of life. In this way the popularization of science had overtones beyond teaching merely that science was useful; indeed, the idea of modernization has come to include as characteristic not only this sense of control but openness to innovation and to science particularly.[47]

The problem with the ante-bellum synthesis of piety and practicality in popular science was that for most purposes piety was not essential, and indeed it was within a generation that "Nature" began to substitute for God. In natural theology itself, nature and God tended to become interchangeable. Religious explanation became natural explanation at one remove.[48] God's general providence—the laws of the universe—remained intact, but the allowances that had been made for God's special providence, with bows to Biblicism and commonsense moral philosophy, faded away. In 1865, the New England thinker Chauncy Wright wrote for both highbrow and other well-educated readers of the *North American Review* a refutation of natural religion. Basing theism upon the idea of design, Wright pointed out, was dangerous because it suggested that the design was an active force that made the world subsidiary to the existence of animals, and particularly humans; but in the case of chemistry, for example, science did not in fact confirm such a hierarchy. Better, said Wright, that religion should stay out of the realm of science, which would help keep superstition at bay:

Progress in science is really a progress in religious truth, not because any new reasons are discovered for the doctrines of religion, but because advancement in knowledge frees us from the errors of both ignorance and superstition, exposing the mistakes of a false religious philosophy as well as those of a false science. If the teachings of natural theology are liable to be refuted or corrected by progress in knowledge, it is legitimate to suppose, not that science is irreligious, but that these teachings are superstitious.[49]

Regardless of Wright's insight, explanation in natural terms proceeded on the popular level both in natural theology and otherwise, helping to demystify the world. The first step was the establishment of facts, the basic element of Baconian science. Whether in the object lessons of the schools or the compilations of scientific and technical progress, facts— acceptable to theologians and scientists alike—marked the era of practicality and piety before the Civil War. The facts, however, increasingly included explanations of how events happened, and the explanations were naturalistic. As early as 1819, for example, the anonymous author of *The Young Florist's Companion* (probably S. G. Goodrich of Hartford, the publisher) invoked "Nature" as the agent who, for example, seemed "intent upon the continuation and increase of the species," and it is as possible to infer nature as to infer God in the protective purpose of the structures of various flowers that the author described teleologically.[50] In terms of popularization, it did not matter, on one level, at least, whether or not the science was of high quality. The explanations even in grotesquely inferior science were still naturalistic.[51]

Whatever the content, then, even in a religious context science was not mystical. Further, as it was evolving, and as Wright saw, with ever new openings for explanation, the scientific enterprise had no need of the supernatural—either theistic or superstitious—to claim both truth and the power to be uplifting. As early as 1819, Denison Olmsted justified teaching chemistry at the University of North Carolina on the basis of "explanation of natural phenomena" and "moral and intellectual advantages arising from the study of the works of Nature." By 1850 W.H.C. Bartlett at West Point was content merely with studying nature, but under that term he included "the assemblage of all the bodies of the universe; it includes whatever exists and is the subject of change. Of the existence of these bodies we are rendered conscious by the impressions they make on our senses."[52] In the midcentury years, popularizers were emphasizing the facts and explanations that were secular. Although Baconian aggregations were not yet ready to replace all of superstition, much less religion, the direction of development was clear.[53]

"American life is crowded with facts," wrote J. G. Holland, discussing popular lectures in 1865—facts, he continued, "to which the daily newspaper gives daily record and diffusion." But then he went on to suggest that mere fact collecting, the naive Baconianism of many of his contemporaries, was insufficient: "Men work for nothing more than to know how to classify their facts, what to do with them, how to govern them, and how far to be governed by them."[54] As Holland sensed in the last year of the Civil War, a new element was coming in to supersede natural theology and fact mongering: the development of a systematic pattern within which the facts would fall. Popularizers began to stress that only with a distinct world picture could they show facts to be distinctively scientific, for otherwise mere facts might serve, indifferently, superstition or religion as well as science.

Besides beginning to pursue explanation, pre–Civil War popularizers took science one further important step toward the era of the men of science and the science of religion. That step was to extend the applicability of explanations. In emphasizing piety and practicality in the first half of the nineteenth century, American popularizers were not distinguishable from those in England. Where Americans did differ in their explication of science was in their more intense interest in self-improvement and in their support of a series of fads, particularly mesmerism, phrenology, and spiritualism, which, as I have indicated, were sometimes part of science—at least applied psychology—and sometimes not. These fads constituted an aspect of the great pre-Civil War reform movements, as was noted, for example, in the case of health popularization. Those reform movements involved more than fads, however, for they were based in large part on environmental assumptions and ideas that human beings could exert a substantial amount of control over the world. Indeed, a large part of the most vigorous popularization of science appeared in activities in and around the reform movements—not least, of course, self-improvement. Mesmerism and phrenology, especially, constituted in nineteenth-century eyes means of changing human behavior. Most important, reformers appealed to the validity of science to argue for the validity of melioristic techniques. In so doing, the reformers extended science into the realm of human activity and essentially pioneered the social sciences, even beyond psychology. In the process they also connected improvement in the world with the validity of scientific explanations. Not only did the reformers reinforce the connection between science and progress, then, but they moved popular science into all human affairs—just in time for the further extension of biology to humankind in the wake of Darwinism.[55]

The Late Nineteenth Century and the Men of Science

The legacy of the early nineteenth-century popularizers was therefore a set of institutions and concern for the meaning, context, and effect of conveying to the public discoveries about nature, especially correcting error and diminishing superstition. In the late nineteenth century, popularization continued to appear in a context of emphasizing facts, progress, and practicality, but popularizing differed in a number of ways from the pioneering period before the Civil War. Not only was science now more intensely applied to human beings and human affairs, but a more systematic secular context crystallized. Above all, the men of science appeared, and a very substantial number of them affected the ordinary course of popularization.[56] In 1863, Oliver Wendell Holmes wrote appreciatively to one of the first of them, Louis Agassiz: "I look with ever increasing admiration on the work you are performing for our civilization. It very rarely happens that the same person can take at once the largest and deepest scientific views and come down without apparent effort to the level of popular intelligence." Within a few years, many more of the men of science had begun popularizing. Moreover, they were not merely diffusing knowledge; they were clearly removed from the amateurs and were translating science for the nonprofessional. They lectured. They wrote. And the change in popularization was obvious. When the International Science Series, a group of books written by the leading experts in their fields, was well under way in 1872, the editor of the *Atlantic Monthly* commented: "The age of crude and inaccurate text-books, prepared by half-educated compilers, seems at last to be passing away."[57]

One sign of the change in popularization that came with the men of science was the fact that they became aggressive in defending science not only from superstition but from poorly qualified writers and speakers and ill-informed journalists, similar to the reaction of the psychologists noted in the previous chapter. In 1872, chemist F. W. Clarke attacked clergymen and journalists, especially, for distorting and passing judgment upon matters about which they were not qualified to speak. "My purpose [in writing] is twofold," noted Clarke. "First, to call attention to the silly character of much of what is called 'popular science;' and, secondly, to urge upon true scientific men the importance of rendering real knowledge more accessible to the masses. There is a demand for science," Clarke concluded, "or the trash which is written would not be read."[58]

The "true scientific men" were separating themselves not only from the masses but from the amateurs. The geologist John C. Branner, for example, was complaining in 1895 that "there are still plenty of persons of intelligence who have no conception whatever of the duties of a scientific man[:] those who imagine that science as a profession can be picked up just as the duties of certain civil offices, or of clerical positions, may be readily learned and performed by any man of ordinary intelligence." Occasionally, as had happened earlier, when the amateurs got control of a publication or organization, their resentment of self-conscious professionals became explicit. For the most part, however, the men of science dominated the American Association for the Advancement of Science (AAAS) and other venues in which amateurs and professionals formerly had shared. Professionals also dominated the leading (that is, the most culturally prestigious) institutions of popularization, such as the *Annual of Scientific Discovery*, the *American Naturalist*, and the *Popular Science Monthly*.[59] For many years, virtually all of the officers of the AAAS had at some time contributed at least one article to the *Popular Science Monthly*. In a similar way, the leading figures in any field tended also to try their hands at textbook writing and some at other popular writing and speaking. Like Clarke, they believed that such activities were part of the duties of a man of science.

Popularization therefore developed into a two-tiered activity, with one part on the high level engendered by the men of science. The other level typically was commercial and typically was "newspaper science," especially at the end of the century. For science, even more than for health, yellow journalism meant that the merely curious tended to give way to the sensational.[60]

Newspaper Science and the Demand for Popular Science

Part of the corruption of newspaper science grew out of the ignorance of journalists, who in the 1870s or the 1890s—or even later—could take the story of a discovery and get it thoroughly confused. The development of liquid air, for example, led to a reporter's stating that an inventor "with three gallons of the liquid . . . had repeatedly made ten gallons," an obvious violation of the law of conservation of matter committed long after the law had become common knowledge. Or, in another case, the editor ran an illustration of a saltwater diatom rather than the pathogenic microbe that was supposed to be depicted. In still another instance, a Boston newspaper reporter asserted that "the size of the molecule is never larger than the five hundred-millionth of an inch, and . . . in some cases it may be found no larger than the thousand-millionth of an inch. *Minute as this last dimension is, the 'second power' of our best microscopes makes the examination of it an easy task.*" For such misleading material, a number of both scientists and journalists blamed editors and reporters who did not verify science stories with reputable scientists. "We read every day," wrote the physicist Trowbridge,

> so-called scientific articles in newspapers and magazines which have evidently never been submitted to competent critics. Have we not read statements of the possibility of exploding powder magazines on board ships by electric waves; of the manufacture of liquid air without expenditure of energy; of electricity direct from coal; papers on the nebular theory more nebulous than any nebula yet discovered?[61]

When errors appeared in the public press, men of science took responsibility to correct them. The pattern showed up clearly, for example, in 1898 when the *Chicago Tribune* carried a story about a Washington, DC, scientist who proposed to stop crime by excising parts of the brain, leading the reporter to say, "The murder in a man's brain can be removed by the surgeon's knife." The somewhat confused explanation involved the ideas of localization of brain function and the physiological effects of emotional states. That the reporter (or his or her editor) was not totally in command of the subject is suggested by a reference to "the vase motor circulation of the blood." No sooner had the story appeared, however, than John A. Benson, a local Chicago physiologist, answered it in a long letter attempting to correct some of the "scientific absurdities" while yet affirming the view inherent in the article that tended to reductionism, if not materialism.[62]

Such incidents illustrate well not only the two tiers of popularization but the way in which men of science sprang to the defense of scientific accuracy and took advantage of every occasion to preach the religion of science—typically now embodying evolution and reductionism—to any available audience. But such incidents also suggest the increasing distance between scientific experts and specialists, on one hand, and even an educated public, to say nothing of the masses, on the other.

The advocates of science of course had another problem, which also plagued health popularizers especially. The source of some of the newspaper science was not infrequently some other scientist. To insist that editors screen such material was really to hold them to a very high standard—as in the case when someone signing himself "Physicist" objected to a magazine article written by Nikola Tesla in 1900. But by that time, specialization among the professional scientists was transforming the meaning of the term, so that "expert" opinion, too, was specialized. "Physicist," however, insisted that members of "the general public [are] helpless before any supposedly scientific statement . . . [because they lack] both knowledge of the relevant facts and training in logical criticism." Only the expert, he concluded, could protect people "against fraudulent medicines, bogus inventions and nonsensical enterprises."[63] And, he could have added, only the expert could protect the reputation of the scientific community. In the 1890s, for example, new observations of Mars proved to be very disappointing to the public, who expected more from astronomers because newspaper stories had led people to expect that human beings would be sighted on that planet.

It was true, as Clarke had said, that the appearance of newspaper science signaled public demand for popularization. All signs pointed to the existence of an audience for good science in the high-Victorian era. Therefore the deterioration at the end of the century was particularly disappointing. By the 1890s, American newspapers had turned scientific developments into "news"—not just interesting or uplifting background or such general stories as might appear in magazines, but "events." The earlier annuals of scientific discovery had not succeeded (nor of course tried) in turning "progress" into events in the way in which the new kind of editor, using telegraphic dispatches, did. The chief example, aside from medical developments, was the Roentgen ray. A few years later, by the time of Marconi's work with wireless, the journalists were fully ready to manufacture an event, giving Marconi credit even when others had actually made prior discoveries. Journalistic events were not thoughtfully compiled events of the year. And they certainly were not the religion of science. But they competed against the evangelizing of the men of science as they tried to answer the demand of the public for science.

Magazines, especially, at a pinnacle in the last decades of the nineteenth century, reflected the continued quest of many Americans for self-improvement.[64] Another conspicuous agency explicitly devoted to self-improvement was the Chautauqua program of lectures and the Chautauqua home study program, but countless other lectures and self-teaching programs continued to flourish as they had in the reform period before the Civil War. The fact that more and better materials were available and the conspicuousness of men of science in adult education efforts was all that distinguished such institutions from those of midcentury and earlier.

Educational Institutions in the Late Nineteenth Century

Adult education during the last three decades of the nineteenth century still was not fully separable from regular educational efforts. For home study programs, for example, the Chautauqua officials often simply reprinted ordinary school textbooks in science, and in general the elementary text often continued to serve adult as well as youthful learners, although now more incidentally than deliberately.[65] By the end of the century, however, popularizing science in the school setting was largely distinct from popularizing among the various American publics—just as other aspects of modern urban civilization fostered specialization in society in general.

Until the very end of the nineteenth century, college instruction in science tended, even more than earlier in the century, to set the standard for science teaching at all levels, especially because most secondary school students were still college-bound. Men of science who worked with this younger public typically had two goals in mind: establishing in American colleges and universities a science training that could produce more and better professional scientists, on the one hand, and, on the other hand, developing instruction in science that would be competitive with the traditional classical curriculum emphasizing Greek and Latin—competitive in that science education would be considered an integral part of a liberal education. The classics-versus-science debate was raging in England throughout the century, where T. H. Huxley and Matthew Arnold clashed. American educators, too, joined in and repeated the arguments that one kind or another of teaching would produce students who were superior thinkers—had developed the best mental discipline or mental cultivation, as the goal was phrased then. This identical argument applied to all levels of education, from the highest to the elementary.[66] Altogether the amount of ink that Victorians spilled on this debate was very great indeed, and the passions aroused on the anticlassical side helped account for the commitment of men of science to science. Moreover, the elevation of science in the curriculum was fundamentally involved in the rise of the graduate school, in which scientific subjects could easily enter on a par with the traditional liberal arts and in which science did not depend upon natural theology for a place in instruction.[67] The scientists and their allies seized every opportunity to ensure the place of the study of nature, natural law, and natural facts on their own terms at all levels in American educational institutions.

In attempting to let the student at any level confront nature rather than memorize didactically, science educators tried to use laboratory instruction, first introduced in midcentury, to modify textbook teaching. The laboratory turned out to have the dual advantage of furthering both specialized training and, it was hoped, the ability of the student to think, and particularly to think in antimystical terms. As soon as European-trained teachers in the colleges were successful in introducing formal laboratory instruction, pressure developed for labs for preparatory students (these were the labs that showed up in the school basements). Harvard authorities started requiring mathematics and physics for admission in the 1870s and by 1886 were recommending strongly some high-school laboratory experience, the very experiments of which were spelled out for physics and chemistry (and which therefore acted as a first national standard, or at least aspiration). By the 1890s, a science laboratory, now sometimes moved out of the basement, was a badge of the modernity of instruction in the leading high schools. As L. L. Conant wrote in 1893, "Empiricism is the watchword of today. 'Read Nature in the language of the experiment,' cries the reformer. The cry has been heard and heeded; and the high school or academy which is not well equipped with laboratories and apparatus is not looked upon as 'progressive,' as 'up to the times.'" Even textbook writers came to assume that there would be hands-on experience beyond reading the text. Moreover, more general popularizers followed the textbook-schoolroom model in suggesting "simple yet instructive experiments," as one author put it.[68]

In the lower schools, an equivalent of the laboratory, hands-on approach developed in the form of nature study, a curricular item of great popularity after the object lesson faded; nature study indeed reached a high point only in the twentieth century. Nature study involved a sentimental and romantic regard for nature, along with as much specific science teaching as the individual teacher could manage. The rise of nature study, however, occurred in an educational system in which administrators of the common schools were responding to a whole series of pressures and currents in the late nineteenth century: community demands that the subject matter be practical and prepare an industrial work force; educational theories that emphasized children's development, interests, and capacities; and internal as well as external pressure to develop a comprehensive, graded science education program—on the presumption that science was an important and necessary part of education. Either independently or following the leadership of the men of science, even on the elementary level teachers and administrators often viewed science as a systematic whole and as a cultural necessity. "The life, health and happiness of the individual is dependent upon his knowledge of the things about him, and upon the understanding that he has of their relations to each other and to himself," wrote Wilbur S. Jackman, a pioneer of modern science teaching, in 1891.[69]

Nature study therefore generated great enthusiasm before 1905 from any number of educators who quoted Agassiz's dictum "Study nature, not books." The movement met some difficulty when teachers turned out to have inadequate training and when the demand in the 1890s led to the publication of a number of inferior and inaccurate textbooks. Only when some eminent research naturalists from the colleges entered the field and provided appropriate textbooks after the turn of the century was nature study rescued and the remarkable momentum resumed. Yet the tradition of rote learning in the schools persisted so strongly that enthusiasm for nature study penetrated into only the better schools.[70]

Even in the last part of the nineteenth century, science instruction in the schools was frequently imperfect and fragmented, if not absent altogether. Nevertheless, in those decades substantial amounts of science teaching did appear in very large numbers of classrooms, primary as well as secondary, if only largely in the form of memorizing texts in temperance physiology and physical geography. Moreover, men of science who were based in higher education wrote the leading textbooks, which, in the decentralized educational system of the United States, standardized the curriculum far more than any other influence—as exemplified most transparently in the spread of nature study. "Within the last ten years," wrote Harvard botanist William G. Farlow in 1886, "a large number of books and papers has appeared in print, intended to show teachers how to teach and students how to study plants and animals. Some of them are excellent, and certainly, as far as books go, they leave little to be desired. They all start with the advice that a beginner should study plants and animals themselves, rather than what has been written about them." In biological subjects, the leading scientists shifted zoology school textbooks from a narrative format to an analytic one, emphasizing first classification and then morphology, that is, the idea of systematic interrelationships. Physical geography was particularly well suited to suggest the pervasive naturalism of the men of science. "Physical Geography," wrote one author, "covers the entire field of nature. It combines the facts and principles established by various natural sciences, and informs us how these facts and principles are exhibited and illustrated on the earth's surface," that is, how nature accounted for the entire world.[71]

This guidance from above in the educational system carried into the twentieth century, even though the domination of the schools by that time by the men of science was beginning to come to an end, particularly as large numbers of students who needed terminal training, not college preparation, began to flood the system and change the mission of the American high school.[72] Coincidentally and contemporaneously, some American scientists increasingly became preoccupied with specialized and advanced training and research and tended to turn aside from their responsibilities to develop science as culture. But before the turn of the century, these trends were only beginning (see chapter 5).

The Quantity and Intensity of Popularizing

Professional educators themselves were particularly active in the 1870s in agitating for more and better science teaching. Outside of the schools, popularization of science reached an unusual peak of intensity in the early part of that decade. As has been suggested, a combination of the reaction of the audience and the activity of popularizers, particularly as was evident in magazines, was noticeable, and people commented on it. At Dartmouth in 1873 Whitelaw Reid observed, "Ten or fifteen years ago, the staple subject here for reading and talk, outside study hours, was English poetry and fiction. Now it is English science. Herbert Spencer, John Stuart Mill, Huxley, Darwin, Tyndall, have usurped the places of Tennyson and Browning, and Matthew Arnold and Dickens." [73]

The spontaneous multiplication of scientific content in many publications early in the 1870s confirmed the existence of a new era. "Within the past three or four years," wrote astronomer Simon Newcomb in 1874, "there has been a large increase in the amount of popular scientific publication in this country." The editors of the *Boston Journal of Chemistry* waited until 1881 to begin to change the name of their magazine into the *Popular Science News*, but they recalled the days after the journal was founded in 1865 as a trade journal, primarily for the purpose of selling chemicals:

> It was soon found that the familiar style adopted in its conduct, and the interesting nature of the articles, had drawn to it a large number of readers from all classes, outside of those directly interested in chemistry. The number of patrons among farmers, horticulturists, teachers, artisans, heads of families, physicians, clergymen, dentists, apothecaries, literary gentlemen, etc., so rapidly increased that it became necessary to change the direction of the JOURNAL in no small degree and give it a more popular character. It became from necessity in its early history a monthly review of *Popular Science*, and has so continued to the present time.

Similarly, the *American Naturalist*, which was founded in the previous decade, in 1867, with a special popular constituency, did not take hold until into the 1870s and after. [74]

The outstanding incident in this rising intensity of popularizing activity was of course E. L. Youmans' founding of the *Popular Science Monthly* in 1872. The magazine was successful from the first; indeed, the first two numbers had to be reprinted. The circulation quickly rose to approximately twelve thousand, an incredible number for that day, and then eighteen thousand in 1886. Meanwhile, other signs, beyond the journals, such as book use in public libraries, also suggested the unusual new intensity in public interest in popular science around 1870. As one orator noted in 1875, "It is plain to all that the marked feature of our modern culture is the enthusiastic study of Nature. . . . This change, even within the last thirty years, is a striking one. . . . It is amusing to meet to-day those who a while ago were talking of the infinite soul in man, and are now quite proud of their pedigree from a West-African ape." [75]

After some years, either the intensity or the obviousness of the interest fell off, and just at the turn of the twentieth century, Americans had less popularization available except insofar as the newspapers carried the burden, which of course meant that the quality was more variable and very much less under the control of the men of science. The signs of some decline around 1900 were various. The *Popular Science Monthly* circulation fell well below ten thousand. The *Atlantic Monthly*, a general magazine that in 1866 had included "science" in the subtitle along with literature and politics, by the end of the century included, in fact, almost no scientific content, whereas in 1872–1874 there had been in addition to articles a special review section labeled science, and even after 1874 the editors continued to notice science books. Or, to use other magazines as gauges, the editor of the reorganized *Cosmopolitan* carried a "Progress of Science" column between 1893 and 1898, but it disappeared, except in a couple of issues in 1902. In a similar way, the *American Catholic Quarterly Review* "Scientific Chronicle" column, begun in 1886, disappeared in 1906. Other magazines, such as *Harper's*, showed similar phenomena— unusual interest that tended to fade just at the end of the 1890s. Indeed, in 1901 the change elicited a defensive comment from the editor of the *Popular Science Monthly*, who insisted that interest in science was still flourishing. Another observer, however, spoke of "the mass of readers, who are void of curiosity for scientific inquiry." And possibly both were right, for to some extent apparent diminutions in various popularizing activities could be deceiving in that they represented more the success of science propagandists, so that people took science for granted, rather than decreases in effort or even interest. In 1891, for example, the Boston Society of Natural History closed the Teachers' School because most teachers were by then sufficiently well educated that they no longer needed the special courses offered by the society.[76]

One particular organization suggests graphically the way in which the impulse to popularize science became institutionalized and, in the process, the popularizers developed a growing constituency in the United States. The organization was the Agassiz Association (AA), which preceded and paralleled nature study in the schools. In concert with the proponents of nature study, the Agassiz Association emphasized studying nature firsthand, as opposed to textbook rote learning. The association was founded in 1875 and within seven years claimed 15,000 members, chiefly in the United States. The main organizing call went out through the children's magazine *St. Nicholas,* which had already organized a society named Bird Defenders (to discourage nest destruction). The international Agassiz organization was based on local AA groups, which usually consisted of children of various ages, for which the association was designed; but a number were adult groups, members of which collected minerals, mosses, and arrowheads and observed fauna, microscopic slides, and the heavens just as the younger members did. The founders of the AA found the enthusiasm that they encountered overwhelming, and they succeeded in enlisting the help of leading scientists:

> A boy in a grammar school in the uttermost parts of Dakota becomes interested in fishes. He finds the common varieties that he knows, and studies them. By and by he takes in his net or on his hook a stranger. . . . He studies the fish with his eyes, examines fins, and scales, and skeleton. Then he prepares a description . . . and sends it with a rude sketch, it may be, to Dr. Holder, of the New York Central Park, who is one of the gentlemen who kindly assist our students. In a few days he receives a letter, giving him the name of his fish, and, what is better, the name of a book from which he can learn much more about fishes than from any volume that ever before found its way into his village.

This idyll from the handbook of the association conveys the spirit of the myriads of people who furthered the work of the Agassiz Association. Their goals were to get young people, especially, "to *observe* accurately" and "*reason* correctly upon the observations which they have made." In the late nineteenth-century context, reasoning correctly would have involved learning to interpret naturalistically, and observing accurately would of course diminish superstition.[77]

From the 1870s to the end of the century, then, in magazines, lectures, books, teaching materials, and other media, working and often eminent scientists took the lead in presenting science in general and individual sciences, too, to students and the more or less educated general public. Neither popularizers nor public doubted that science was part of culture, the high culture that was the aspiration of both the upwardly mobile and those who were already in the cultured classes.[78]

Standard Scientism

The science that popularizers so confidently taught was based upon the idea that investigators were rapidly establishing the details of scientific truth, which was that certainty which explained all phenomena in terms of the laws of science, now most conspicuously the conservation of energy and Darwinian evolution. The firmness of that knowledge, the trust in facts, provided an important part of the fundamental appeal of the religion of science. In this spirit, for example, a writer in the *Popular Science News* in 1895 exulted over a report of liquifying hydrogen: "At last hydrogen is liquified. What was once pure theory is now an established, substantial fact. Every known gas has been forced from invisibility to visibility."[79] In part, emphasis upon fact continued earlier Baconian attitudes, and in practice a substantial part of popularization consisted of trying to get an audience to learn facts and get them straight, whether a description of the way colors appeared in the rainbow or knowledge of the way in which a species of fish managed to survive. To love science is to love truth, wrote Frank Sargent Hoffman of Union College in 1898: "The more patiently and persistently you observe, the more carefully you experiment, the more logically you arrange and systematize,—in other words, the more scientific you make your knowledge,—the more quickly will ignorance and superstition vanish, and the earth be prepared for the reign of righteousness and peace."[80]

Just as earlier, when facts continually illustrated the work of an awesome Great Designer, so in the late nineteenth century facts also appeared in a tendentious context. Even when popularization appeared to consist of simply amassing one fact after another, popularizers continued to send additional messages that were frequently explicit. In the later period, facts were to function in three ways. First, they explained the otherwise inexplicable, even more so than earlier. Second, they illustrated discovery, the idea that new scientific information was always forthcoming if only scientists and public alike remained open-minded. Mark Sullivan in reading science books of the 1870s was struck that authors "had a manner of saying: 'It was once thought . . . but we now know.' Doubtless," commented Sullivan, "the process is not ended." Facts in the third place showed the contributions of scientific discovery to material and practical improvement, for even as pure science and application tended to separate among professionals, the traditional view of practicality was reaffirmed publicly.[81] Altogether, popularizers over and over contrasted their happy times of explanation and open-mindedness with the benighted past when explanation was neither available nor welcome.

This tendentious context distinguished an era. Even though Tyndall died in 1893 and T. H. Huxley in 1895, others continued to argue their viewpoint, and David Starr Jordan, the American ichthyologist and university president, had already begun to take the place that they had held in the pages of the *Popular Science Monthly*. The changes of the 1890s, coincident with the rise of the yellow press, signaled the beginning of the end, however, even though the late nineteenth century was truly the time when the religion of science flourished and even overflowed from the realm of popularization.

The Religion of Science

Although the religion of science drew on earlier tradition—particularly the idea of culture and the belief that science was practical—yet the high-Victorian version was distinct. The openness of the scientific partisans' declaration of the warfare of science and religion contrasted markedly with the just-departed era of natural theology. Although many thinkers decried the conflict and tried to reconcile religion and science, many others followed Youmans when he asserted, "We consider this conflict to be natural and inevitable, to be wholesome rather than mischievous." Youmans of course believed that religion had a legitimate function but also that that function should not impinge on the domain of science. Religion, he wrote in 1874, "has no enemies so dangerous as those who insist upon staking its truth upon any conditions or results into which it is the legitimate business of Science to inquire."[82]

Youmans probably was unaware of the extent to which he in fact supported an aggressive campaign against conventional religion. He, like a number of his colleagues, customarily capitalized the word "Nature" (as well as "Science") in a worshipful way. The tendency of such partisans to substitute Nature for God, even implicitly anthropomorphizing natural explanation, elicited comment at the time. Already in 1858, theologian Horace Bushnell had denounced the new infidelity, in which explanation was kept "within the terms of mere nature itself." "I suspect," wrote a Unitarian critic in 1883, "no little latent, insidious power of deception in the word 'Nature.' One of the most patent *idols* of the present generation is this very 'Nature,' undefined, generally, and often meaningless." He went on to observe that "very often nearly all the content of 'God' is smuggled into 'Nature.'" In either case, he warned, "personification is the thief of sense."[83]

The subject matter that the men of science popularized in those decades reinforced their enthusiasm for propagating the religion of science. The negative campaign against superstition and superstitious religion consisted to a very large extent of making observations, as has already been noted. By the late nineteenth century, explanations were far more numerous and far more intellectually satisfying—dramatically so—than had been the case earlier; everyone was aware of the exciting discoveries of those years, and the demystification so prominent in psychology was also a feature of the other sciences. Readers of popularized science knew that an article entitled "The Mysteries of Plant-Growth," probably would explain why it was not mysterious at all. Some of this persistent negative campaign was very direct. It was not just showing that a bat was not a bird, nor even unmasking—giving material explanations for—mysterious phenomena. After photography became common, for example, scientific editors delighted in printing deceptive photos, including mirages or people who looked like giants, and so forth, and then explaining how the effect had been achieved—hoping in the process of explaining to undermine credulity.[84]

Typically popularization, such as that in magazine articles, opened with the observation that a popular belief was not so, or that a simple observation had much more to it. Explanation of course followed. Such explaining as an activity gathered momentum and carried popularizers along. Writing of meteorites and comets, for example, Lewis Swift of Warner Observatory told his readers, "As study and observation in the past have dissipated the mysteries of the comets, we may confidently hope that, by the same means, the meteors may be forced, in the future, to disclose their marvelous secrets." Or, as the editor of the *Popular Science News* commented upon announcing that an English researcher had found the secret of the "singing sands," which give a musical note when rubbed, the findings "will undoubtedly be of the greatest interest and importance, and furnish a solution of a problem which has hitherto baffled investigators." [85]

The general tendency of popularizers' explanations was toward an ever more rigorous reductionism. Intelligent readers were well aware of the tendency. E. A. Washburn, a New York theologian, declared in 1876, for example, that the "unreasonable" conflict between religion and science had "been forced on religion by a school of naturalists, who mask[ed] their materialism under the name of science, and because nature teaches only phenomena, den[ied] all knowledge of God beyond force, or a life beyond that of these physical atoms." Reductionists could draw not only on increasingly sophisticated physics and chemistry—especially organic chemistry—but on a mode of scientific explanation endowed with new power by Darwinism, that is, the developmental. Writers could, beyond describing life phenomena in physicalistic terms, go on and read nature, or Nature, as regression and progression, where primitive elements explained present-day events, even in humankind. "The ultimate object of geology," wrote Johns Hopkins geologist George H. Williams in 1889, "is to decipher the complete life-history of our planet." [86]

In one particular area, reductionism took on a compelling salience in both technical and popular science: neurophysiology. More aggressive popularizers simply ignored the soul and instead pictured human thought and behavior as an aspect of physical processes. As an anonymous reviewer of 1880 put it, "We know nothing of mind except as an organic manifestation. Throughout the entire scale of animate nature, intelligence is an endowment of a nervous mechanism. . . . The laws of mind have their basis in this material substratum, and mental operations are conditioned upon physiological processes." Despite some thinkers both inside and outside of science who objected to excessive materialism (but with the assumption that some was acceptable), enthusiasts tended to ally American popular science with both mechanism and materialism, provided only that neither one was dogmatic but, rather, emphasized the openness of science to new discoveries. By 1900, when E. B. Rosa wrote "The Human Body as an Engine" for readers of the *Popular Science Monthly*, he could have surprised no general reader. He in fact used the idea of evolution and the law of the conservation of energy to conclude that animals, including humans, were more complicated than locomotives but operated on the same principles. Among men of science, questions of materialism and determinism that had troubled careful thinkers tended to give way to "purely scientific" accounts by the end of the century.[87]

In pursuing reductive explanations, proponents of the religion of science developed a functional equivalent of monotheism, that is, a unitary system within which all of nature fitted. Physicist Trowbridge, for example, in 1884 explained how the principle of the conservation of energy liberated scientists from metaphysics and other complicating contexts: "The ancients had a god for every manifestation of Nature—a god of peace, a god of the land, a god of the sea. Fifty years ago scientific men were like the ancients. There was a force attached to every phenomenon of Nature. Thus, there were the forces of electricity and magnetism, the vital forces, and the chemical forces." Trowbridge of course went on to observe that now the physical forces were reduced to "a mechanical system" that permitted prediction. By bringing biology, including human nerve processes, into this same mechanical schema by reductionistic explanation, the late nineteenth-century men of science had a universal view into which any observed phenomenon could and would fit. They believed that alternative or special explanations—whether superstitious, metaphysical, or religious—were no longer necessary, any more than the specialized gods of the ancients were. Scientist popularizers instead tended to insist on unifying explanations.[88] In Arthur W. Wright's department, "Scientific Progress," in each issue of the *International Review* in 1876–1877, for example, he showed how each little fact or discovery of the day contributed to a general set of orderly, nonmysterious beliefs in a natural view of the universe.

Even the popularizers at the most rudimentary level could maintain the overall viewpoint of "Nature" into which all knowledge could fit. "There should be no aimless work in the elementary schools," wrote educator John W. Dickinson of Massachusetts in 1873. "Every fact that is taught and learned should have a well known relation to scientific knowledge." Readers of the *Popular Science News* in 1885 were not permitted merely to enjoy the novelty of growing a lead-tree in a bottle; "This experiment," wrote the anonymous author, "illustrates very prettily the laws of chemical reaction," and he mentioned specifically affinity and exact proportions. Another educator, William G. Peck of Columbia, appealed in his *Elementary Treatise on Mechanics* to observation, experience, and what was generally believed in mechanics, but nevertheless made his presentation in an orderly context, starting with atoms and coming out at the end of the book with locomotives, hoping, he said, to help students and others "keep pace with the discoveries of modern science."[89]

The progress of scientific explanation was altogether inexorable, at least in popularization. At midcentury, it had still been possible to cite phrenology as the form in which "psychology and physiology, marching hand in hand, left metaphysics at a remote distance . . . the light of modern civilization succeeding to the darkness of the middle ages." In subsequent decades, far more precise and satisfying terms of explanation, such as electrical activity and nerve force, substituted not only for metaphysics but for soul or ghost or nonmechanical entity of any kind.[90]

The Scientific Method

By the end of the century, the influx of new information and concepts in all fields of natural science was so rapid that proponents of the religion of science worked very hard to include in the systematic context of nature and naturalistic explanation the idea that science constituted method as much as facts; and it was just in this period that the idea of method developed a critical role in popularization. "The whole body of modern scientific truth, disclosing the order of Nature and guiding the development of civilization," reported a committee headed by Youmans, "must be taken as an attestation of the validity of the scientific method of thought."[91] The ultimate certitudes of science turned out, then, in the religion of science, to be those of the open-ended nature of scientists' quests for truth— a truth that could never be absolute, because the search was increasingly an end in itself. Findings along the way, although certain, represented but incidental stopping places as the progress of science proceeded. In high culture, one version of this attitude became known as pragmatism, which was tellingly satirized as adopting a method in lieu of a philosophy.

But popularizers of science made additional uses of the apotheosis of the scientific method, or what was often called the scientific spirit. First, following such thinkers as Karl Pearson, they used the scientific attitude to justify their expanding the realm of science to all areas of life—not just to conventional natural phenomena, not even to humans and their psychology, but to literature, culture, and religion, the very places that formerly had been reserved for another kind of truth. Now science, or Science, claimed all. "The legitimate offspring of the laboratory is the seminar," wrote botanist John M. Coulter in 1900. John Brisben Walker, editor of *Cosmopolitan*, in 1904 asserted that "a good knowledge of science, if they are to hold their own," was essential for engineers, clergymen, lawyers, manufacturers, merchants, businessmen, farmers, physicians, artists, and literary men. Extending the realm of science was the ultimate secularization of the religion of science: those who admitted the validity of science in one area were asked to surrender all realms to the same source of knowledge, to a new reality. Youmans after just a year of the *Popular Science Monthly* pointed out that he was giving "especial prominence" in popularizing to material bearing on social policy. The religion of science was in fact often aggressively controversial.[92]

Partisans of science in the late nineteenth century therefore made many claims for science. For the world, science promised material and social improvement. "Scientific progress," wrote W J McGee in 1898, "especially in a land of free institutions, is so closely interwoven with industrial and social progress that the advance of one cannot be traced without constant reference to the other." For the individual, science promised culture and morality. The editor of the *Popular Science News* in 1884 noted, "Rarely or perhaps never has there been an instance of a boy becoming dissipated or bad who, from reading a journal like the [POPULAR] SCIENCE NEWS, acquired a taste for scientific investigation and experiment." Altogether, the program of popularizers added up to, on the one hand, faith that humans could progress and, on the other hand, a commitment to civilization as it was understood then and as it galvanized aspirations in American culture for generations.[93] Most controversy then and later centered around the issue whether science was fully adequate for civilization or, indeed, if in undesirable, reductionistic, or skeptical forms science was inimical to civilization.[94]

In this context of science as civilizer, the emphasis that popularizers put on the scientific method or the scientific spirit took on significance beyond training children's minds or purifying democratic processes. The significance went even beyond the late nineteenth-century idea of the scientist as the objective, self-denying puritan of the laboratory.[95] By the opening of the twentieth century, the advocates of science in their explicit statements were emphasizing the skeptical and open-minded nature of scientific inquiry—not only to expand the territory of science but increasingly to portray the uncertainty of exactly what the method might turn up. Where earlier, for example, Americans had wanted facts so that they could demonstrate the wonders of God's world, now facts tended to be explanatory and appeared in explanatory contexts, so much so as to tend toward reductionism. But the reductionism as well as the facts led only to a constantly changing view of nature. The anonymous author of "The Mysteries of Chemistry" in 1889, for instance, noted that "the existence of atoms cannot be proved, and even if it could there would still remain many questions to be answered and phenomena to be explained." Projecting the progress of chemistry from the past into the future, the writer expected results before very long, but only on these open-ended terms: "Our conception of the nature and action of matter will be much clearer than at present."[96] And people at the time contrasted this constant change, dictated by facts, with dogma. The uncertainty of which way new developments would go, however, was not yet the uncertainty that was popularized two or three decades later.

Discovery of facts was fundamental to the negative element of science as the men of science translated it. As early as 1875, Trowbridge had noted the criticism that Tyndall had set off when he tried to defend science from hostile clergymen. Tyndall had, noted Trowbridge, "a certain want of reverence characteristic of many scientific men." No doubt, said Trowbridge, "this deficiency in reverence is to be lamented, but," he added, "the attitude of an investigator is generally one of irreverence."[97] That irreverence was the direct descendant of earlier varieties of skepticism. Evangels of the religion of science presented the public not only with a well articulated viewpoint of negative opposition to superstition—involving an emphasis on method—but with a world view in which facts led to naturalistic explanation. By the end of the nineteenth century, the religion of science had developed great momentum in American culture, momentum that carried over in the face of the powerful new forces of change that the next century brought.

Chapter 5

Popularizing the Natural Sciences in the Twentieth Century

IN THE NINETEENTH century, popular science came to stand for the mission of converting people to the scientific way of life. After 1900, many scientists, teachers, and amateurs continued to evangelize for the unity of nature, reductionism, and explanation. As popularization evolved further, however, what the public heard, instead of translation, condensation, and explanation, was a series of events and products—presented not with an eye to upgrading humanity and society but written in terms of personal interest and payoff for each consumer—or of public relations.

This chapter does not just document the change; my intention is to explain how and why the transformation occurred. Examination of the events will therefore proceed by uncovering a series of layers. I shall start with a quantitative chronological profile and then expand the superficial profile into a narrative to suggest the flow of events as well as to serve as a reference point for the rest of the analysis. The next layer consists of an investigation into the ways in which educators, a crucial group, attempted to accommodate the vast changes that occurred in their circumstances. Next to be examined will be the changing roles of the various types of media, printed and electronic, and the functioning of the science writers. Still another layer will consist of the decline of amateurs and the rise of specialized popular audiences. The deepest layers will appear in a review of the way in which popularizers started with a naturalistic world but came to emphasize not only the products of science but science as a policy and image—almost anything, in short, but science as a way of life.

The particular content of popularizations did not usually distinguish the twentieth century. Halley's comet, the Scopes trial, the discovery of

Pluto, radar and the atomic bomb, space, and the environment did not in and of themselves demand any special treatment or emphasis in presentation to the public. From the nineteenth century (not to mention the Enlightenment), everyone knew that science was itself progressing and, for the most part, bringing about progress. As in the popularizing of health and psychology, the format of the popularization of science, the kinds of people who undertook the task, and the significance of it distinguished the twentieth century.

The Quantitative Profile

In the twentieth as in the nineteenth century, peaks of activity in popularization of science appeared in the record. The basic outline has been established by Marcel C. La Follette, who sampled popular magazines for the incidence of science articles between 1910 and 1955, and other evidence extends the validity of her findings. A generally low level of activity existed in the 1910s, but beginning just about 1920 an extraordinary upsurge in science content appeared. Then with the coming of the Great Depression, the amount of science popularization fell again to the low, 1910–1920 level—with the exception of a brief mid-1930s flurry related to accounts of the Mt. Palomar Observatory. After 1945, the volume increased again, to a level making the 1950s comparable to the 1920s. Numerous surveys by other scholars suggest that into the 1960s, signs of popularizing activity continued to grow. No doubt the high point came in 1961, when the editors of *Time* chose fifteen U.S. scientists as its "men of the year." Just at the end of that decade, however, the intensity of activity began to falter, and by the mid-1970s, popularized science shared in what later came to be recognized as "the science slump." Then at the end of the 1970s, a series of specialty magazines appeared and heralded a resurgence in popularized science as a number of Americans found that they suffered from "sci anxiety," as a series of ads labeled it—the lack of knowledge about what was going on in the world of science.[1]

The high points, in the 1920s, the 1950s and 1960s, and the end of the 1970s and early 1980s, along with the low points (the opening years of the century, the 1930s and World War II, and the 1970s), provide a framework, as I have suggested, within which to begin to understand popularization in the twentieth century. Did high and low points reflect consumer demand or popularizers' enthusiasm—or cultural and institutional context? Beyond a framework, the quantitative narrative establishes a basis for discerning the factors involved in the transformations of the twentieth century.[2]

The decline of science in both specialized and general magazines of the late 1890s (noted in the previous chapter) continued into the twentieth century, as did a relative scarcity of books on popular science subjects. In 1905, the University of Chicago botanist Coulter remarked of newspaper and magazine coverage of science, "The material they furnish, which may be said to deal with research . . . is scant in amount, sensational in form, and usually wide of the mark. The fact that it is scant in amount is a cause for congratulation if it must involve the two other features. The sensational form is a concession to what is conceived to be public taste." Coulter was not a neutral observer, yet other evidence confirms his observations. In the depression of the 1890s, the *Popular Science News* alone absorbed seventeen other, mostly failing, special-interest publications and then itself expired in 1902. *Discovery*, the next major magazine to attempt to reach the public with science, lasted for only six issues in 1907. The *Popular Science Monthly*, which, by contrast, did persist—but at a loss for some years—finally in 1915 was transformed into the *Scientific Monthly*, without the word "popular" in the title, although the owner, psychologist J. McKeen Cattell, was still attempting to popularize at least down to the level of highbrows and school teachers. In general, the very term "popular science" carried negative connotations around the turn of the century, and for good reason.[3]

Newspaper science reached its nadir at that time, as yellow journalism continued to flourish before World War I, particularly in the notorious Sunday supplements. The idea of the journalists then, Will Irwin recalled, was to make the reader look at the paper and say, "Gee whiz!" It was in this context, he continued, that editors made a "surprising discovery: the public liked science or pseudo science! So in tabloid doses, the yellows gave them archaeology, gave them medical discovery—always jazzed up to the emotional point." (Irwin went on to recall fondly how on one occasion the Sunday supplements reported the finding of "the germ of baldness.") Hillier Krieghbaum, looking back in 1941, concluded that "science reporting before the World War was a combination of editorial whim, hoax, newspaper-financed stunts, garbling and faking of details when truthful information was scarce, plus an occasional job well done."

Hearst, for example, was responsible for the headline, "X Rays for the Battlefield," of an 1898 story in fact about the possible medical applications of roentgenograms during the Spanish-American War, and a rival editor printed such material as "Rain Made to Order," a story about the claims of a weather faker. La Follette found that much of a brief flurry of science in the magazines around 1910 could be accounted for almost entirely by exciting astronomical items from the Mt. Wilson Observatory, following the period when Halley's Comet had made good newspaper copy—that is, sound science that was treated in a sensational way.[4]

The generally low level of popularizing at the opening of the twentieth century is baffling because the prestige of science was so high at that time. Progressive reformers held the dispassionate professional scientist up as a model for emulation in other areas of life. The boys' adventure book hero, as Russel Nye points out, was Tom Swift in his laboratory. And yet not only did measures of public interest decline, but the percentage of high-school students electing science courses declined precipitously and did not increase much even in absolute numbers.[5]

The keys to this seeming paradox of low quantity combined with high esteem can be found in the changing nature of popularizing science and in institutional circumstances. As scientists increasingly devoted themselves to the ideal of pure research, writers in the popular media directed attention less to science than to technology. In what Lawrence Badash calls "the radium craze," which hit just after 1900, for example, the wonders of radioactivity were overshadowed by the practical results that journalists thought up or publicized. An ounce of radium would drive a fifty-horsepower car clear around the globe at thirty miles an hour, or radium mixed with chicken feed might result in eggs that would hardboil themselves or hatch chicks without an incubator.[6]

Whereas in the nineteenth century popularizers drew few distinctions between science and technology, by the 1900s members of the public increasingly respected research but gave their attention to application and development. With a large part of what had been thought of as science, that is, technology, removed from the concept in popularization, the perceived decline is not surprising. Moreover, the news of contrivances, gadgets, and projects, such as attempts to fly heavier-than-air machines, was taken up appropriately and effectively by newspapers. In 1921, when the publishers of the *Scientific American*, which for decades had been directed toward mechanics and inventors, closed down their supplement and definitively shifted from a weekly to a monthly format, they noted that because the daily press covered so thoroughly "every scientific advance, . . . every invention of importance," the function of factual news dissemination that the *Scientific American* had earlier served was now superseded.[7]

Although World War I effectively reduced the amount of science popularization (with the notable exception of that concerning the area of chemistry), the role that applied science played in that war for both good and evil made a deep impression on scientists and members of the public alike. The result was a series of institutional developments that led to a very large increase in popularization. In addition, radio appeared, to supplement or displace printed media, and, as will be noted more fully below, changes in education led to a new course in the schools, general science, particularly for the millions of new high-school students, and a new curriculum came in to go with general science, also in the 1920s. Altogether the enthusiasm of scientists for what Ronald Tobey has called an ideology of science, plus the institutional changes, greatly increased and upgraded the popularization of science.[8]

Events of the 1920s also lent themselves to popularization—such items as the opening of King Tut's tomb and airplane feats and arctic explorations. Perhaps the most effective incident was the Scopes trial of 1925, which led to a great deal of thoughtful writing in magazines as well as extensive news coverage. The actual broadcast of the trial over clear-channel station WGN of Chicago was so widely heard that people later assumed that it was a pioneer network broadcast. Finally, journalists ingeniously made Albert Einstein and his ideas noteworthy, indeed, common currency on the descriptive level. Altogether the media furor caused a wit to pun, "According to the scientists we may suppose our first ancestors were Atom and Eveolution."[9]

Newspaper science reporting as such changed suddenly at the beginning of the 1920s. Between 1920 and 1925, the volume of science news doubled in major papers. The coincidence of a number of events in 1920–1921 suggested the magnitude of the change, which signaled not only quantitative increases but a remarkable improvement in the quality of science news as reporters and editors became conscious of new standards of accuracy and responsibility. The most notable development was the appearance of the special science reporters and even the special subsidized news service, Science Service, directed by chemist-journalist Edwin E. Slosson. Alva Johnston became the science writer for the *New*

York Times and David Dietz the same for all of the Scripps-Howard newspapers. John J. O'Neill appeared as a science writer with a series in the *Brooklyn Eagle*, and Watson Davis began a daily science column in the Washington *Herald*. These events inspired many others; by 1927, for example, the Associated Press had two writers and a special science news service.[10]

This momentum from newspaper science carried over into other media. E. T. Bell, of California Institute of Technology, commenting on the new popularization, observed, "Science has at last become articulate, not to say garrulous." Although the subject of science was slower than that of health to be presented on the radio, numerous radio talks on science—many republished in the *Scientific Monthly* and elsewhere—flourished from the late 1920s into the 1930s and even 1940s. Moreover, popular science writers also produced not only magazine articles but books, and at the end of the 1920s the Scientific Book Club appeared. In all of these efforts Science Service was often central. *Science News-Letter* (founded in 1921–1922) embodied many of the Science Service press releases and by the late 1920s was standing on its own as a regular magazine, with a circulation of 10,000 (30,000 by 1940).[11]

Probably 1930, with stories about the discovery of Pluto, represented a high point for science in the media.[12] After 1930, the erosion consequent to the Great Depression was decisive in journalism. In 1936, O'Neill, now of the New York *Herald-Tribune*, noted in a letter that even the Sunday editions of the leading New York papers carried less than one percent in the field of science: "There has been a decrease in the space devoted to science and technical subjects since 1931. In my most hopeful moments," he continued, obviously disheartened, "I like to think of this as a transient drop, due to economic conditions." In other areas, the Scientific Book Club faded out, and popularization of science on the radio, too, never recovered the level of the early 1930s. By 1941, foreign and national events had largely replaced local as well as science news in the newspapers.[13]

Events in the Last Half of the Century

The Great Depression had nevertheless brought into popularization of science a new element: the argument that everyone should understand science because of the social impact of research coming from the laboratory.

Technological unemployment, as it was known then, was the basis of a substantial amount of negative comment on the social effects of science (still confused with technology), contrasting with the usual optimistic, futuristic popularization, which of course persisted, and not only in connection with the 1939 New York's World Fair theme, "The World of Tomorrow."[14] With the advent of the atomic bomb in 1945, the social responsibility argument became very conspicuous indeed. This concern for social responsibility combined with interest in atomics and medicine to cause the high incidence of science in the 1950s and early 1960s. As early as 1951, a survey of newspaper editors indicated that the amount of science news that they printed had doubled over a very few years. Only space, the editors asserted, limited the amount of science news that they would publish; the increase was impressive, despite the fact that their citing space limitations meant that editors did not habitually displace other news for science, regardless of their verbal enthusiasm.[15]

By the 1950s, a number of forces had combined to suggest to opinion leaders that all Americans, young and old, needed to know much more about science than they did. Talk about social responsibility reinforced the customary arguments, and then Cold War fears that Americans were lagging in technological development compounded leaders' concerns. Americans' reactions to Sputnik in 1957 embodied all of these tendencies; science popularizing programs that had appeared successful suddenly were perceived as failures. The so-called space race that subsequently developed did not necessarily increase the popularization of science in the press or in the schools immediately. But in the long run, the space race did help accelerate the activities of science writers and educators. Fred L. Whipple, director of the Smithsonian Astrophysical Laboratory, for example, within just a few weeks took advantage of the commotion over Sputnik to call on newspaper editors to take responsibility for creating an intellectual climate in which American science could flourish and so win out over Russian science. Such pressures may have had some effect. By the mid-1960s, newspaper editors again claimed to have increased greatly the amount of science news that they were running, this time since Sputnik. The very numbers of identifiable science writers, too, confirmed that there was a new wave of popularization. The National Association of Science Writers, founded in 1934 with twelve members, had 61 in 1945 but over 300 in the 1960s as a third wave of recruits joined. And, finally, at the same time, a vigorous program to inspire science teaching penetrated into the schools (as will be described below).[16]

Nevertheless, the outlook for science popularization weakened during the 1960s. Whereas some measures showed a steady increase of science news, the general magazines that had carried important articles, magazines such as the *Saturday Evening Post*, tended to disappear, and specialized magazines did not fully replace them. The *Scientific Monthly* expired in 1957, almost in effect having been already reincarnated in 1948, however, by a new, high-level "popular" science magazine using an old title, *Scientific American*. It is true that the newspapers expanded magazine and general cultural coverage as the old universal magazines expired and television began to shape the modern function of a newspaper. Science popularization benefitted to some extent along with the arts in this shift, which in effect made science news relatively more prominent. That prominence culminated at the time of the moon landing in 1969, already after decline had started to set in. In any event, exactly how much the content of space coverage was science and how much just events on television was unclear.[17]

A number of factors conditioned the retrogression of the late 1960s and 1970s. To begin with, the increasing presence of television after the 1950s oppressed and counteracted all serious attempts to popularize science. From the very beginning, successful educational television programs tried on one level or another to popularize science. They sometimes had a devoted following, but always a small one, which although representing one kind of success nevertheless rendered them ephemeral. Moreover, as will be noted below, such programs did not succeed in developing in their audiences either scientific literacy, as it came to be called, or, apparently, attitudes toward science that made any difference in the way in which members of the audience viewed the world.

During the 1960s and especially in the 1970s, "environmental" issues, which could pass for science, did appear frequently in the press and elsewhere. These issues represented various groups' criticisms of the effects of science and technology, which built on the earlier idea that popular knowledge about science was necessary for an informed citizenry to control science. The act of learning about ecology and the environment, as will be suggested below, often appeared in a guise hostile to science. Hence some of what appeared as discussions of science not only had little scientific content but undermined traditional popularization, which had, of course, been friendly. "Environmental education" sometimes displaced regular science instruction in the schools. And whereas even negative material did in fact embody science popularization when it raised issues of interaction and effect, that potential for teaching members of the public about science was blunted because economic and political considerations caused mass media controllers to play down environmental issues as much as possible.[18]

It was, then, just as the space race peaked and as science writers improved in portraying complexity in the wake of such sensitizing forces as Earth Day that science popularization tended to diminish quantitatively. A projected science daily, to serve science as the *Wall Street Journal* did business, never materialized. In existing general newspapers of the 1970s, economic forces tended actually to reduce special science assignments for reporters. By 1974, even the press corps covering space events at Cape Canaveral had broken up. Concerned scientists commented even more than usual on the miniscule level of science content in the media. As noted in chapter 2, medical stories flourished in the era of narcissism, and cancer stories were especially good press when celebrities Happy Rockefeller and Betty Ford underwent breast surgery. But natural science was not, usually, finding a major place in the media. Even sociologists' and journalists' interest in science reporting and science reporters, an interest that had grown and thrived for a generation, shriveled in the 1970s.[19]

The best indication of the low level of popularizing activity in the 1970s was the contrast of the mid-decade lack of activity with the stir at the end, when the new popular science magazines suddenly appeared and some older ones were retitled (*Chemistry*, for example, became *SciQuest*). The rush was so great that a first wave of magazines at the end of the 1970s was followed by a second wave in the early 1980s. Altogether, the number was sufficient that in many newsstands a special "science" section (often, of course, including astrology) appeared. The inspiration for the new magazines was largely the success of *Psychology Today* as well as the continued financial and intellectual well-being of the highbrow *Scientific American* (circulation 700,000). Some of the late 1970s magazines also gained circulations of 500,000 or more. These periodicals, large and small, ranged from *Science 80*, an official publication of the American Association for the Advancement of Science, down to *Science and Living Tomorrow*, which had a substantial sex content. Meanwhile, in a parallel development, following the success of environmental and medical stories and columns, a number of newspapers added popular science supplements and columns as regular features. Even on television the number of "science" programs increased.[20]

All of this activity suggests that the self-appointed popularizers and "gatekeepers" of the media had misjudged the extent of a market for popularized science. As John Henahan pointed out in 1974, the supermarket tabloid the *National Enquirer*, which was by any other standard irresponsible, had already for years been doing well by incorporating a substantial number of science stories—almost always sensationalized (as has been noted particularly in connection with health and psychology). The demand seemed to exist, but what was it a demand for?[21] Was all of it popular science? Were the *National Enquirer* sensations, Earth Day reporting, *Science 80*, *Physics Today*, and television shots of space events all properly part of the same social and intellectual process, even if it still had two tiers? The institutions of the twentieth century—books, magazines, newspapers, lectures, and schools—which had started out familiar and more or less unambiguous, had evolved in only a few decades into a confusing set of mediators that raised more than routine questions about the popularization of science—questions not only of institution and audience but, as has been suggested, of the act of popularizing itself.

Science Education

One of the major and most persistent findings of sociologists who studied popularization of science in the second half of the twentieth century was the fact that a person's education controlled to a remarkable extent how and how much the person sought out and understood popularized material, whatever the medium. For the twentieth century, at least, then, science education was a necessary preliminary to further popularization as well as a popularizing institution in itself.[22]

The findings of the sociologists suggested that in modern America one of the functions of popularization—to educate the already educated—became the dominant activity, a finding that, as will be remarked, the new science magazines and features of the late 1970s seemed to confirm. Another possible conclusion was that for the ignorant or unschooled adult, most, if not all, science popularizing was therefore a waste of time or a function of the lower tier, the yellow press and later the *National Enquirer*. But such a conclusion then put on the schools almost the entire responsibility for the level of "scientific literacy" and understanding of science—a position not uncommon, nor unexpressed, in the last half of the twentieth century. If the surveys pinpointed schooling, so did common sense. In 1954, for example, a public relations educator predicted that as the level of education increased, so would the demand for popular science. Thirty years later, in the midst of another science "crisis," a leading intellectual similarly concluded that only schools, not the media, could increase Americans' scientific competence and appreciation of the scientific enterprise—what physicist Cecily Cannan Selby called "turning people on to science."[23] In contrast to other campaigns to blame the schools for social ills, this attribution of responsibility had substantial merit.

During the twentieth century, circumstances and institutional changes had transformed parts of the popularization of science in the schools. The major new external constraint was simply that more young Americans attended school and stayed in school longer. In 1900, about six percent of the youngsters of appropriate age graduated from high school; half a century later, the figure was about 60 percent. The change was so massive that at one point early in the century, an average of one thousand new high schools opened each year. Simultaneously, elementary school and college attendance also went up. This increased aggregate amount of school experience eventually recast what many popularizers were attempting to do; they had to adapt to changes in the educational background of both school and nonschool audiences.

Those who worked with school children had therefore to cope with large numbers of students as well as to develop curriculums and teaching materials. Meantime, the growing numbers of educators were themselves professionalizing and specializing and asserting their competence and independence. By 1901, a special-interest journal, *School Science and Mathematics*, was in existence, and when an umbrella national organization of science educators finally came together in 1944, the constituent societies, some of which dated back to the nineteenth century, were numerous indeed.[24]

Despite institutional and other changes, however, long-lived observers in the field of science education often had a sense of déjà vu. Generation after generation, the same problems and solutions seemed to recur in science education. One educator in 1964, for example, did not know whether he was seeing cycles or pendulums, but he was certain that linear progress was elusive. Another midcentury writer contended that after 75 years of the same questions, no answers were forthcoming for secondary-level educators: "What knowledge at the high-school level is best for college preparation? Should this knowledge differ for the vocational or business student? Is the laboratory method of teaching really fruitful for the high-school student? Are any useful techniques transferred? . . . How can high-school students be motivated to elect physics and chemistry courses?"[25]

One conclusion that seemed clear throughout the twentieth century was that students had to be compelled to study science in order to diffuse it effectively. As I pointed out in chapter 1, science content in the area of pedagogy that was aimed at adults (who had a choice) did not flourish, from "university extension" of the 1890s to "adult education" decades later. In contrast to nineteenth-century self-improvement efforts, the place of scientific subjects in adult education diminished remarkably in the twentieth century, to perhaps the five percent level noted earlier. In substantial part, of course, regular schools by then had already met some of the demand for learning that earlier brought adults into classes.[26] Even Sputnik caused only a slight break in the adult educators' pattern of avoiding the natural sciences in voluntary programs, and then the few new courses dealt with understanding the place of science in society, not scientific knowledge for the older learner.[27]

Educational Restructuring during the Early Twentieth Century

For teachers at the elementary and secondary levels, whose students had but few choices, the problems were very different. The new century opened not only with extraordinary growth but with the curriculum in turmoil. Elementary school students in the lower grades had little instruction other than an occasional object lesson or, now, nature study, depending upon the training of the teacher. In the upper elementary grades, physiology, with an emphasis on alcohol education, was still frequently mandated and taught out of a textbook. As more and more teachers received normal-school training, two changes occurred. The first was the continued dramatic growth of the nature study movement that had begun in the 1890s. The second was the increasingly successful attempt to introduce a systematic, cumulating curriculum.[28]

Nature study changed in the twentieth century in that the emphasis shifted from organisms (objects—not unlike the older object lesson) to relationships in nature (what was coming to be called ecology). Nature study in either guise still had the advantage that teachers could stress the more poetic and less rigorous aspects of science. Moreover, nature study embodied the new pedagogic goal of making children, rather than subject matter, the point of departure for study. Science for the elite students had a place, wrote Liberty Hyde Bailey of Cornell in his definitive statement on nature study, but for all children he advocated a nature study in which the child learned to observe closely and to appreciate natural phenomena of all kinds. "Nature-study is not science," Bailey wrote. "It is not knowledge. It is not facts," he continued, still alluding to the rote learning of texts against which many educators (not to mention students) were rebelling then. "It is spirit. It is concerned with the child's outlook on the world." Many science proponents of the early twentieth century also praised nature study because in it children dealt with the tangible, practical environment, and nature study had the additional value of helping children appreciate the rural way of life, which was vanishing rapidly. Altogether the subject had great advantages in the elementary school.[29]

But nature study was frequently still unsystematic. In the new professionalism of education, some leaders were working hard to get a compulsory set of graded science subjects, beyond physiology, into all of education, including the lower grades. Nature study of course at first continued to offer the best opportunities. Edward Gardinier Howe, for example, in his *Systematic Science Teaching* of 1894 utilized the natural framework of "the stars and earth," "minerals and rocks," "plants," and "animals," the latter of course including boys and girls (but little material was needed for studying them, he noted, "as live specimens are common!"). The physics and chemistry in Howe's curriculum was minimal, but in the age of nature study, that could wait for high school.[30] Despite such efforts as Howe's, as it turned out, the elementary curriculum could not be settled until that in the high school was.

The influence of nature study in the schools spilled over into other aspects of American life. In extracurricular endeavors similar to those of the Agassiz Association (which continued for a few years after 1900) and especially in the Boy Scouts, Girl Scouts, Campfire Girls, and similar youth organizations that flourished for several decades, the programs and leaders carried the message and the enthusiasm of the nature study movement. They also picked up and furthered the conservation movement, which in turn encouraged appreciation of nature and knowledge about it.

Although nature study in the schools was designed for the elementary students, in fact the movement affected many older youth and even adults.[31]

In contrast to the grade school programs, the American high-school science curriculum underwent a veritable revolution in the first quarter century of rapidly expanding enrollments. As mandated by colleges or state legislatures, in 1900 a surprising number of students were taking physiology and physics, and a very large number continued to take physical geography. At the same time, physics, chemistry, zoology, and botany, not to mention mathematics, were increasingly coming into the domain of the specialist teachers and educators. Each field therefore tended to have a separate history as well as a distinct group of advocates. Chemistry teachers, for example, early in the century revolted against college leadership and modified their courses because students could not master the abstract material that colleges had required. High-school chemistry courses therefore became more elementary and practical. Although the physics teachers did not change their orientation toward college preparation, they did challenge the usefulness of the set laboratory exercises; still, by 1920 laboratories in both physics and chemistry were seemingly immutably in place.[32]

Laboratories were also in place in the biological sciences in high school, but there, within only a few years, zoology and botany disappeared from most school systems, and physiology as well (in 1910–1915 alone, physiology courses lost twenty-five thousand students despite the overall rising school enrollments). Instead, a new course, general biology, came to dominate that area of instruction, and eventually more high-school students elected biology than any science course. This new course fitted in with a shift in college and research biology to focusing on physiological functioning. And general biology also embodied the practical emphasis of the Progressive period. Textbooks appeared with such titles as *Civic Biology*. The New York 1910 syllabus, for example, emphasized that children should know common plants and animals, the common functions of living things, their economic and ecological importance, and individual and public health.[33]

Before general biology was established, however, another course, and this one often required, appeared in the secondary schools. In this case, the educators broke away entirely from the collegiate model, and what they developed was "general science." As the numbers of students in high schools expanded and patronage of traditional science courses dropped, science educators reacted to this really alarming erosion—part of the first low point of popularization in the 1900s—by joining in the movement to have a more general course in science that would be appropriate for students who were not preparing for college. The tendency to abandon preparatory courses and to use the high school as a common school with practical training peaked around 1917, when the federal government began financing vocational schools.[34]

Physics and chemistry courses as well as those in biology therefore also tended to shift to a more practical orientation, but general science courses were extreme in practicality. Such courses helped to suggest to students the tangibility of the benefits of science that so many scientists and other enthusiasts had promised in previous years—and they also reinforced the popular science technology described in the newspapers. Textbooks had titles like *Civic Science in the Home*. Generations of students learned particularly about pumps and sewage and other hygienic and engineering matters as part of general science, in which transportation, health, and conservation were important topics. Educators had as their goal to get the students to learn about and master their immediate environments— "heating, lighting, ventilation . . . sanitation . . . obtaining food and clothing"—but at the same time to learn the process by which people gain scientific knowledge. Altogether the aim, as a Minnesota teacher put it in 1917, was in this latter area to teach "the scientific attitude" rather than "a '*bunch*' of facts."[35] Progressive-era educators thus consciously invoked simultaneously the new research ideal and practicality, thereby reshaping not just general science but the whole curriculum in the light of the "great growth of science in research and in affairs," as one pioneer put it.[36]

By the early 1920s, then, a new pattern of science courses was fixed in American education. At the ninth grade level, students took general science. Moreover, general science tended to reach down into the seventh and eighth grades, leaving nature study for the earlier years. For those who elected more courses, usually for college preparation purposes, biology came in the tenth grade, chemistry in the eleventh, and physics in the twelfth. This pattern lasted for more than half a century. The only major change came in the 1930s, when a truly graded elementary school general science curriculum became available in several series of widely used textbooks, usually displacing nature study.[37]

The Struggle of Content versus Pupil Development

Physical geography therefore virtually disappeared from the curriculum, even more decisively than physiology, which was absorbed into both general science and biology. For generations thereafter, educators had no motive to try to change the new sequence. What they did do was to attempt to improve each of the courses in the sequence and the teaching of science in general, with the usual debate about "laboratory" versus "demonstration." Typically, educators reduced formal and mathematical content to gain more understanding from a definitely nonelite population. The purpose of their book, wrote the authors of an important text, was "to create a preliminary widespread interest in science as a thing of personal importance," and they hoped in this way to break down students' resistance to further study of science. By the 1940s, "double tracking" in mathematics and science was common, with traditional, college-oriented courses for some students—courses invigorated by college entrance examinations—and a more general and practical curriculum for the generality of students.[38]

Finally, the goals of leading science educators changed, and along with them, of course, textbook content. The shift in goals became acute because, beginning in the 1920s, for the first time science and mathematics teachers no longer justified their work in terms of "mental discipline." Research suggested that "transfer of training" really did not work, and so disciplining the mind, the bugaboo of Victorians, gave way to "pupil development" and, especially after the advent of the Great Depression, social usefulness; the new slogan was "life enrichment through participation in a democratic social order." The life enrichment often showed up in attempts to base curriculum content on student interests, as in the best-known textbook series, and the rest of the slogan reflected the social concerns of the 1930s. Focusing on the student led further to an emphasis on thinking and discovering (as opposed to formal discipline) and on the scientific method and the scientific attitude—the opposite, of course, of superstition. This scientific attitude was an important positive goal as information, observation, and morals diminished as educational objectives. Although in fact knowledge continued to dominate in the classrooms, educators were talking, as earlier in the century, about adaptation to the environment, adaptation that they interpreted as applying to everyday life. "The science of the high school," wrote an educator in 1933, "needs to be taught as preparation for life, as a consumer science rather than a producer science."[39]

Following the soul searching that the atomic bomb induced, rather suddenly, beginning in the 1950s, important figures in American science, almost all of them college and especially graduate school teachers, introduced major changes into American science teaching on the elementary and secondary level. "For the first time in over a generation," remarked one educator, "a number of research scientists have assumed a major share of the work."[40] Several factors came together to facilitate changes that were the more impressive because American educational institutions were so decentralized. To begin with, the prestige of the scientists after 1945 was very great.[41] They were, moreover, by the 1950s able to mobilize first foundation and then federal funding on a massive scale ($117 million was spent by the National Science Foundation alone). Finally, the educators themselves had long talked about the importance of teaching the scientific method, and one survey, for example, showed that this concern was showing up in chemistry and biology curricular discussions with greater frequency after 1945.[42]

The university-based scientists had long been dissatisfied with their students' precollege preparation, and they had already developed momentum in attempting to effect changes in the schools when the orbiting of Sputnik provided an opportunity to push massive curricular changes and introduce new ways of thinking that they believed were appropriate for students in the atomic age. The new curriculums emphasized basic patterns in various sciences—what later educators, following psychologist Jerome Bruner, called the "structure" of scientific disciplines. These basic patterns could be taught to all students, but they would enable those destined for science to go on and enter modern conceptual courses with much better preparation. The research scientists believed that they could develop instead a universal cognitive progression for each science, and it soon became clear that scientists and educators alike believed that they were working with the essence of scientific thinking.[43]

Mathematics provided an excellent example of what happened. Throughout the twentieth century, mathematics teachers had been teaching traditional arithmetic and the higher branches. The great transformation of mathematics in the nineteenth century—to say nothing of further developments in the twentieth—simply did not affect the school curriculum, and math teachers tended to group with specialists in teaching, not with research workers or even college teachers. The mathematical logic, statistics, and other material that was exciting leading American mathematicians was therefore truly alien and unknown to a freshman entering college who, because of constantly improving traditional teaching, had been good at arithmetic and algebra. With vigorous promotion in the media and National Science Foundation funding, however, in the late 1950s and early 1960s, following the lead of a new physics curriculum, the "new math" came in, drawing additionally on momentum generated by "operations research" of World War II and then the computerization of the postwar period.[44]

The first scientists to attempt curricular reform, the physicists, had argued as early as the 1940s that the consequences of their research were so momentous that popular understanding of the new ideas in physics was a necessity in a democracy. And, as has been noted, most observers agreed that the school system was the place to start. So was born that first curriculum, but very shortly afterward the other scientists, like the mathematicians, had analogous programs, with comparable funding. The proponents had real talent and a strong sense of urgency. "For the first time in human history," wrote the biology curriculum project director, "we must fashion public policies for which a fundamental knowledge of science is central and imperative."[45]

But once they had developed curricular and course materials, the university scientists withdrew. The new materials affected instruction into the 1980s, especially the continuing emphasis on concepts and inquiry. But before the 1960s were over, the new movement was beginning to wither away. The professors' efforts were, in the end, aimed at future scientists, or at least science majors, and both teachers and more general observers (including many parents) believed that the materials were too difficult.[46] Therefore educators began again to emphasize pupil development, as opposed to knowledge—an emphasis that was soon reinforced by new studies in the psychology of cognition. "The question in the . . . curriculum can never be what is 'best' for science," wrote Gerald S. Craig of Teachers College, responding to the first of the new curriculums; "rather the question must be what is 'best' for children. The teacher must recognize always that children are greater than science." Moreover, it was just as doubts about the curriculums matured that environmental concerns gave science negative connotations. Between the difficulty of science courses and questions about the consequences of science that students learned from the media as well as the classroom, young people did not respond well to science instruction. By the 1980s, scientists and science teachers had good reason to lament their unpopularity and to try once again to tie funding for science education into Cold War fears.[47]

The basic problem in science education therefore remained the same throughout the century and over the years underlay the shifts in content and rationale. The problem was that grounding in science required tedious memorizing and thinking that no pedagogical innovation, from the laboratory exercise to the discovery method of the Deweyites and the inquiry method of a later day, ever succeeded in easing. As late as 1983 an educator was lamenting, "High-school science texts average between seven and ten new concepts, terms, or symbols per page. Typically, the 300 to 350 pages assigned during a school year means that students are expected to learn between 2,400 and 3,000 terms and symbols per science course . . . in class periods of approximately fifty-five minutes each, twenty concepts would have to be covered per period, an average of one every two minutes."[48] As the century wore on, this type of educational experience was more and more what controlled the kind of popularization of science a high-school graduate might choose and enjoy.

The Media Hierarchy

In an increasingly urban, specialized, bureaucratic society, people specialized. So, at least on the secondary level, science teachers specialized in their concerns and their roles. For popularization of science for the general public, the science writers materialized. But their functioning as translators of science occurred within the context of the mass media institutions, and those institutions influenced profoundly the ways in which the writers popularized science and unwittingly opened the door to superstition.

The mass media, starting with yellow journalism and some books and magazines, came in with the twentieth century and have already been alluded to above in other connections. In the 1930s and after, radio became very important. By the 1950s, comic books were a sufficiently important medium for some population elements that popularizers had put science educational material in some of them. Soon even the comic books were overshadowed by television, as has been noted in discussions of health and psychology.[49]

These media were not insulated, but affected one another. To begin with, people who wrote for one medium often also appeared in another. Or, beyond cultural lag on the part of media consumers, for example, midcentury studies showed that what science writers wrote was filtered through various editors, a group of people who in turn were often not well informed or even cultured. One key group of these so-called gate-keepers—people who decided what stories a newspaper did and did not print, for instance—had for their main source of perspective on the world such mass media publications as the *Reader's Digest.* Therefore what the *Reader's Digest* and similar mass media magazines carried in the way of popular science was important in shaping what went into the news-papers. Moreover, contrary to many expectations, what appeared in newspapers continued to set the agenda for all public affairs, even long after television became dominant.[50] Such interrelations as these of course help explain why science popularization appeared with similar intensity in various parts of the culture at about the same time and why the media are lumped together as a social unit.

Traditionally, the highest element in the hierarchy of media was the book, even though in fact the quality of books varied as much as presentations in most of the other media. As in the nineteenth century, so in the twentieth: the appearance of a book often led to magazine or even news-paper (and, later, television) notices. And, as has been suggested, the rate of publication and circulation of comparable books paralleled magazine articles throughout the twentieth century, except that markedly important volumes still continued to appear, however infrequently, in periods of quantitative decline such as the 1930s and the 1970s. Even before the 1920s, for example, plenty of popular science books were available. All science books, popular and technical, together constituted less than ten percent of library circulation—and popular science therefore held a quantitative place in libraries comparable to its place in newspapers.[51]

Books were particularly important because they underlined two fundamentals of science popularization. First, consumers of popular science books tended to consist of a special-interest group, made up largely of people in or about the scientific-technical community, a number of whom had in fact been recruited into science by means of popular science books. The Scientific Book Club, for example, originated when a group of scientists "found that they were besought persistently by associates, students, and friends for information about the newest scientific books." In the 1960s and 1970s, the combination of affluence and numbers of such Americans begat similar book clubs, for popular science was an important publishing area, even if the audience was limited in numbers. The second fundamental that showed up in the books was that Americans well into the 1930s continued to depend upon English popularizers to a substantial extent. At one point, for example, perhaps half of the most strongly recommended selections of the Scientific Book Club were written by British authors such as Sir James Jeans and J. G. Crowther. Only in the post–World War II period did American authors tend to predominate in book publication. Regardless of origin or time period, however, content did not differ substantially from that of other types of publications except for the incidence of lowbrow science—and pseudoscience—books: the number of such books decreased early in the century but thrived in the 1970s, when, as I have suggested, science was in retreat. Even in the best years, different authors of popular science books aimed at various audiences and translated at various levels.[52]

Science in the Magazines

Typically the next medium below books in the hierarchy was the magazine. In terms of the grand quarterlies and monthlies, the *North American Review*, *Harper's*, the *Atlantic*, *Century*, and so on, the magazines did operate on a very high level, with long essays and thoughtful reviews. But by the turn of the century, the rise of inexpensive magazines brought a number of them into direct competition with the new yellow press, and editors responded with newsy and sensationalistic approaches. The change was particularly noticeable in the area of science. Moreover, the newspapers in turn competed with magazines by developing the notorious Sunday supplements, notable not only because of sensationalism but because writers in this part of the newspaper followed a magazine and not a news format. It was these magazine supplements, as I have already suggested, that were the source of the most anguished complaints about "newspaper science."[53]

By the turn of the century, the issue for editors and publishers was whether or not the magazines would all succumb to the news format in which writers treated science as just another event. As early as 1901, the editor of the *Popular Science Monthly* noted that "the daily press now publishes articles everywhere of a readable and light character on scientific topics, and no monthly magazine is complete without one or two such articles. What the country needs is a journal that will set a standard of accuracy and weight, and will separate the real advances of science from the vagaries of the charlatan." Naturally the *Popular Science Monthly* was that journal. "Such a journal," the editor continued, "obviously does not appeal to children or to superficial readers."[54] And, in fact, the editor was carrying some stories with complex steps or diagrams and mathematics that would have appealed only to people who were used to that kind of thinking already. When the *Scientific Monthly* succeeded the *Popular Science Monthly*, the *Scientific Monthly* carried essays and in each issue only a few brief items of recent developments of science such as were symptomatic of the redefinition of science by the purists. Short reports of new inventions were left to the new *Popular Science Monthly* (formerly *World's Advance*) and its competitors in the applied science and invention field like *Popular Mechanics* (founded 1902). Many of the more general magazines, like the high-circulation *Saturday Evening Post*, followed the *Scientific Monthly* format for science stories.

By the 1920s, the market had established a stratified pattern of magazine publishing that included general journals, digests like the newly founded *Reader's Digest*, news magazines like *Time*, and pulps, as well as, for special-interest constituencies, the tinkerers' magazines. In each kind of magazine, science played a particular part. Meanwhile the founding of Science Service had not only led to *Science News-Letter* but affected even the *Scientific Monthly*, in which Science Service material now filled the news segment, "The Progress of Science." At that point, the magazine format was distinguished primarily by length and by the amount of "untimely" (as opposed to "timely") background included, as well as the author's effort to contrive reader interest. Unlike the newspaper feature article, in which the journalist often carried his reader away from the subject, magazine articles tended to maintain an essay on just one subject.[55]

By the time of World War II, general magazines were increasingly carrying nonfiction material, including science, which of course demanded even more attention from the editors in the 1940s and 1950s. The most influential magazine—after the *Reader's Digest*—was now *Life*, which featured photojournalism, including many outstanding illustrated popular science expositions, some of which were noted in chapters 2 and 3. At the same time, articles in general magazines were running longer. Science popularization, as La Follette notes, flourished in both the longer format and the persistent newsmagazines, the editors of which from time to time added science sections of one kind or another, sometimes particularized, like the psychology headings, or more general, like "Space and the Atom" (*Newsweek*, 1958). The specialized science newsmagazine, *Science Digest*, had begun publishing as early as 1937 and had 85,000 readers by 1945.[56]

Then as television rose, the general magazines—even *Life* and the *Saturday Evening Post*, and, not least, the *Scientific Monthly*—tended to die out (the *Scientific Monthly* had a circulation of 15,000 in 1947), while specialized magazines thrived. As recounted in chapter 4, there had been specialized magazines in the popular science field from early in the nineteenth century, conspicuously at first in mathematics and then particularly in natural history. The area of astronomy was the most promising during the early twentieth century (with, for example, *Sky and Telescope*), supplemented by magazines aimed especially at teachers, such as *Chemistry* and its predecessors. These journals persisted because they could draw on amateur and student audiences that the *Scientific Monthly* also drew on until it faded away with other general magazines.[57]

The refounding of the *Scientific American* as a "popular" science journal in the late 1940s set the stage for the next period of popularizing in magazines. Once again, as would be expected in a highly organized society, specialization explains in large part what happened, and magazines provided an index to general trends. As early as 1898, the editor of the *American Naturalist* was attempting to find a new mission for his journal now that natural history was giving way to biological specialists: "Instead of the general scientific journals and societies of natural history of former times," he wrote, "these conditions have called into life and elevated to the highest prominence societies and journals dealing with the special problems of restricted lines of research." The solution for the editors of the *American Naturalist* was to try to inform the specialist about developments in neighboring fields, a function ever more important as ecological and biochemical questions became increasingly urgent. "Physiologists," continued the editor in 1898, "in studying the functions of the nervous system, for example, have found it possible to draw important conclusions from data furnished by morphology. The geologist supplies the biologist with information concerning the conditions that have influenced the geographical distribution of organisms, and learns from him in turn."[58] With this insight, the *American Naturalist* evolved into a professional biologists' journal, parallel to but even more technical than *Science*, which served all of the sciences. At about the same time, *Popular Astronomy* developed a parallel function for both amateur and professional astronomers. For more general audiences, by contrast, there was, beyond the higher class of journals, little except the *Scientific Monthly* to try to meet the demand for the science knowledge that any cultured person ought to possess. These general journals were the ones that faded out in the mid-twentieth century, and along with them, to a substantial extent, the cultural ideal that in the nineteenth century had shaped the *Popular Science Monthly*.

The *Scientific American* of 1948 and after was indeed also aimed at popularizing in a more general way, but, as it turned out, not for the public or even for the well-educated person; rather the target audience was the growing community of specialists in science and engineering. The shock to some technical readers was immediate and unmistakable. One unhappy subscriber wrote, "You have ruined the finest shop and hobby magazine in the world. Gone high-brow."[59] And, in fact, readers of the magazine included dramatically higher percentages of college graduates than even the better general journals. The *Scientific American* approach was basically intellectual, and authors did not have to lure readers with human interest and the like, although stories of discovery appeared often as lead-ins.

Yet the *Scientific American* did not meet the needs of all of the growing midcentury sci-tech population. Even though the editors eschewed mathematical formulas, for a number of years a market was developing for a far more vulgarized account of science. There were many signs besides the success of *Psychology Today*. General newspaper readers, as we shall note, claimed that they wanted more science news. In the specialized magazines market, applied science and mechanics magazines did very well (although they did not quite keep up with the outdoors and leisure group). The *Smithsonian* and other magazines were immensely successful with affluent, upwardly mobile people who frequently worked in technical industries. Even the publishers of *Time* found that issues with science on the cover sold better than any others except those featuring drugs, sex, and rock music celebrities. It was against this background, then, that spontaneously several publishers in the late 1970s tried to tap a new market for popularized science. But they all strongly emphasized making that science palatable. When the American Chemical Society converted *Chemistry* to *SciQuest*, the publisher admitted that one reason was that "the word 'chemistry' is identified in the minds of many students and lay people alike with a subject that has no excitement and little relevance to their lives." Jean Pradal, in one of the few modern works on popularization, had already concluded that translating the work of specialists for the truly non-scientific public involved distortion: "This is why it is virtually impossible to envisage a scientific periodical for the general public. Most readers of popular science periodicals are people who already have some connection, even if only indirectly, with science in their own occupation. Whenever a periodical tries to lower its level to reach a wider public, it is likely to lose more readers in the upper categories than it gains in the lower." He was in part mistaken. The late 1970s market appeared to include sufficient readers of both kinds, but publishers of the new magazines either addressed people within the sci-tech community or else, like the *National Enquirer*, they engaged in marketing what might not be fully recognizable as science.[60]

The magazines therefore showed that by midcentury a number of audiences for science existed, most of them still apparently in the upper tier of the public. The most conspicuous audience, the sci-tech community, was very large and in turn contained several overlapping elements. One group of readers wanted popular science with substantial scientific content. Another wanted more general material about the technical results of science. And there were various types of science buffs, some organized by subject matter and amateur interests, others by interest in the drama of scientific discovery or scientists' lives, and still others by a persistent interest in tinkering. Above all, the magazines, regardless of audiences, underlined the difference between popularization of science and science news. It is this distinction that became so important in the twentieth century as science news tended to function as traditional obscurantism.

Science Journalism

The chief institutions involved in science news were the newspaper and the science writer. Science writers were primarily reporters but often also wrote magazine articles and books. The astonishingly large amount of study devoted to science journalism, science in the newspapers, and particularly the science writers caused many people to identify popularization of science with the writers and newspapers and, furthermore, to confuse the development of institutions with substantive popularization. In fact, of course, regular, unspecialized journalists also continued to report about scientific matters, without regard for institutional constraints.[61]

The founding of Science Service was the overwhelming event in institutionalizing. Science Service was an agency so successful that competitors soon appeared syndicating science stories. By 1937, Watson Davis, then director of Science Service, could conclude, "In a sense the essential effort to put science into the American press has been successful." Nor did succeeding years diminish this achievement. In 1950, leading American daily papers carried an average of two columns of science each day, and virtually none of it was sensational in the old sense.[62]

But the truth was, that institutional or "bureaucratic" achievement did not represent accurately the effective popularization that occurred. As early as 1931, for example, an anonymous writer in the *Nation* made fun of the new cult of science news. "It is a very poor meeting of any scientific body," he or she wrote, "which cannot produce at least one new dimension and a couple of original theories concerning either the origin or the end of the cosmos." The writer went on to suggest that science news was often reported solemnly but as an empty exercise without real communication. Among other quoted examples of incomprehensibility (from the *New York Times*) was this summary of some of the implications of Einstein's new ideas: "By applying relativity to thermodynamics, we can no longer speak of energy in terms of up or down or of intensities." "While we are not sure just what this means," commented the *Nation* writer, "we see no reason why a universe which Einstein has deprived of a past and a present should not get along very well without an up and a down also." There was much similar evidence over the years that science news was often ceremonial rather than substantive. When events called for really serious science reporting, for example in the case particularly of the post–World War II atomic bomb and atomic energy discussions, the urgent and important messages and news from scientists got lost in the usual political-romantic-ideological journalism that dominated the American press.[63]

Not even in the age of Science Service was the old problem of the accuracy of reporting solved. Perhaps the most hilarious example of chronic journalistic confusion was George Gaylord Simpson's account of a news story about his research into the paleontology of Montana. He saw stories that had been printed in almost one hundred newspapers, out of which only "about one tenth had reports that were neither seriously wrong scientifically nor obnoxious to me personally." Writers took the press release and both garbled and sensationalized it, making Simpson say that man was descended from mice and not primates, that Kodiak bear-sized dogs used to live in North America, and many other amusing inaccuracies.[64]

But until the 1970s, few skeptics complained about the science writers, for the two relevant specialized groups in American society had co-opted each other: the scientists and the journalists. For years, the two took turns singing each other's praises. Before, newspaper reporters wrote ignorant and sensational copy; now, as the younger of the Drs. Mayo put it in 1931, "The medical meetings . . . last week were covered by the best men on the staffs of metropolitan newspaper and press services, and while their reports had to carry headlines, there was in the headlines none of the false rainbows that used to make conservative doctors grind their teeth." On the other side, the eminent scientists who used to be so difficult be-cause of almost universally bad experiences with the press drew praise when they worked with the journalists, first notably in the American Chemical Society publicity program and then Science Service. The praise of course included, incidentally, favorable newspaper attention. The mu-tual admiration grew saccharine; yet it did serve to draw together scien-tists who were conscious of the requirements of public relations and newswriters who served them, altogether a tour de force. As a later middleman of science news commented, "Few newspapermen are inter-ested in a scientific finding unless it can cure cancer while in orbit. This could be called the 'rocket-scalpel complex.'" Likewise, he noted, "few academicians are interested in press coverage unless the facts are expressed in mathematical Latin and are heavily qualified to prove that nothing really important happened. This is, of course, the 'scientific dignity-protective obscurity syndrome.'" But for decades the two in fact often worked to-gether. Together they communed cosily, bemoaning to each other the antijournalistic holdouts in science and the editors who still did not understand that science was important and interesting. Both sides agreed with Dr. Mayo: a lively headline need not be inaccurate.[65]

The actual process by which the scientists consciously obtained the co-operation of the newspapers through Science Service has been told often in positive terms, as if the relatively sudden enlightenment of both parties were a natural development. The fact was that leading American scientists, as has been suggested, repeatedly pressured the writers and editors to upgrade their treatment of science. As the public relations of science became remarkably deeply enmeshed in research-funding efforts, a special urgency crept into the scientists' hectoring of journalists to give science a good press. The campaign utilized particularly the professional pride of journalists in motivating them to improve their performance. Thus one critic in 1901 noted that "a few, a very few, newspapers—exceptions but prove the rule—reflect expertness and evince common-sense accuracy, still at the same time losing nothing in the way of presenting the subject in an interesting and attractive manner." Another—in 1908—needled those responsible for ignoring an important zoological congress by observing that it did not "make an impression on the public mind at all comparable to that ordinarily produced by any serious crime." The campaign further involved arguments that scientists indeed deserved a place in the media. Even before the atomic bomb, for example, G. Edward Pendray of Westinghouse made the interest group argument, pointing out to a meeting of important journalists that the number of people employed in industrial laboratories had doubled since 1931 and constituted with other scientists an important segment of the public. Finally, as has been suggested, there was just plain flattery. An officer of the AAAS remarked in 1935 that inexperienced reporters did badly at scientific meetings because they did not understand what was going on. "So they take refuge in ridiculing or distorting the proceedings. Aggravating as this is to the victims, any attempts to exclude such reporters, or to have them reprimanded, would only make matters worse. The only way to achieve results in press relations work is to show appreciation of the good work done, and ignore the bad." [66]

But it would be unrealistic to ignore the effects of the relentless negative campaign of the scientists who over the years ridiculed "newspaper science" and, at least for some decades, held the feet of the writers and editors to the fire when a popularizer or reporter deviated from the scientists' standards. In 1903, for example, the editor of the *Popular Science Monthly* in a single page destroyed the credibility of Carl Snyder, a science popularizer, with examples of his ignorance and errors from articles in leading magazines such as *McClure's*, *Scribner's*, and *Harper's*, the latter of which had just carried "a potpourri of truth, half-truth and falsehood concerning chemistry, physics, anatomy, physiology and psychology," including the suggestion that members of the public could get their brains measured, which as the *Popular Science Monthly* editor pointed out laughingly, could be done in fact only post mortem. Even Science Service included among its agency functions that of helping editors check stories, and in 1929, Davis, the director, began sending editors each year a list of "Stories to Be Careful of," such as cancer cures and man-eating trees. For many years, then, spokespersons for science did not let up. As late as 1954 a leading journalism educator was reminding writers and editors that scientists would be offended by sensational and inaccurate writing.[67] (Of course in thus continuing to pursue the traditional campaign against superstition and error, scientists were working unwittingly to increase the credibility of the media, in which, however excellent the content, the form was subversive of the many traditional goals of popularizing, as will be described further in chapter 6.)

What the scientists came to want, and frequently got from the editors, was not just proper coverage but coverage by the sympathetic special science writers—typically reporters who received a special assignment. As these writers developed their symbiotic relationship with scientists, the journalists on their parts gloried in sharing the high prestige of science and in advancing the cause of science. "A few science writers," complained the president of the National Association of Science Writers in 1949, "have acquired so much knowledge of science that they seem to have lost the layman's approach. They get too technical. I read one article by such a science writer that was so obscure in its meaning that I had to get a physicist to explain it to me."[68] The science writers not only praised and imitated scientists but took on certain of their values, to an extent that became obvious in the 1970s when a number of journalists broke ranks and were among the leaders who raised questions about the benefits of scientific activity; it was only then that some reporters explicitly expressed doubt that a science writer necessarily had to be the scientists' advocate.[69]

The fact was that science writers enjoyed a special status, not only before the public but in the newspaper offices where they worked. Other staff members deferred to them and, because they had access to the latest medical findings, called on the science writers for advice on all personal medical matters, so that typically these writers came to be known in the office as "Doc." Editors, too, deferred, giving science writers far more latitude with regard to length and deadlines than other reporters enjoyed. "Are we getting some reputation as snobs?" asked the president of the science writers' organization in 1955, urging his colleagues not to treat their colleagues so patronizingly. By organizing in 1934, the science writers confirmed their move toward professionalization as such. Moreover, unlike other reporters, they cooperated with each other, some of them eventually forming what Sharon Dunwoody has called the "inner club" of science writers. And by cooperating with each other, members of the club set their own standards for science writing, standards by which even their editors judged them, standards that were found only in the work of the other members of the club. The scientists helped confirm the writers' special status, for the scientists had every reason to give friendly aid and support to writers who of course tended to report favorably as well as relatively reliably about science.[70]

Without really intending to, then, leading American natural scientists, like those in psychology and the health fields, increasingly left popularizing to nonscientist specialists, the science writers. One survey showed that the science writers were indeed nonscientists; only about nine percent of them had science training even at the B.A. level or had come into the field from science.[71] From the point of view of the public relations of science, the journalists served well. Nevertheless, the journalistic dominance had shortcomings. First was a tendency, already noted, for both scientists and writers to assume that ceremonial reporting of science news constituted or substituted for popularization. Second was the fact that the science writers were not themselves able to control what the editors—gatekeepers—printed, the most notorious instance coming in 1940, when the editor of the New York *Herald-Tribune* killed a story on nuclear fission that the rival *New York Times* ran. The author of the *Times* story, William L. Laurence, told of another pre-atomic bomb event, when an important editor explained to his reporter why he turned down a story on cosmic rays: "The publisher doesn't like cosmic rays, and neither do I. Furthermore, let me tell you, I don't believe in atoms and have but slight faith in molecules."[72] Beyond the fallibility of gatekeepers, a third shortcoming was the continuing tendency I have already stressed for journalists' "science" to consist of medicine, psychology, and sex to the exclusion of the natural sciences per se—the skewing that all professionals recognized and regretted.

The fact was that the newspapers set the agendas for popularization on the basis of what was news; that is, the story had to be timely in some sense to get by an editor. When atomic energy was first science news, for example, editors and writers emphasized its political and applied aspects overwhelmingly. As with the later space race, any really scientific material was a fortuitous by-product.[73] Moreover, by abandoning the field to journalists, scientists again opened the door to sensationalism. The small world of the scientists and science writers did not encompass all of science journalism. Everyone in that world tried to ignore the unspecialized and often undocile reporters who occasionally got into the field (especially noticeably in the 1970s) and also the disreputable pulps such as the *National Enquirer* that, as has been noted, carried a substantial amount of science misinformation. By the 1970s, in any event, political and social developments forced journalists of many kinds to deal with science, and the science writers' monopoly was partially broken. Moreover, the development of citizens' groups set up alternative sources of science news. Altogether the coalition between the science writers and science establishment was not as effective in American society as it had been earlier.[74]

One instructive way to view what happened is to see that the gatekeepers and journalists throughout the twentieth century published science news beyond the sensational and political only when they answered pressure from various media constituencies, just as newspaper editors in the nineteenth century had responded to groups of science amateurs. The midcentury research on science journalism symbolizes the concern: the research was almost always on the question of quantity—what percentage of space was devoted to science subjects—rather than content or quality. As early as 1914, for example, J. A. Udden of the University of Texas identified this confusion of quantity with content. He found that extensive local press coverage of a geological congress, coverage that passed for science news, consisted almost entirely of descriptions of formalities, including personalities and social events, rather than knowledge or even discovery, much less intellectual excitement.[75]

The Other Popularizing Media

The pressures on the nonprint media mirrored those on the newspapers and magazines, and sometimes the science proponents were very effective in obtaining the substantial popularization that they wanted. Lectures continued for cultured people, and both popularizer and content often were the best that science had to offer. For the perhaps slightly less dedicated, the Chautauqua lectures reached a high point in the 1920s, after which radio put them out of business.[76] Museums and fairs and expositions continued, including science fairs for children. In general, the displays were graphic, and, as in the science fairs and some museum programs, having visitors participate in doing science in one way or another, if only by pushing a button, was responsible for many successful programs. Not only was museum attendance constant, but science museums at one point after midcentury accounted for 40 percent of all museum attendance.[77] Altogether, the pressures on all of these traditional means of popularization kept the level up to at least that of contemporary educators, and sometimes well above that.

Quite different were radio and television, in which the gatekeepers at first resembled those of the newspapers. The radio science talks of the 1920s to 1940s, usually in a lecture format, have already been noted. They, and in fact all cultural content of radio, peaked in the mid-1930s, and science, along with the rest of culture, was never again a substantial element in radio programming, despite many efforts to preserve its educational content. Radio dramas did, of course, convey a great deal of pseudoscience.[78] Like the moguls of the radio industry, the motion picture executives, who were always in the business of entertainment, had no motivation to attempt to carry any science content even in their pretelevision newsreel programs, unless of course the science was novel or amusing; in actuality, science content in newsreels was less than one percent and at some points far less than that.[79] Altogether, the promise of the pioneer health movies was never fulfilled.

The fate of science on the radio and in motion picture newsreels foretold what happened later on television: like the most superficial newspaper reporting, science was reduced to a short presentation involving little or no explanation. At first there were some attempts in the lecture format, as in the radio science talks, but, in general, science programs where they existed could not draw any audience but one already committed to science or culture in the nineteenth-century sense. Science news did not do better on television than in the newsreels; all of the problems of the newspaper were greatly increased, almost to the point of parody, so as to diminish both quantity and quality. "Science," as La Follette summarized it in 1982, "when it appeared on television at all, was most likely becalmed within a Sunday afternoon segment of 'Omnibus,' ridiculed in science fiction comedy, confined to a lecture, or hidden in a 'nature' program."[80]

Television had great potential for popularizing some types of science, as long as the material did not include sustained hypothesis or analysis. Yet the mass audience that might have patronized science, and even still yearned a little for self-improvement, in actuality devoted itself instead to "pure" entertainment. Through advertising and drama, the television gatekeepers not only did not popularize science but pushed pseudoscience and often portrayed science unfavorably. Even when a few "good" science series, especially in the 1970s, caught public attention, they tended to focus on personalities of scientists or great scientists rather than science content. And critics continued to comment that such programs very seldom reached beyond the already dedicated science audience.[81]

Workers in any pictorial medium found the temptation to trivialize science overwhelming. The fragmenting effect of the picture magazine of the early century and midcentury prepared the way for the loss of science content and sequence in motion pictures and television. Shortly after World War II, for example, a movie maker was touring an applied science laboratory at MIT, where investigators told him they were attempting to develop a new product. "Hit by an inspiration," according to a report of the event, the producer wanted to mount "a motion picture camera in the corner all set up and ready to roll so that when the New Product was discovered, the moment could be recorded for posterity."[82]

Amateur Science

The patterns in all of these institutions, from the schools to the media, show that in the years around the turn of the century the audience for popularized science as well as the type of person who was popularizing changed. The first step came when the amateur scientists tended to drop out of the audience for popular science. As Charles W. Heywood has pointed out, the young people of the late nineteenth century, perhaps after an apprenticeship in the Agassiz Association, often continued to study nature in the field or with microscopes or telescopes, constituting a major popular science constituency. They hoped perhaps to discover a new fossil or to amaze their friends with apparatus. Then relatively suddenly, around 1900, young Americans turned in a different direction, to mechanics. Again, the record of the magazines shows the trends. It was no coincidence that the *Popular Science News* disappeared by merging into the *American Inventor*, that the title of the *Popular Science Monthly* was transferred to a tinkerer's and handyman's journal. The new publisher of the latter commented in 1916: "There are now a thousand laboratories where there was one in the days when Youmans was a student. Instead of propaganda for laboratories, The Popular Science Monthly now gives the news that comes from these laboratories it helped to establish." The editor went on to note that the journal was not ashamed to feature interesting material and would not hesitate to publish "mechanical vaudville." Obviously entertainment, news, and products were a far cry from Youmans' work, as will be remarked below. But the emphasis on mechanics was the fundamental sign of audience shift. In a sense, the bicycle and the Model T—along with specialization within science—killed off the most important amateur constituency. It is true that many Americans continued to take an interest in nature, and nature study persisted for a time in the lower grades in school. Science, however, no longer engendered participation as it once had, although gadgets and consumption did; and, as has been remarked, the change was reflected in an institutional way in the rise of mechanics and vocational education in the high-school curriculum.[83]

To some extent this shift at the turn of the century was not entirely anti-scientific, especially insofar as applied science had scientific content. Photography, with chemistry and physics content, engaged people's attention along with auto mechanics. But before many years had passed, the movies and radio had devastating effects upon patterns of leisure pursuits. Whereas electronics and other technology spawned sizable amateur movements after World War II, not until the computer craze took hold in the late 1970s did an amateur movement crystallize that was at all comparable to those of the nineteenth century, and then the emphasis was still upon technology and science products (if not consumption) rather than scientific method, thinking, or understanding.[84]

Throughout the century, a number of science enthusiasts regretted that amateur science was on the wane, and they tried to revive at least young Americans' independent and group science activities. The enthusiasts particularly encouraged science clubs in secondary schools, tying their work into curriculum makers' emphases on the child's interests. Many evangels also tried to revive the natural history tradition through Boy Scouts and Girl Scouts and kindred youth movements—with some success before World War II. Museums and other institutions continued to serve as centers for amateur science activities for both youth and adults, and as late as the 1930s amateur scientists persisted as an important element in popularizing science. In the Philadelphia area, for example, a survey found 287 clubs and societies, with 32,000 members. As earlier, amateurs did frequently group into clubs, but now they had newsletters instead of formal publications, a change that tended to reinforce and symbolize their shift to marginality.[85]

The other element that all but eliminated the amateur, the growing dominance of specialized professionals in all fields, as noted in the case of the *American Naturalist*, was a circumstance about which many observers commented.[86] In the 1890s, it was not yet obvious that widespread popular participation in science was doomed. At the 1890 meetings of the American Society of Microscopists, for example, a witness reported, "On the one hand it is held that the society is only for amateurs, and that nothing is likely to be brought forward worthy of the attention of a professional worker; on the other, that among an assembly of professional workers the amateur and the beginner would be out of place. For either of these prejudices the best cure is attendance at one of the annual meetings." Despite these cheerful words, the society members held their last microscopical soiree in 1895. Amateurs did linger on in some fields, as the astronomy magazines' example showed, but sometimes almost as an underground. When in 1939 the American Philosophical Society appointed a group to study amateur scientists, it was as if they were an endangered species. The committee found both "a large general public with some interest in the sciences" and "a smaller and more select group of laymen who actively pursue scientific interests as hobbies." But this finding had no national impact. Popularization of science by then was proceeding on the basis of new clienteles.[87]

For some years, early in the century, it appeared that mechanics, instead of killing it off, might provide a substantial basis for popular interest in science. After all, traditionally from the nineteenth century, science embraced all engineering improvements as well as natural phenomena. Surveys of consumers of popularization found that they emphasized the importance of applied science and took interest in such science subjects as "aviation" and "electricity." Attendees at the New York Museum of Science and Industry in 1937 wanted to know, "How does it work?" as well as "What is new in science?" and "What does it mean to me?" But no matter to what extent Einstein was good press, it was hard to confuse the kind of activity he represented with a new combination automobile and airplane. And it was just in these early twentieth-century decades that the scientists increasingly came to support the ideal of pure science, as part of the process of specialization. Moreover, as educational standards rose, larger parts of the population could respond to science that was not applied.[88]

The Rise of Specialized Audiences

As the development of popularizing institutions shows, the popularizers targeted three groups: children, through the schools; the sci-tech community, through media with restricted audiences; and the masses, through journalism. With the demise of the Chautauqua and the general magazine, and the rise of the electronic media, the popularization that had once been directed to cultured people or constituted an important part of adult education almost disappeared. Instead the pattern found in the magazines dominated the popularization of science: the sci-tech community provided the most conspicuous consumers. The *Scientific Monthly*, successor to the cultured *Popular Science Monthly*, evolved into a magazine written by scientists for members of the larger scientific community, including teachers, but never found a definite audience. By contrast, the renascent *Scientific American* successfully tapped the new technical public: at one point, 85.5 percent of the readers were in technical occupations.[89]

The work of the editors and writers of the *Scientific American* nonetheless constituted genuine popularization. Just as the editors of the *American Naturalist* had perceived, what had happened was that scientists had become so specialized that outside of their narrow subspecialties they functioned as lay persons. "Almost every day," wrote the editors of *Science Conspectus* in 1914, "there are new developments in special lines of research, any one of which may lead to fundamental discoveries, but, although these matters would be of general interest if they could be understood, their significance is often obscure, even to scientific workers in not dissimilar lines."[90] *Science Conspectus* represented a short-lived attempt to inform specialists about other scientific specialties, either closely related, as, say, within the biological sciences, or in completely different fields but within science. By midcentury, popularizing science for other scientists was a major aspect of science popularizing, whether the focus was that of *Physics Today*, for example, or the *American Scientist* or the *Scientific American*, all of which were midcentury products. So tied into the scientific community were these efforts at disseminating science among scientists that eventually publishing in them brought rewards within the professional reward system, in the form of recognition and prestige.[91]

Insofar as members of the technical community succeeded in pressuring mass media gatekeepers and writers into presenting popularized science, again the audience specialized. Typically those with technical background appreciated the content of the presentations, while those without tended to ignore material that did not have extraneous interest. While the potential for understanding was low in a general audience, even mass media presentations, it turned out, played an important part in the functioning of the technical community by sensitizing scientists to developments in science. Altogether popularizing science for the scientists, while not perhaps popularization in the traditional sense, was nevertheless popularization, and it played a not insignificant role in the culture.[92]

Popularization aimed at the masses also changed as the late Victorian high-culture consumer receded in importance. The growth of newspaper science and then the science writer worked out so that popularizers were challenged, above all else, to interest the reader or listener or viewer, rather than letting science content and individual curiosity and initiative act as the attraction (as it still in part did within the sci-tech community). Where once discussions of the applications of science served to explain how some scientific principle worked as well as to interest the audience, now they functioned merely to make science attractive. In the more recent period, popularizers conceptualized interest, as has been suggested, in terms of what science could do for a person, and it was no wonder that medicine and psychology, which could contribute to individual ease and comfort, loomed large in science popularization. In the 1959–1969 period, for example, Ann Roberta Larson found that *Newsweek* and *Today's Health* writers, who had to deal with technically uninformed audiences, utilized a variety of techniques to gain and maintain interest—such techniques as personalizing researchers or even objects, dramatizing, and even bringing in traditional human interest as well as relating results immediately to the reader. She found that writers in the *Scientific American*, by contrast, assuming already motivated readers, emphasized summaries of material and explanatory style to attract and involve the receptive audience.[93]

The Change in Popularizing Personnel

The change in the personnel of the popularizers that was so strikingly parallel to that in health and psychology was obviously one of the major causes of the change in content and approach of popular science. Whereas in the late nineteenth century, scientists—and often leading scientists— themselves translated and explained science to the lay audiences, increasingly in the twentieth century the scientists turned the job over to someone else—"the entrepreneurs of science," as one group of researchers designated them.[94] Under Cattell, the *Popular Science Monthly* and the *Scientific Monthly* tried to continue to have eminent scientists as authors. In response, some of the best researchers did at least indulge in popularizing to the extent of addressing that highbrow audience; for example, T. H. Morgan himself wrote on genetics for the 1918 *Scientific Monthly*. Others, too, were active, at least in those days. Major investigators wrote school as well as college textbooks. Simon Newcomb, for example, produced *Astronomy for Schools and Colleges* (1879; last edition, 1893). Moreover, university scientists took an active interest in education at all levels, some of them appearing very prominently as authors of papers in the opening volumes of *School Science and Mathematics*. Later editors attempted to keep major investigators active in popularizing, as in the 1947 volume edited by Warren Weaver, *The Scientists Speak*, as well as in the magazines popularizing for scientists. But the overwhelming momentum continued in the direction of letting nonscientists do the work. As Associated Press science writer Frank Carey said in 1952, he was a lay person writing about items that would interest a lay person.[95]

Scientists dropped out to begin with because so many of them had had such bad experiences with the yellow press. This circumstance led to a vicious circle of events; as Arthur E. Bostwick pointed out in 1929, when an investigator had informed his colleagues of his findings, he left

the task of informing the general public to uninformed writers, or to scientific quacks, or to journalists in search of sensations. This style of 'popular science' does more harm than good; and its greatest harm perhaps, is its reaction on the mind of the real scientific investigator, whose impatience at it and contempt of it show themselves in the hasty conclusion that all attempts to interest the general reader in scientific work must necessarily be of the same kind.[96]

The other major reason that scientists tended not to popularize was, as already noted in connection with psychology and elsewhere, that the reward system in science, especially by the midcentury period, not only did not encourage popularizing but stigmatized it. The lack of scientists' follow-through on the science curriculums of the 1960s reflected particularly graphically how relentlessly the system worked.[97]

Popularization therefore did pass into the hands of specialists in popularization in not only health and psychology but also the natural sciences. Most scientists were glad to be free of the responsibility. Except for the curricular efforts of the post-Sputnik period and the training workshops that went with them, the scientists even forsook a role in training the specialists in interpretation. The specialist in science, wrote Columbia economist Wesley C. Mitchell in 1939, "should welcome help from people more skilled than themselves in the arts of popular presentation."[98] Moreover, as will be noted elsewhere, specialist scientists themselves came to depend upon journalistic sources for information.

The process by which educators took science education over from the scientists was, as the evidence presented above shows, a slow one, but the revolt of the teachers against the rigid college curriculums early in the twentieth century (alluded to above) was obvious to everyone. In 1915, in justifying one of the major texts that introduced general science, the principal of William Penn High School, W. D. Lewis, recalled,

> When the colleges agreed to accept science for entrance on the same basis as mathematics and the foreign languages, they prescribed the content of the science courses and totally changed their character.
> The new syllabi were determined by college professors who had in mind only the needs of the pupils destined to go to college. For these reasons, without real blame being attributable to any one, the proper aim of the study of science in the high schools was defeated.

Lewis and other educators did succeed in reclaiming the right to set the content and method of science education, as I have suggested, so much so that almost forty years later, in the midst of the new curricular reform,

Johns Hopkins biologist Bentley Glass believed that "for the first time in the history of American education we now see a large number of research scientists, from the colleges and universities, taking part in a co-operative effort with high-school teachers of science and science supervisors."[99] Such naive evidence as this, offered by participant witnesses, suggests the validity of the hypothesis of an alternating dominance of educators and scientists.

But another personnel factor suggests instead that the intervention of the scientists in the 1950s and 1960s was an aberration, not least because the educators reasserted themselves in the 1970s. The authorship of school science textbooks reveals most clearly what occurred. In the nineteenth century, as in the case of Newcomb, authors of textbooks tended to be leading men of science—usually college or university subject specialists. In the early twentieth century, the authors were typically active school teachers. Many school textbooks (almost half), particularly in the fields of physics and chemistry, continued in midcentury to list scientists as at least coauthors. But educators persistently encroached even on that proportion, and ultimately the number of outstanding scientists involved in school textbooks declined markedly. Perhaps even more noticeable was the way in which the scientists disappeared from the professional science education literature. Moreover, whereas once teachers had predominated as authors in works on science education—teachers who often considered themselves part of the scientific community—later the pages of the journals were dominated by science education specialists, that is, teacher trainers whose ties to science were more tenuous.[100] This shift by which the major force in the popularization of science through the schools had become specialists in curriculum and teacher training was, as I have suggested, only one element in transforming popularizing. The other was, of course, the parallel change in the realm of popular writing.

That change, from the pure scientists to the science writers, was even more stark than that in education. As early as 1926, Austin H. Clark of the Smithsonian could conclude hopefully, "Progress in science has resulted from popular appreciation of its interest and value. This has been brought about through the work of intermediaries able to explain it to the populace at large . . . . by publicists rather than by research workers."[101] It was not many years later that scientists were in fact systematically insulated from "the populace at large" by public relations personnel, typically those employed by the great universities.

Did it really make any difference if educators and journalists came to do most of the popularizing? There is evidence, to start with, that makes it doubtful that popularized science improved markedly or inevitably just because a specialist in popularizing produced it. It is at least arguable that in fact educators and science writers were not noticeably more adept at communicating with the public than were researchers, and the at least partial success of the scientists' school curriculums of the new math era provides obvious evidence for that contention. Or, to cite other evidence, a researcher in 1950 found that in science journalists' work in major U.S. newspapers there was for every 600 words of science coverage—a typical story—still an average of two "fog words," such as "ion-exchange" or "ergotomine," suggesting that scientists would not have done much worse in "translating."[102]

The answer is, nevertheless, that it did make a great deal of difference who did the popularizing. Scientists continued to complain about the low quality of educators. In 1930, Benjamin C. Gruenberg uncovered from science teaching material a scandalous amount of anthropomorphizing of nature, of teleology ("husks are developed to protect the corn ear"), of animism ("roots search for water"), of defective experimental models (without full consideration of what was and what was not shown), and of other types of what he called "unscientific thinking." In 1968, a study found that students often did better on a test of understanding science than did their teachers. Another study, from the 1970s, showed that students exposed to science teaching tended to be more negative about science than the general public. A number of other investigators tried to find out why science writing, despite the specialists who did it, generated continual problems with accuracy; one of the studies showed that the simpler the material, the better the accuracy, regardless of the prestige of the science writer involved. Altogether, there should have been real doubts about these specialists. In 1938, for example, David Dietz, the pioneer Scripps-Howard science writer, described Gayle B. Pickwell's *Weather* as "One of the most attractive books about the weather ever put together. . . . The information presented is clear and complete." A reviewer in *Science Education* likewise described it as attractive and recommended it for all teachers. But the professional scientist reviewing the book independently in the *Scientific Monthly* noted that while it was a beautiful book physically, it needed to be revised completely. "Its errors are far too numerous to discuss in detail," he continued, and he used such phrasing as "it is erroneously stated," "the absurd statement," "the exceedingly misleading idea," and "the explanation of 'black lightning . . . is quite the worst I have seen." As this and other evidence shows, then, entrusting science to specialists in translation exacted a high price in terms of accuracy and comprehension.[103]

Yet the important issue in who did popularizing was not so much the content as what popularization was about. Even in the 1970s, scientists disagreed with the popularizer specialists about what the public ought to hear and read. As two researchers reported in their study, "A basic divergence was clear throughout: [science writers] wrote what they believed would interest their audience, while scientists held to the academic tradition of trying to teach people what they believed was new and important . . . whether the audience was willing to listen or not." The scientists' goals were simply not honored by either writers or gatekeepers. In 1957, a science writer declared to a group of scientists, "You think science writing should be educational for the public, primarily. But no newspaper editor expects to publish science stories because they are primarily educational. They are published because they are news. If we can educate the public along the way, we're doing well. We can't always do it."[104]

The problem therefore was not just that, as another pair of researchers concluded, journalists took liberties "with the substance and perspectives of science." That was bad enough. The problem was also that the specialists' priorities of entertainment and news clashed with those of enlightenment. "Good science reporting is impossible as long as its purpose is assumed to be entertainment and not education," noted the editor of the *Bulletin of the Atomic Scientists*. Even though the best science writers might have striven to educate, their editors as a group judged stories on the basis of color and excitement. Benjamin T. Brooks, a New York chemist, in 1928 denounced "'tabloid' science" and asked directly, "Must morons be supplied with moron science?" For generations in the twentieth century, many editors (and, later, producers) seemed to think so.[105]

Finally, it should be reiterated how deeply the standards of journalists and educators affected the scientists who did try to popularize. There were many evidences beyond the curriculum planners' retreat in the 1960s in the face of educators' imperatives. The most suggestive early instance was the way in which the level of discussion in the *Scientific Monthly* shifted markedly to a more elementary level just after the advent of Science Service. Moreover, even though Cattell, the editor, persuaded eminent scientists to publish in the *Scientific Monthly*, the subject matter was very frequently set by journalistic priorities and in the 1920s included such topics as vitamins, Madame Curie, relativity, eugenics, and the endocrines. As late as the 1980s, June Goodfield was complaining about the similar influence of media fads on the presentation of science and health.[106] But there is occasion below to note further what happened when specialists in popularization set the standards for the popularization of science.

Public Relations and Image

The scientists' move into actual, overt public relations came in several stages. After the attempts of the American Chemical Society and Science Service to mediate directly to the press, in the 1920s, as Ronald C. Tobey has shown, the leaders of American science continued their public relations efforts to improve the place of science in American social priorities. At that time, everyone tended to depict such activities as popularization of science. The 1920s upsurge in amount of popularization, as I have suggested, was, in fact, in part a result of that campaign.[107] Only thereafter, but particularly by midcentury, did the public relations office become a standard part of the bureaucratic matrix, institution by institution, within which most American scientists functioned.[108]

Public relations was not new in that throughout the twentieth century research scientists frequently had shown interest in having at least some part of the general public appreciate their work. It also turned out after World War II that in practice researchers often worked with journalists directly as well as through the institutional public relations officers. The direct contacts typically took place on the initiative of the journalists, however.[109]

Public relations was, of course, not necessarily popularization, in the 1920s or after. Sometimes public relations did represent an attempt to popularize a particular scientific development. At other times, public relations consisted merely of publicizing an individual, not to mention an institution. And sometimes public relations was soliciting funding or perhaps, at best, just recruiting able young people into research and teaching careers.[110] As in popularization in general, it was always hard to distinguish the real activity from programmatic statements, from self-justification, and from propaganda for funding. But overt public relations work—even aside from other attempts to manipulate the press—was a major factor in science popularization throughout most of the century.

Beyond funding and recruitment, the public relations of science helped determine the way in which science functioned in society, as La Follette points out, by shaping social expectations.[111] Early in the century, popularizers tended to feature the potential benefits of science, chiefly the advantage of using reason to solve problems, together of course with the material products of science. After World War II, especially, another theme became prominent: how science could prevent evil—particularly in the form of pollution—mainly through a quick "technological fix."

But instead of focusing on content or message, Americans conceptualized the function of the public relations of science in terms of the general "image" of science (using a midcentury term first applied to individual business firms). Image was a version of the earlier idea of the public's "attitude" toward science; moreover, in the last half of the century, social scientists in substantial numbers measured those attitudes, and the success of the public relations of science—if not all popularizing—frequently was gauged in terms of attitude and image. By the 1970s, particularly, many leaders were concerned because they detected a decline in the public image of science and scientists. "The Image of the Scientist Is Bad," announced a headline in *Science* in 1978. Most observers assumed that it was undesirable for the public image of science to be less favorable than in an earlier period, ignoring the fact that all institutions and professions had declining image scores.[112] And many of those observers believed that a defective image represented a failure of popularization.

The fact that the image of science had important social consequences underlined the concern of statespersons of science—and other Americans. To begin with, recruiting scientists was a constant problem, and young people's attitudes were therefore a special focus of inquiry—why at any given time were they not becoming scientists, or at least taking science courses? Closely connected to recruiting was salary level. Already in 1874, government astronomer Simon Newcomb had connected image to salary level and recruitment, and a century later, social scientists could still demonstrate a statistical connection between remuneration and recruitment. Everyone concerned was aware, too, of a connection between funding for research and the well-being of science in the areas of recruiting and salaries as well as research productivity. But the image also had more general implications for the freedom of scientists and even, as one of them put it in the days of McCarthyism, in 1954, for "our basic philosophy." Observers detected then a "revulsion" from science, and scientists found themselves characterized as "valuable but untrustworthy."[113]

In searching out how public relations and image affected the politics of American science, political scientists of midcentury and after eventually identified in the population a critical element who concerned themselves with science issues. They were the "attentive," or knowledgeable, public, along with a second element, the interested public, who were not so knowledgeable. In 1957 the attentive public was but one percent of the population, but by 1981 it had grown to twenty percent; the interested public at the same time grew from eight percent to 19 percent. The extent to which these politically concerned segments of the population were identical to the sci-tech public involved in consuming most of mid- and late twentieth-century popularization was not fully known, but the suggestion was that the overlap was substantial indeed, and one of the defining characteristics of the "attentives" was consumption of popular science. Between educational preparation and concern, observed two researchers in 1981, about half of the population could and would benefit from more popular science—in addition, of course, to serving as a political base for science issues.[114]

From Complexity to Products

One reason that nineteenth-century evangelical popularization of science receded in the twentieth century was that what scientists had to communicate—beyond image and attitude—grew much more difficult to put into popular form after 1900. At one time, the task of popular science had been to clear up mysteries. Indeed, as late as 1924, Slosson, the voice of Science Service, was still denouncing false beliefs and commercial distortions by saying that "the test of real science" was "its honesty" in attacking "the real mysteries of nature." Explanation was for him, as it had been earlier for "men of science," the essence of popularizing. But by the midcentury period, popularizers of all varieties were bemoaning the fact that pure science had become so complicated that they could hardly explain it. The science of the new century did not necessarily confirm the gospel of certain progress, unity, and reductionism of an earlier day. Biologist Francis Sumner of the University of California in 1937 summarized the dilemma for example of those who read about the new physics: "There would seem to be a vast inconsistency between the traditional notion of the man of science, with his uncompromising insistence on evidence and his lofty scorn of guesses and unproved assumptions, and the quasi-mystic who tells us all these strange things about space and infinity and who describes with such assurance the detailed intricacies of an infinitesimal world forever beyond the range of human observation."[115]

While innumerable newspapermen of the 1920s tried to explain relativity, and in later years other baffling ideas, or to explain why something could not be explained, only a few scientists attempted to draw conclusions for the public from the unsettling findings of the new physics and other mathematical or abstract studies. Popularizers of every stripe found themselves instead portraying confusion. They therefore often had to readjust what they were doing, because they could no longer appeal to the paradigmatic act of explaining mystery. They were, rather, being called upon to explain the confusion, which was particularly difficult without the vision of ultimate unity that earlier popularizers had enjoyed and exploited. The newspapers were not to blame, insisted the editor of the *New York Times* in 1935: "The function of the newspaper is primarily to report what the leading scientists do and say. If they contradict each other, and there is confusion, the newspapers merely picture the confusion and do not create it."[116]

The result of this challenge to the unity of science was to encourage popularizers to redouble the emphasis that had been developing on portraying the results, rather than the ideas, of science. *The Science Year Book* published in the 1940s, for example, usually had "aviation" as a major category and consisted almost entirely of articles about applied science developments. As early as 1903, W. S. Franklin, a physicist at Lehigh, observed: "Everything that appears in the name of science in our newspapers and magazines relates only to results. Have any of you seen in our newspapers or popular magazines any detailed description of the principles and methods used by Marconi in his wireless telegraphy?" More than half a century later, Palmer Wright, a Dow Chemical chemist, wondered if popularizers should not build on applied science for understanding. "The popular thrust," he observed, "is toward the what, not the why of science."[117]

So it was that popularized science in the twentieth century continued as in the nineteenth to emphasize progress—but progress now in terms more exclusively of the "applications mankind can make from [the] marvelous findings" of "pure science," as a 1926 writer put it. But the new context of progress had further implications. Any facts at all could be digested into the popular science of results; they needed no further context than that they were part of the advance of science. Thus a discovery at any level of science reported in the 1920s was a fact and a part of the progress of science; so, too, was a machine of the 1930s or a cure of the 1940s a fact and a part of the progress of science. This approach to popularizing was compatible with the rise of general science in the schools, in which teachers emphasized application and turned away from the work of researchers that was abstract and unpopular. Even in the 1960s, reported Howard E. Gruber, "high school teachers generally approach[ed] science teaching as a matter of conveying science as established facts and doctrines" rather than "science teaching in which science [was] treated as a way of thought."[118] In the more general popularizing of the twentieth century, audiences would have been lucky to get doctrines in addition to lists of products.

This shift away from the ethos and content of science appeared also in another arena through which science, as has been suggested, often reached at least some popular audiences: science fiction. As Joseph F. Patrouch, Jr., points out, most of science fiction gets the name because it depends not upon science per se or the scientific method but rather the technological products of science and invention. Science fiction originally drew upon both the Gothic tradition of the mad scientists and the realists' adulation of the scientist and the objective approach. The modern version of science fiction, which developed in the 1920s and 1930s, continued to draw upon the nineteenth-century synthesis of science and technology, and for a long time the audience was based in the sci-tech population. But the plots came increasingly to depend upon magical intervention of nonhuman (and nonworldly, i.e., exceptional) beings; and, especially as science fiction spread into television, the genre failed markedly to propagandize for the scientific solution of problems or even for scientists as heroes. The attraction lay rather in clichéd escapism decked out in various, often purely incidental and unreal, technologies. The content in this type of popularization was at best on a par with that of the *National Enquirer*. Defenders of science fiction as a popularizing tool pointed out that it at least encouraged readers to maintain open minds and be receptive to innovation. Such comments led one critic to wish for "more science-fiction stories that dramatize the virtues of tough-mindedness as well as open-mindedness."[119]

In confronting these varieties of popularization, Matthew Whalen has differentiated popular scientism—the products and appearance of science—from popular science proper—translating the scientists' science. The differentiation is the more urgent because throughout the twentieth century, most observers and popularizers confused the two. Some observers insisted that the barebone facts and especially the products of science did not represent the influence of science, that is, scientific thinking. At most, observed I. Bernard Cohen in 1948, useful things were but the "by-products of the search for fundamental truth."[120] But most members of the public, like my airline attendant, made an artificial and tenuous but persistent connection between technological plenty and the defeat of superstition (a defeat that everyone knew was connected to science).

Nor, as events of World War I and the Great Depression showed, was the product interpretation of science always favorable. I have already suggested that the environmental movement in part embodied recognition that the products of science can be negative, or at least mixed. And there was much additional evidence. By 1964–1968, for example, motion picture portrayals of innovation, chiefly science and technology, showed innovation to be a failure in about forty percent of the instances in which it was pictured, whereas in 1939–1952 it was never shown as a failure. But even with the negative possibilities, the public still tended to react favorably toward items that they perceived, usually with the aid of the media, as new and better products of science.[121]

In later decades, products worked into one other theme that popularizers used—what will science do for me?—a theme particularly well suited, as noted above, to the post-World War II age of narcissism and concern about health. "There is," noted a science writer in the early 1970s, "an emphasis away from cold, indifferent science to that which produces some gain in the quality of life." It was in these circumstances that emphasizing the personal application of the advances of science became so hackneyed that the science writers joked about the "new hope" school. In the environmental era, negative popularizers emphasized the personal effects of science products, and all of this appeal to self-involvement in science products, along with dramatic involvement with events reported from space activities, led to a new kind of sensationalism in science popularization as the Gee Whiz! school came back to life.[122]

From Products to Policy

The products of science gave not only personal interest but social urgency to popularization. As early as 1946 W. C. Van Deventer of Stephens College observed that "science teaching has changed progressively in the direction of greater attention to individual and social needs." In sensitizing Americans to the social effects of science, the impact of World War I and the Great Depression, as has been noted, were greatly intensified by the spectacular product of natural science, the atomic bomb. Physicist Harold C. Urey explained what he was doing: "I have dropped everything to try to carry the message of the bomb's power to the people because if we can't control this thing there won't be any science worthy of the name in the future." And then the space race and the social aspects of environmental problems intensified many Americans' concern even further as they argued that the public had to be educated.[123] These citizens therefore developed motives for popularizing science far beyond the personal interest typically found in health and psychology.

Arguing social effects and social responsibility greatly confused the role of popularization. As in public relations, popularization was in fact often muddled with scientists' political activism, which was not usually directly connected with conveying the content or spirit of science, although, as in psychology and health, it could be. Nor were the scientists the only ones involved. At one point, at the end of World War II, both "the liberal, with the public behind him, and the reactionary, with support from the armed forces and potentially from other federal sources," as a bemused educator reported, favored more science education. The *Bulletin of the Atomic Scientists*, which for decades carried a mix of messages, symbolized the confusion. By the time of environmental awareness and the distancing of science writers from the scientific establishment, there was even talk of the social responsibility of the popularizers, particularly since the power of the press, as noted above, extended to determining what issues would be raised in the public forum. Moreover, as journalist John Lear observed in 1970, "The present situation never would have come about if science reporters had presented developments in their true perspective as the events occurred." Lear was not alone, by that era, in believing that popularizing was close to policymaking. The educator-statesman Robert M. Hutchins summarized the change in 1969 (parallel to that noted in psychology in chapter 3): "Science began as part of the search for understanding. Now it is part of the search for power."[124]

One sign of the confusion in popularization was the rise of the idea of scientific literacy, a phrase that has already been alluded to. "Scientific literacy" in practice tended to mean that what passed for popularization had science policy at the top of the agenda. In the last half of the century, beginning especially in the 1960s, educators began to use the phrase to describe goals in science education and ultimately promoted the idea as the key to industrial productivity in a technical world. Two aspects of the idea soon became clear. First, both adults and children needed scientific literacy. And, second, no one was exactly sure what it was, nor was agreement forthcoming. Most commentators described scientific literacy as analogous to literacy in reading and writing—an ability to understand and take appropriate action, or, as Herbert J. Walberg put it in 1983, "mastery of the basic knowledge and skills of communication in science." Many writers hearkened back to James B. Conant's original description of scientific literacy as the ability to judge experts in a world increasingly based on expertise. A scientifically literate person, Conant wrote, could "communicate intelligently with men who were advancing science and applying it." In practical terms, the idea was complex indeed, as suggested by one observer, who called it "knowing how to know."[125]

Educators wanted to test scientific literacy by whether or not the student behaved in certain ways—joined science clubs, accepted science as a part of modern living, showed confidence in scientists and the scientific method—goals that could for the most part have come out of the nineteenth century (in contrast to the idea of the limitations of science). But agreement on scientific literacy was elusive because advocates did not all agree on all goals, particularly the extent to which everyone needed to know the actual content of the various natural sciences.[126] Whereas the emphasis on products of science could appear in the form of facts without context or meaning, scientific literacy in some hands had a tendency to consist of attitudes without content.[127]

Scientific Attitudes

The idea of scientific attitudes had an honorable history in popularization, from the late nineteenth-century emphasis on scientific method to what later came to be called scientific thinking. The scientific method (noted in chapter 4) was particularly important in popularizing because method, as I have suggested, offered a practical way to combat superstition directly, to find the natural law that could explain any phenomenon. "How few there are among us," lamented E. N. Transeau in 1913, "who can carry the idea of natural law into all of their thinking and who are willing to accept the consequences of a natural explanation for natural phenomena. The clairvoyant and the charlatan . . . the healer . . . the astrologic weather prophet, and the promoters of something for nothing . . . enjoy the confidence and respect of a majority." [128]

As science continued after 1900 to become more and more complicated, serious popularization in the *Popular Science Monthly* and then the *Scientific Monthly* contained an unusual incidence of discussions of what science was. More than ever, the method, or the approach, distinguished science and particularly set it in opposition to various kinds of credulousness. But these discussions of the scientific method were taking place in a context in which newspaper and other writers were putting increasing emphasis on the products of science. Between the method emphasis and the applied science progress, it was no wonder that educators combined the two in general science courses. Moreover, central intellectuals of the early twentieth century found that the scientific approach promised a better road to reality, a method, called pragmatism or not, to ascertain facts to which one could adjust even while preserving rationality, as opposed to the formalism of logic and tradition that was passing away in those years. [129]

Events in the realm of education reflected developments everywhere in the world of popularization. In 1900, although textbook authors were now committed to investigative formats, still they did not often talk about the scientific method. Educators listed as their goals not only inculcating a naturalistic view of the world but more particularly providing useful information, developing ideals and good character, and training powers of observation. By the 1920s and 1930s, however, the scientific method showed up particularly conspicuously as the goal of instruction, along with development of "scientific attitudes." "This method of science," wrote the authors of a general science textbook in 1921, "should become a part of the daily life of every educated person. It should become a habit of mind, a way of thinking." And they proceeded to show how to use a rational and experimental approach in so homely a matter as fitting a rug to a room. [130]

One of the major departures that post–World War I educators made away from many college and research scientists was to abandon the latter's assumption that exposure to science subject matter, especially in the laboratory, would automatically cause a person to know and use a scientific approach to all problems. In the *Scientific Monthly*, for example, it was possible to discuss "interesting" phenomena, readers presumably understanding that "interesting" material would show how nature and natural law functioned. The educators discovered instead that it was both necessary and possible to teach the scientific method directly—without any particular subject matter, and also without any particular product, either (although of course the accidental association of method with products, as in general science, continued). Educators began to speak of the "habit of scientific thinking." The particular advantage of the habit of scientific thinking was that it could be applied both to one's personal problems and to social problems as well. "It is not too much to say," Victor H. Noll began his classic 1933 paper on the subject of scientific thinking, "that a large proportion of our present-day ills and troubles is directly traceable to false, prejudiced, and generally unscientific thinking."[131]

At that point—and particularly in the 1930s—one more element entered into educators' discussions, and now by name: the scientific attitude. ("Contemporary trends in natural science teaching place a new emphasis on beliefs and attitudes," reported one educator in 1934.) The scientific attitude differed from the method in that it represented an inclination to action, as opposed to the merely instrumental method. Under the guise of teaching science, then, educators tried to inculcate a whole series of attitudes, including such items as "readiness to control all conditions" in an experiment and a more general "readiness to be open-minded." In practice, and still in harmony with traditional advocacy of science, a large part of the scientific attitude turned out to be negative— "readiness to avoid being swayed by the mere novelty or sensationalism of an idea" and "readiness to discredit and abandon superstitious belief." The teachers were in fact directly teaching naturalism, engendering opposition to superstitious or dogmatic authority and simultaneously building character.[132] Their program came from the late nineteenth-century men of science, but it operated in a twentieth-century context.

Part of that context was liberalism. The better thinkers in education, often quoting John Dewey on the value of a scientific approach in both teaching and solving social problems, used scientific habits of thinking and later, and more directly, scientific attitudes to teach tentativeness, tolerance, adjustment, naturalism, and receptiveness to social reform. Nor was this context for science limited to education. By going beyond the "halfway and accidental use of science," wrote George Gray, using Dewey's words in *The Advancing Front of Science* in 1937, one could attain peace, plenty, security, and health. But the scientific method was not enough for many such thinkers. "The scientific method has become the shibboleth of our times," proclaimed Haym Kruglak, a physicist at the Univeristy of Minnesota. To capture the openness of science, such writers talked about the scientific attitude as well as adaptability and pragmatism. And it was in this context, too, that by the 1950s many advocates of science had identified unscientific thinking with maladjustment and neurosis as well as superstition. "What is the answer to . . . emotional instability?" asked one science educator in 1944. "It is the use of habitual intelligence that is best taught and understood by the study of science." [133]

Although not so prominent in general popularization, all such rationales to some degree did affect writers such as Gray, especially as the social scientists developed their emphasis on scientific method and in turn affected education and more general intellectual fields. In education, after World War II began, the social importance of science obscured educational leaders' emphases on method and attitude. As the educators discussed what they could teach of science, however, method and attitude continued to look important to them. Those who had tried to teach a scientific way of viewing life began to inquire what social factors affected those who, in the end, could not solve life problems in the scientific way. By 1965, when two educators wanted to convey how to "teach the pursuit of science," they were still reduced to character building by means of setting forth "the characteristics of scientists"—who turned out to be curious, independent, imaginative, inventive, prudent, informed, and hard working. In subsequent years, educators confirmed the idea that individual teachers' own attitudes determined the fate of science in their classrooms. [134]

By the time that the idea of scientific literacy became prominent, then, it could draw on a number of concerns, from esthetics to character, that represented science without any particular content. "The preoccupation with information should give way to popularization of the objectives, the method and spirit of science," declared the cofounder of the new *Scientific American*, Gerard Piel, in 1957. [135] All of these concerns, with programmatic statements typical of science educators, therefore showed up also in statements of other kinds of popularizers, as part of the context of the material that they were translating for the public. Emphasis on process and "structure" appeared not only in the works of midcentury curriculum reformers but in general science writing, often in connection with more traditional content. "The gee whiz story," noted one writer in 1974, "has taken a back seat to interpretative pieces that view science as process."[136]

The Passing of Science as a Way of Life

But for the most part, during the first half of the twentieth century, the initiative in advocating the religion of science, or "science as a way of life," passed from the dwindling ranks of men of science to the educators. Whereas in the nineteenth century research scientists viewed popularization of their findings as part of their scientific evangelism, in the years after 1900 it was increasingly the educators, often following Dewey, who crusaded for the scientific attitude and extended the scientific method to all of life—as a New York City schools official put it, "Since it is only mind, intelligence, and reasoning which solve problems, there is fair justification for the assertion that the method of science can be applied to other fields." And one of his subordinates spelled out the fact that, just as fifty years earlier, character formation was involved in the scientific way of life in the form of love of truth and hard work as well as an ethic of human service.[137]

After World War II, the social idealism of the educators died out, and with it much of what was left of the science of religion. Increasingly, the scientific method—or process or structure—in the schools translated into an idealism dominated by "beating the Russians" with science feats and products or controlling technology, not defeating superstition and solving the problems of civilization. At best, the new goal was scientific literacy. Where once natural science findings were "interesting" because of the naturalism and intellectual excitement that they fostered, now the media demanded personal relevance. Even the notably elevated intensity of interest in science in the early 1980s was based on the products and practical effects of science, far more than on curiosity about nature and the scientific method.[138]

As the foregoing narrative has suggested, beginning in the 1920s, especially, scientists tended to play roles other than that of the old-fashioned man of science. Now researchers ever more frequently spoke to the public through various kinds of journalists, who translated science, and when scientists themselves did undertake to address a popular audience, the rules that they followed were not those of the evangelists of the religion of science but rather the rules of the journalists: the agenda was timeliness, the mode of discourse was "news writing."[139] Like the educators who tried to develop a scientifically literate population of citizens to deal with the products of science, so the researchers in their public discussions generally also spoke of the products of science, in the form of either technology or public relations and the bureaucratic consequences of it.

By the 1960s, internal growth and external interconnections with the rest of society had transformed the American scientific community. The most obvious change was an extreme fragmentation of the different research specialists.[140] Popularization with real content—typically that in the new *Scientific American* or *Physics Today*—as discussed above was aimed at the sci-tech public and was part of an immediately scientific context, not part of an evangelism or even a world view that all scientists could subscribe to or participate in. The word "interesting" was not part of the vocabulary of the contributors to such magazines.

Particularly just around mid twentieth century, there was an attempt to provide still another context for popularizing science: the history of science. Evangelists of science had long used the heroes and history of scientific discoveries to dramatize the battle against superstition and intolerance as well as to suggest that progress made in the past could be projected into the future.[141] The new approach was to insist that science was part of civilization and that every cultured person, benefiting from the "general education" movement of the midcentury period, ought to be able to understand science without having to learn vast amounts of content. The history of science, advocates argued, could convey understanding. And others, especially after the "two-cultures" debate flared up in 1959 (the scientific versus the humanistic), contended that the natural sciences and the humanities both were humanistic and rational and should be learned and viewed in a context of culture—history—rather than of application and technology.[142]

History of science was always effective in popularizing in that a popularizer could humanize a discovery by tying it to a possibly interesting discoverer; and in the classic popularizations, the heroes tended to be

Galileo and then Darwin, both of whom suffered at the hands of the despised forces of obscurantism. As the twentieth century wore on, many potential heroic figures tended to remain aloof or to bring complications into the account. Instead, the media played up the "visible scientists," as Rae Goodell named them—not heroes but media celebrities whose mission was changing science policy, not popularizing scientific discoveries, much less advocating reductionist thinking or campaigns against superstition.[143] The end product, then, was the twentieth-century scientist celebrity and his or her products, in place of the man of science.

Both the context and the actual popularization of natural sciences changed in the course of the twentieth century, beyond the personnel and the nature of the leadership. Science itself evolved from an understandable system to a body of complexity difficult to grasp; instead of explaining mystery, popularizers had to contain confusion. Instead of offering reductionism and the unity of nature, the purveyors of science tended to embrace romanticism and pluralism. The confidence and certainty of the religion of science got lost in the products of science, in timeliness— indeed, in fear. The mission of the scientist shrank down to public relations and propaganda for funding or, sometimes, political or consumer activism.[144]

Not everything changed from the nineteenth century. The orientation toward both health and psychology of much of popular science persisted. Some of the high-culture tradition in popularizing persisted, as in the writings of Lewis Thomas in the 1970s. The idea of order in the universe still lurked in popularizations, as, for example, in the search for symmetry in nature that was a theme in *New York Times* stories in the 1960s. Above all, science continued to appear in the guise of progress, whether in the form of products or as a rationale for talking about knowledge about nature. And, here and there, skepticism survived in small corners, as in "Skeptical Eye," a regular feature that served as a tie to traditional popularizing in *Discover*, one of the new slick magazines of the early 1980s.[145]

Chapter 6

The Pattern of Popularization and

the Victory of Superstition

IN THE CHAOS of history, patterns in the events are difficult to discern, and repeated patterns appear only rarely. It is striking, therefore, that in the United States, the popularization of health, psychology, and the natural sciences all followed courses that in basic outline were parallel. Timing and emphasis varied, as I have observed, but each went through a series of stages:

1) Diffusion—when science did not need condensation, simplification, and translation;

2) Popularization—when men of science tried to share their vision of the religion of science;

3) Dilution—when popularization passed into the hands of educators, who represented science only at second hand, and, simultaneously, journalists;

4) Trivialization—when popular science consisted of impotent snippets of news, the product of authority figures.[1]

The Negative Forces

These stages were, from at least one point of view, the culmination of forces unleashed near the beginning of Western civilization. One of the fundamental sets of forces was negative; popularizing science and health always had negative motives, from the beginnings of skepticism down to the 1920s. Indeed, as late as 1940, psychologist Knight Dunlap could expostulate, "I must insist that at the present time one of the major duties of psychologists, in the service of society, is to combat the popular superstitions about heredity" (at other times he mentioned other credulities).[2]

Over a long period of time, the enemy was superstition allied with mystery. But one of the animating motives for opposing superstition and superstitious mysticism was that they were corrupt: both could be and were used to manipulate people for private gain, be it money or power. Attacking corrupt motives was therefore a commonplace of the campaign against superstition, whether in the early hygiene writing, in Draper's and White's classics, or in science advocacy of the twentieth century.[3]

In the Enlightenment period and the nineteenth century, still another negative focus of popular science developed explicitly: old, outdated teachings. As I noted particularly in chapter 1, the idea of progress, and most specifically progress in science, meant that yesterday's discoveries and teachings were a potent source of error and had to be combatted just as superstition was. It made no difference whether outdated science took the form of folk beliefs or more authoritative teachings that had simply been superseded: error and superstition together constituted the enemy against which men of science mobilized. In 1896, for example, William Wells Newell defined a superstition as "a belief respecting causal sequence, depending on reasoning proper to an outgrown culture," neatly combining obsolescence and irrationality. E. T. Bell in 1930 noted, "The public interested in science is entitled to know at the earliest possible moment what things science has abandoned, what it regards with reasonable suspicion, and exactly how far it can go by its own methods, with those things it retains. . . . To be worthy of its public, science must be debunked."[4]

Closely allied to old science was another source of error, pseudoscience. Pseudoscience differed from discarded science because it was never respectable but merely took on the forms of science. Unlike folk beliefs, pseudoscience has a basis in the authority of only the scientific forms, not tradition. By the twentieth century, as has been suggested above, Americans in their increasingly bureaucratic society found that the forms of science in pseudoscience commanded more respect than conventional superstition, but the two were often lumped together along with outdated science.[5]

Pseudoscience is of particular interest because in the late 1970s it occasioned the rise of a special, organized group of self-proclaimed skeptics.

Their particular targets were the new occult practitioners using scientific forms—astrologers, psychics, and telepathists in particular. The skeptics reacted especially against the media promotion of fraud and nonsense, and although the skeptics concentrated on overt pseudoscience, they incidentally also sometimes attacked superstitious thinking and credulity in general. Within a few years, they had attracted 17,000 members. These specialists in doubt helped symbolize their generation's quota of skeptics, but their conventional and restricted definition of their concerns greatly limited their impact.[6]

One important aspect of the struggle to bring new science to the public was that, since the substance of popular science—not to mention science itself—was continually changing, what was constant was discovery, or science as process, or, as the men of science formulated it, the scientific method. Keeping up with the findings and ideas of scientists therefore led away from past misconceptions and toward scientific activity, not toward any particular content. As an enthusiast wrote in 1911, "The physical sciences will solve the problems of environment, the biological sciences the problems of life, and the social sciences the problems of society."[7]

The negative animus against superstition, commercial exploitation, and outdated beliefs therefore had positive aspects, and these positive aspects, too, had roots in ancient times. Scientific method in practice linked with naturalistic explanation. Popularized science involved not only ardent naturalism, then, but also the genuine fascination that can arise in a person who suddenly catches a glimpse of a coherent and orderly world view. One of the reasons that the nineteenth-century giant of popularization, Herbert Spencer, had important effects on Americans was that his works provided such a glimpse for a sizable segment of the public, members of which had not theretofore confronted abstract thinking, much less an organized viewpoint.[8] Large numbers of people were entranced by learning about nature, by discovering natural, scientific explanations, and by being able to put all of nature and man into a satisfying context, with the knowledge that better views were constantly opening up. This confidence in their objective world view made these people moralists, for they felt that they had enough authority to prescribe rules for living—in accord with nature—for their fellow citizens.[9]

This vision of the negative and positive roles of popularized science in American culture faded away during the twentieth century not only in health, in psychology, and in the natural sciences, but also in other divisions of society.[10] The reason for the defeat was not the message of the popularizers but, rather, two other factors, as I suggested in the introduction and here and there in my substantive narratives. The first factor was institutional change, and the second was a shift, reinforcing the institutional change, in the forms that superstition took.

What was new was an aspect of superstition noted before: it involved authority, an authority alternative to science (and, originally, at least, to religion). But in the twentieth century, as I shall explain, the new authority was imposed through the media and advertising, thus uniting the two most traditional enemies of science in the popular sphere: superstitious authority and commercial interest.

The Destructive Effect of Facts

The first step in destroying the classic uplift popularization of science was the phenomenon that I have described in health, psychology, and the natural sciences alike, namely, reducing the context of science in popularizing and at the same time emphasizing "facts" so that "science" in the new mode of popularization consisted of isolated bits and pieces. As early as 1920, the editor of *Modern Medicine* complained that such knowledge of scientific investigations as was "current among the general public [was] fragmentary, unrelated, and, for the most part, acquired through spectacular accounts of the Sunday newspaper," leading, he thought, to "the tendency to mysticism in the absence of definite knowledge."[11]

From earliest times, science was distinctive in part because, in contrast to superstition, science was part of a system. In 1830, the editor of the *Mechanics' & Farmers' Magazine of Useful Knowledge* assured readers that scientific subjects would "be treated systematically, no part being omitted that [might] be deemed essential to a right understanding of them," hoping, he said, to "succeed in arresting the attention of those who . . . read, but read to no purpose."[12]

Throughout the nineteenth century, as science showed up in other magazines (as well as newspapers), often the form that it took was indeed an isolated, short summary, as in, for example, the "Bits of Science" that appeared in *Godey's Lady's Book* in the 1880s. Yet even in such brief notes it was possible to suggest a wider context, as in, for instance, this sample from *Harper's Weekly* in 1857 in which one type of naturalistic causation was extended to another in a social activity that involved both excellence and tentativeness:

> *Cause of Earthquakes*—M. Perrey—a distinguished European savant, has been engaged in late years, in a learned investigation of earthquakes. . . . From a careful discussion of several thousand of these phenomena, which have been recorded between the years 1801 and 1850, and a comparison of the periods at which they occurred, with the position of the moon in relation to the earth, M. Perrey infers that earthquakes may possibly be the result of an action of attraction exercised by that body on the supposed fluid centre of our globe, somewhat similar to that which she exercises on the waters of the ocean.[13]

As late as the 1930s—as Jennie Mohr shows in her careful analysis of popular books on science—authors, whatever their credentials, tried not only to convey to readers an appreciation for the scientific way of thinking but "to enable the layman to see the world as the scientist sees it; to show him that the world is not chaotic, but ordered, and that apparently discrete and unrelated events follow a regular and understandable pattern." A few years later an Illinois librarian noted that popular books that were successful succeeded because the authors took the trouble to explain fully each step in thinking and how it connected to others.[14]

The danger of unconnected facts outside of a systematic context was recognized early in all fields. In 1901, Stratton D. Brooks, who taught pedagogy at the University of Illinois, criticized untrained science teachers who, lacking "the spirit of scientific investigation," taught useless facts unrelated to the body of science. More than thirty years later, another educator was still denouncing "giving the world *facts* without teaching it how to think about those facts and how to use them properly." Nor was this phenomenon merely an aspect of bad teaching. F. C. Robinson of Bowdoin in 1905 denounced "scraps of health knowledge . . .— predigested knowledge brought on with one's predigested breakfast food," facts that could entertain but not influence. By 1945, Carl J. Potthoff of the University of Minnesota was still saying, "Health education today emphasizes facts; its contribution otherwise to the thinking discipline appears to be fragmentary," and in 1972 the authors of a Food and Drug Administration report found that most Americans did not have a systematic approach to health but rather used a "rampant empiricism" based upon isolated facts and personal "experience." In 1947, historian of science I. Bernard Cohen was observing that specialization had broken popular science presentations into fragments: "The average reader is not at fault for having little feeling for the life of science as a whole," because modern popularization "has introduced him to unconnected scientific achievements," mostly, of course, practical. And in 1981, Leon Tractman of Purdue was complaining that he was so overcome by the facts of popularized science that he doubted their utility for anything.[15]

All of these witnesses were commenting on a tendency that became more and more pronounced in the twentieth century as the mass media grew in importance in popularization. Producers of facts flooded the public with "a glut of occurrences," as Herbert Brucker pointed out in 1937, occurrences out of many special fields and not just science. The illogical associations that the mass media induce from the overwhelming volume of information, Daniel Lawrence O'Keefe points out, "naturalize a crazy world." Paul F. Lazarsfeld and Robert K. Merton in 1948 named the effects of being swamped by media facts "narcotizing dysfunction": "Exposure to this flood of information may serve to narcotize rather than to energize the average reader."[16]

Science Service was only the most obvious example of a science fact producer. A magazine that started as *Science Facts* in 1938, for instance, in a few years became *Science and Discovery* and then merged into *Fact Digest*. Versions of this type of popularization indeed fulfilled the aims of some consumers of popularization, including some with the best interests, such as readers of *Popular Astronomy* for whom mere technical information fueled interest because the facts fed into hobby activities, that is, by telling readers what they could look for in the sky. But that was a special context for facts. Mostly purveyors of facts did simplify and even translate, but in their works the other usual purposes of popularization got lost in aggregations of information. As physicist R. B. Lindsay wrote in 1952, the loss opened the door to cranks and worse:

> In spite of our vaunted educational system, it is all too clear that to most elements of the population scientists . . . are merely people who collect facts about all sorts of queer things and then use the facts to make all kinds of materials and gadgets. By analogy, it follows (so goes the argument) that any other presumably learned person who also announces "facts" about nature and the world becomes a scientist if he can only get enough people to believe what he has to say.[17]

Lindsay was describing implicitly how the man of science lost his force and distinction when he turned into a fact monger.

Sometimes, as in the *Popular Science Monthly* in the nineteenth century or in the *Scientific Monthly* in the twentieth, a popularizer could give facts and assume some of the context, such as the promise that every isolated "discovery" was a contribution to "progress"—especially if the reader might know what had gone before. Any educated person should have known, therefore, at least some of the significance of a new chemical element or a fossil anthropoid. But the emphasis on snippets without context, often presented in the name of objectivity, ultimately was subversive not only of the religion of science but of popularization itself. The moral superiority of objectivity derived from the method and attitude, not particular findings. The benign "facts" of science in the nineteenth century heyday of Baconianism did not have the restricted connotations of mid-twentieth-century snippets.

The brief snippet misled because of deliberate delimitation. Leaving out qualifications and context not only in itself impoverished information but often distorted it.[18] But the subversive element in bits-and-pieces, contextless popularization of science and health was the circumstance that the reader, or "consumer," was left to make his or her own sense of it. With a well-informed reader, the result might not be deleterious except in terms of eliciting boredom or satiation. But with relatively naive members of the public, the context could be, and often was, simply magic or meaninglessness, an effect that intensified as specialization increased. The original popularizers did not intend to let the public degrade science by furnishing the meaning of it; meaning instead came as part of the popularization, the translation that accompanied simplification.[19] As I. Bernard Cohen wrote in 1952, "The dissemination of information, however interesting and useful it may be, does not provide a better understanding of science."[20]

Bits-and-pieces communication was characteristic of mid- and especially late twentieth-century American media and culture in general and was not limited to science and health popularization. In part the abbreviation of communications was a result of technological change. As early as 1873, one popular science editor noted, "This is the age of telegrams. The public is accustomed to the consideration of useful facts set forth in the briefest terms." Numerous commentators of a century later noticed that television had intensified to an extreme the fragmented nature of

American life so that people thought of reality in terms of "chunks" or otherwise isolated episodes.[21]

Consequences of Bits-and-Pieces Popularization

Other commentators have observed how mass, urban society spawned a "bewildering sense of purposeless energy, abundance, and diversity, operating without plan or pattern, divorced from human or divine reason." Within that context, an educator at New York University, George E. Axtelle, deplored the specialization that had compartmentalized science to the disadvantage of teaching: "Unless the specialization can be grasped in the context of the whole, its own meaning is seen as little more than the part. . . . The whole is nothing less than the whole of nature and culture." What Axtelle and others concerned with popularization objected to was not only the segmentation and lack of context but the fact that the bits-and-pieces format furnished its own closure, as if the fact were an end in itself. Any uplift, much less the missionary zeal of the primitive popularizers, was completely defeated.[22]

As the contextless fact variety of popularizing science evolved, innumerable commentators noted the way in which such a variety of science encouraged the tendency of "folk" to believe in magic. "We live in the 'scientific age,' to be sure," wrote Everett Dean Martin in 1926, "but it is the *fruits* of science rather than its methods and discipline which the majority possess. The 'wonders' of science are to many minds, the miracles of science. Mankind at large still believes in miracles and magic. Science has not dispelled this superstition. Science itself becomes accepted as a new kind of magic." Journalists in particular utilized the equating of magic and science as a metaphor, but the metaphor came to represent substantial reality in many Americans' understanding of science. As a writer in the *Nation* noted in 1902, "Something of the mediaeval notion of science as a variant of the black arts seems to survive in certain popular modes of speaking of modern scientists. Marconi is a 'magician'; Edison, a 'wizard.' Nor are these phrases purely chance-sown. They well express the real mental attitude of millions of honest folk towards science. To them it remains a region of wonder and mystery. Any miracle may come out of it any day."[23]

Other popularizers joined the journalists in unwittingly encouraging this way of thinking as they described mysteries that science had explained or would in the future. Particularly when only facts or findings were described as science, there was no reason for members of the popular audience to think of the solutions as other than mysterious. In this way magical science could function as a substitute for other magics. At the same time, so were created the circumstances that permitted pseudo-science to flourish, when consumers could not identify imposters, whether in science, technology, health, or psychology—if Marconi or Edison, why not Keely? Or Velikovsky? One wizard (or authority) was as good as another. By the mid-twentieth century, popularizer Isaac Asimov undertook his work, he said, specifically because science had "increasingly lost touch with nonscientists. Under such circumstances scientists [had] come to be regarded almost as magicians." He therefore wrote, Asimov continued, in the traditional popularizing way to remove some of the mystery from science and at the same time to help create a taste for it.[24] To remove mystery of course meant to provide a meaningful context for facts and findings. But Asimov was already one of a dying breed.

Facts and Sensationalism in Journalism

The bits-and-pieces strategy of presenting science derived from American journalism, and this circumstance helps explain the great significance of the ingress of journalists and the journalistic mode into the popularization of science and health. The change in types of agents of popularization, especially the rise of the science writer, as opposed to the scientist-popularizer, in essence provided the means for moving the format of popularization toward unrelated fragments, regardless of which of the media was concerned. When Science Service developed a popular magazine, for example (indeed, Science Service in part came into being at first in lieu of a popular magazine), the magazine was significantly titled *Science News-Letter*, in which the controlling word was "news" (which shows again the distinction between the fragmentary news format and that of the classic magazine). George W. Gray in 1937, to cite another example, described his widely read book *The Advancing Front of Science* as "an attempt to report news."[25] The news standard, in short, overwhelmed all popularizing.

High regard for facts was in itself the rationale for the news format for popularized science. The format in journalism in general attracted the attention of commentators of many varieties, who made fun of facts that turned out not to be true as well as of information that, in the "information society," did not inform—a society in which knowledge could even be intellectual, but not necessarily rational.[26] One of the reasons that some of the better journalists tried to avoid the "new hope" style of science reporting was that they realized that reporting isolated "discoveries" was misleading. One widely cited statistic was that 90 percent of the medical "discoveries" reported in the media in fact did not work out— but of course the deflating word of ultimate failure virtually never showed up in the news. How different was the nineteenth century world of, for example, the editors of the *Popular Science News*, who in 1885 took the responsibility to correct a report that they had carried of "a remedy for the phylloxera," which proved "entirely worthless" with the result that "an effective remedy for this pest yet remain[ed] to be discovered."[27]

The journalistic model contained, beyond emphasis on fact, another element that affected the presentation of science and health in the twentieth century: traditional sensationalism. From the nineteenth century on, newspaper editors had always had a prejudice in favor of the wonderful and exciting, not to mention disease scare and cure, and many editors were vigorous sensationalists even before yellow journalism made such an approach standard and acceptable in most newspapers and some magazines. At all times, then, science and health were subject to sensationalizing, which caused consternation, as I have indicated, among good scientists and practitioners. As late as the 1980s, one unfortunate researcher had her debunking work reported in a tabloid under the headline "Horoscopes Really True, Says Psychologist," with the findings precisely reversed from the published article. (The enterprising reporter had made generous use of the simple device of dropping the word "not" out of sentences when quoting the technical report.)[28] Clearly not even a century had mellowed yellow journalism.

By the 1970s, however, under the influence of television's relentless promotion of so-called entertainment, respectable sensationalism appeared in two further guises. First, reformers, especially environmental reformers, pointed out that they could not do any good unless they attracted media attention to their statements, which they did by playing up emotional content in the customary way of more traditional sensationalizers. But still other writers took the second approach. Readers, these journalists held, not only should gain information from journalistic presentations but should enjoy them beyond mere intellectual content. Researchers in the field started measuring the pleasures of reading science articles (chiefly those pleasures typical of the laziest and most self-centered readers). The new standard, then, became "Enjoyment and Information Gain in Science Articles," joining concrete factual material with a watered-down sensationalism appropriate for an entertainment medium. But this was, of course, only the latest production of one side in the debate over how much emotional appeal had to be mixed in with popular presentations in order to attract an audience for popularization.[29]

A structural element in news reporting also intensified the sensationalism issue in science popularization throughout the twentieth century. Journalistic reports almost always started with conclusions and implications and then were filled out with supporting detail—exactly the opposite format from the restrained scientific report in which conclusions and discussion came only after the methodology and findings were fully set forth. The news format therefore put great emphasis on the journalists' interpretations. The whole problem was exacerbated by the fact that news items tended to be short—in contrast to the longer magazine format—and so journalists cut the scientific context at the same time that they played up attention-grabbing elements and products.[30] Again, a combination of sensationalism with the briefly stated facts removed science news substantially from older standards of responsible popularizing.

What was new in twentieth-century popularizing of science and health, then, was not sensationalism but the bits-and-pieces format, and the early to mid-century timing of the coming of journalists and their format explains when and why they had such an impact. Journalism itself, as Michael Schudson has pointed out, developed, around the 1930s especially, a strategy to strive for objectivity, whereby fact and opinion were separated—opinion to go into signed columns and objective fact into the news columns. This development, Schudson shows, was the end product of the nineteenth-century belief in objective reality, when the daily flow of events came to constitute a reality in itself. For most news, then, the interpretive signed column served to provide a context, so that the endless flow of bits and pieces was at least given a place within the sociopolitical world of the journalists.[31]

For science and health, however, only half of this journalistic strategy was effective. By and large, columnists in those fields, when such columns existed, merely multiplied facts—as typically, and best known, in the health columns of newspapers or in Science Service syndications.

Such columnists did not provide context. And ordinary journalistic columnists were not competent to act the part of men of science. The only interpreters of science who had any impact, then, were the advertisers. The result was that sports journalism became the most recognizable model for all reporting, including science and health—a kaleidescope, as Gilman Ostrander puts it, "a jarring and distracting montage of unrelated pictures and news items and advertisements, all competing for attention and most of them immediately forgotten." Science, health, and psychology were incidental elements in this twentieth-century torrent of items, and when they occurred in a sensationalist guise, they became just one of the "tremendous trifles," media fads that Frederick Lewis Allen described as characteristic of the 1920s—insignificant items given emotional appeal, rapidly becoming known to everyone who shared the mass media world and then passing into oblivion.[32]

Customs in Journalism

One of the other strategies that modern journalists devised in order to escape taking responsibility for substantive interpretation was the attribution. A reporter typically first found someone who could be quoted on the subject at hand and then, pretending not to be biasing presentation, merely stated a fact, namely, that some person or other had made a statement or claim. The reporter then did not need to vouch for or judge the statement or claim. This notorious practice was utilized not only to escape responsibility for science and health reporting but in the most irresponsible and socially obnoxious way to continue to encourage superstition and its close relatives. Throughout the twentieth century, journalists quoted and played up the claims of the purveyors of superstition and then claimed only to be reporting facts. Men of science were continually outraged by this type of performance. In 1916 the editor of the *Scientific American* denounced the Washington newspaper editor who gave the same prominence to a soothsayer's predicting the outcome of World War I as to a story about the Pan-American Scientific Congress. Sixty-five years later, two California psychologists blamed the lords of the media for fostering belief in the occult, citing research that showed how important the media actually were as a source of occult beliefs (a demonstration hardly necessary for any reasonably up-to-date American at any time during those decades).[33] If the playful element in journalists' treatment of the occult revival of the latter half of the century (remarked on in chapter 1) did not suffice to legitimate news coverage, they simply labeled any claims "controversial"—which was understood to give license to remove the deviant stigma from the most irresponsible fakers or mentally ill publicity hounds.

Other twentieth-century journalistic customs not only fostered the promotion of superstition but undermined positive attempts to present popularized science in a meaningful context. Many years ago, Daniel Boorstin described the tactics of creating pseudoevents, particularly when a public relations person could manipulate journalists into using press releases. So in health, psychology, and the natural sciences alike, increasingly science became news rather than even progress, something to be forgotten along with any possible implications when the created event—like a discovery, or a publication, or, in recent times, a rocket launch—ceased to be news. Created science events thus could fade away along with all other disconnected information in the continual "collapse of meaning" in modern culture.[34]

One variety of the pseudoevent was of particular importance in the field of science and health: the media celebrity. Boorstin contrasts the celebrity, whose fame is fleeting and, more important, who has no importance in history, with the enduring impact of a truly great person; indeed, just by converting someone into a celebrity, the media denied any greater significance to the person. Various figures from science and medicine suffered prominence in the media (including some whose reputations were nevertheless substantial and lasting), from Albert Einstein, Bernarr Macfadden, and Madame Curie to Joyce Brothers, Linus Pauling, Carl Sagan, and various astronauts. As the achievements of each figure diminished in relevance to the media agenda, the personality and quotability often continued, at times aided by the omnipresent public relations personnel. The entire process of exploiting celebrities served to emphasize personalities at the expense of ideas. The editors of the *New York Magazine of Mysteries* (1901–1914), for instance, had no fear that glorifying real scientists as personalities would detract from stories about occult events and miracles that, with patent medicine and other ads, filled the rest of the pages of the publication. By the 1960s a prominent feature of *Science Digest* was "Personality of the Month," not unlike the corresponding approach of *Psychology Today*. Playing up prominent figures was of course a traditional tactic in popularizing science, but with the celebrity mode, journalists were creating "image" rather than attempting as in earlier years to anthropomorphize an idea, as in the Health Heroes series of the early twentieth century or the glorification of martyrs of science in the nineteenth-century *Popular Science Monthly*. Moreover, a superficially positive image easily transformed into a negative one, and even the extreme of media image—for example, Bob Newhart as a psychologist—did not, in the end, further communicating ideas from psychology.[35]

One important by-product of the personality or celebrity to whom journalists could attribute opinions was that the media established an image of science as the pronouncement of authorities. And, of course, since all facts were equally acceptable, reporters tried to interview authorities who would contradict each other—and, as the notorious polywater debate showed at the end of the 1960s, this pattern (noted in chapter 3) held true not just in the field of psychology. The media winner usually turned out to be the most photogenic or articulate, or both, or the most cooperative with the press, rather than the best exponent of research, much less the religion of science (many scientists were outraged by the prominence the media of the 1970s gave to some of the less acceptable of astronomer Carl Sagan's views, for example). Thus by the late twentieth century, authority in popular science led far away from the scientific way of thinking and even, for authority, was based more on media standards than on peer review. Journalists handled the authorities' opinions not only as inconsequential facts but as productions of scientists, with the result that the media workers treated even the best opinion in the same way that they treated a new cure.[36]

All of these phenomena—fragmentation, pseudoevents, personalities, and authorities—developed in exaggerated form in the increasingly dominant medium, television. Television served particularly to subvert the popularization of science and health. Not only was sustained argument incompatible with even good television programming, but the entire medium disparaged the written word, and, as I noted above, influenced journalism to shift subject matter and ways of appealing to an audience. As one cable network executive observed of the television generation: "Their thinking is non-linear . . . non-narrative. Images, sense impressions are what count—not words."[37] By the late twentieth century, the largest-selling magazine was no longer even the *Reader's Digest*, with sensationalized health and science, but *TV Guide*, with nothing substantial at all. Critics and researchers have commented at length on the deleterious influences of television. From them all, it is clear that responsible popularization of science and health suffered quantitative diminution and qualitative degradation and, further, that the content of television on the balance contributed to unfavorable attitudes toward science. These conclusions, as Neil Postman points out, are not mere elitist critiques of uninspiring activities; rather they focus on what was lost in the shift to new public media and the world that came with them.[38]

Distortion by the Media

One of the myths of the twentieth century was that the media controllers were passive vessels through which science popularization passed and that any distortions were mere institutional by-products or even accidents. The truth was otherwise, well beyond the journalists' disposition to sensationalize. Even the best reporters asserted their viewpoints under the guise of news expertise. The first method of distortion was of course to set the agenda. Editors and gatekeepers showed strong hands, as I have suggested. Repeated mid- and late twentieth-century studies demonstrated that editorial personnel had a contemptuous opinion of media consumers—the people in Boston who would not read about rats or the New Yorkers who did not believe in radioactivity. "I can't conceive what kind of science we could have that would be interesting to the average newspaper reader," said a 1947 editor. The gatekeepers persistently provided the sensational in lieu of the uplifting, and specifically more superstition than science. When the astronomer Otto Struve was giving a radio talk in 1941, the National Broadcasting Company director insisted that Struve omit disparaging comments that he was going to make about astrology, "which I characterized," Struve recalled, "as a menace to sound thinking. But of course more fundamental power was involved in choosing what the public would hear about." Or, to cite a different kind of example, in 1953, well into the science writer era, the stories that appeared in the newspapers about the AAAS annual meetings were about bats as rabies carriers and a suggestion of using rats for food, neither item from among the most significant papers presented there. In setting agendas, the controllers at all levels indulged in both personal prejudice and commercial advantage; perhaps the best instance is found in Arnold J. Meltsner's evidence of the suppression of seismology in popular media in California throughout the twentieth century.[39]

The media distortion of science not only went well beyond sensationalism, then; it went beyond setting an agenda and telling the public what was important. Some late twentieth-century studies revealed what was involved when journalists were translators, in addition to the distortion that I noted in chapter 5. Precisely the elements to which scientists most objected in journalists' reportage were the implications, emphases, and conclusions. The factual presentations usually did not greatly upset the technical personnel, but the phrasing and inferences did. Or, indeed, the scientists who were the sources disagreed with the whole approach to a story. Like the reporter who did not want doctors using him to tell people how to live, other mid- and late twentieth-century journalists resented any man or woman of science who wanted to tell people what to do or believe. That prerogative of the media workers was what militated actively against the religion of science, even though the "facts" of science and health may have been acceptable or useful to the journalists.[40]

The reason that the agenda and value system of the media personnel was competitive with even diluted forms of the religion of science was that the goal of the writers and gatekeepers was acceptance of not the world of science but rather the world of the media. The success of the journalistic mode therefore meant that much of the popularization of science and health was drawn into the orbit of media reality and standards. The influence went far beyond changing popularization of science into science news or science "information." The most dramatic early example of extensive influence was the attempt of a number of well-meaning science educators to tailor science curriculums not to research findings, much less to the religion of science, but to the task of preparing students to read the science stories that commonly appeared in the newspapers. By the late twentieth century, journalists had so channeled science popularization that they had made the best elements in American society anxious not to push a naturalistic view of the world. Now, rather, media praise went to those who used scientific literacy to teach that science was political, that the focus of science popularization should be science policy—which lay, of course, in the media world, where scientific findings could be "controversial."[41]

Advertising

The media world, as numerous commentators have shown, was but a subset in the new consumer culture of the United States in the twentieth century. It is easy to see that science functioned well in a sensationalized form as well as in the form of a producer of things or as a packaged—fragmented—product itself that the public could consume—and throw away—rather than understand. This function was adaptive to what Warren Susman has called "the new world of abundance-leisure-consumer-pleasure orientation." Whereas science once had been symbolic of the power of humans to transform their world, now they were supposed to take a passive attitude toward this entity that was producing products. A 1978 book, for example, was entitled *Science Fact: Astounding and Exciting Developments That Will Transform Your Life*—reflecting the common belief that one just sat back and waited for the facts to make the transformation.[42] In this world of pleasures and consumers, advertising set standards, and it was advertising with which the popularization of science and health had a special relationship.

Advertising was the ultimate form of fragmented fact plus sensationalism, with, of course, pecuniarily interested interpretation. Many commentators throughout the twentieth century remarked on the way in which journalism and advertising interacted harmoniously and simultaneously as national advertising and yellow journalism rose together as fundamental elements in the mass media. Quentin James Schultze has even identified the shift from products to the motivations of consumers as the event that introduced sensationalism systematically into advertising. A writer in the *Nation* in 1905 observed ironically "that the editorial policy of nearly all the magazines we know is happily approximating the advertising policy. In a superb miscellaneousness, in timeliness, in direct and vociferous appeal to the reader, the editors are, after all, not lagging so much behind." Moreover, in the field of science and health particularly, advertising functioned as popularization. When the substance of popularized science consisted of facts or information without context, advertisers could contribute equally with the best-qualified researchers. "The quest for information is universal and unending," wrote the ingenuous editor of *Modern Medicine* in 1951; "in *Modern Medicine* . . . the advertising as well as the editorial material brings news of advances in medicine."[43] Probably the most transparent instance of such conflation was *Science Pictorial*. This magazine started out in 1946 as an apparently slick paper magazine emphasizing the products of science—only a few of the articles were about cells or molecules or any subject involving abstract scientific principles. It soon became clear that the major source of content was the promotional material of various corporations, and in 1948 finally the editors began a "Personal Shopping Service" for gadgets, as an integral part of each issue, suggesting the extent to which science "facts" and advertising had coalesced.[44] The direction of development is particularly telling as a contrast to the *Boston Journal of Chemistry*, which had exactly the opposite evolution in the nineteenth century when this house organ featuring products for sale became the *Popular Science News*.

Popularizers of science and particularly of health watched the successes of the advertisers and tried, for a better cause, to emulate the methods of the merchandizers. Popularizers found, however, that such efforts had limited success. In 1916, for example, a New York state charity worker regretted the ineffectiveness of well-meaning but fragmented public health publicity: "A group that receives a pamphlet today on child hygiene, and one tomorrow on sanitary toilets, and one the day following on the fly menace, will scarcely be in a receptive mood," he concluded, to support general programs or campaigns. As the century went on, popularizers discovered that one way to correct the ineffectiveness of their miscellaneous efforts was to go even further in using advertising as an organizing principle, to sell not content so much as symbolic elements of their expertise—in other words, to appeal to emotional elements rather than rationality and science, at first with bright posters and eventually with cartoon mascots.[45]

Those who even before the era of "health marketing" imitated the advertisers did not see that they were in any way compromising with the kinds of commercial forces that had traditionally been anathema to popularizers, right back to the self-interest that they had detected in superstition and occultism. In the nineteenth century, men of science denounced the publicity given promoters whose inventions defied the laws of physics—notoriously the Keely motor—and similarly in the early twentieth century the American Medical Association led the fight against nostrums. When researchers and practitioners left the arena, the consumer advocates moved in, and therefore, by the mid-twentieth century, scientists who wanted to work in the anticommercial tradition of popularizing tended to join with the consumer movement, in which others were leading the opposition to advertising and business exploitation.[46] In the late twentieth century, parts of the environmental movement enlisted scientists who lined up to oppose commercial activity that rested upon self-interested assertions about natural events, assertions that often appeared in the media as advertised "facts."

Advertising, as it developed, was essentially antirational, indeed, untruthful.[47] In the ultimate form of television advertising, the anti-rational elements were frequently not even masked, as numerous commentators at the time observed and as researchers confirmed. Mere repetition of an assertion could actually reorganize viewers' perceptions, for example. But the most astounding development was the discovery that consumers liked being deceived. They enjoyed the fantasy that was involved in the world of commercials, in which advertisers emphasized illusion, not product. Viewers entered into a special world of illogical discourse, a world in which they acted upon the stimulus of messages that they knew were not true.[48]

The Cultural Function of Advertising

Advertising thus increasingly established a powerful cultural authority in twentieth-century America. Even people who claimed to get health information from the best sources had items in their medicine cabinets that clearly were there because of advertising. Part of the authority ironically derived from advertisers' use of the name and even regalia of science, and therefore of the prestige of scientific authority (just as in the realm of pseudoscience). The most obvious and notorious examples occurred in the area of health; in magazine ads, at one point, characters dressed as doctors recommended brands of cigarettes. In the 1930s, for instance, there was "no mystery about pink toothbrush. Dental science has recorded these facts," went the advertising copy of one toothpaste maker. But science was also invoked more broadly, as when "scientific" tests by dealers presumably validated the superiority of Exide batteries in 1940; indeed, T. J. Jackson Lears shows that for generations a major element in the authority of both health advertising and general advertising was scientism.[49]

Advertising, as Roland Marchand has shown, even took from science the authority to define that which was "new" and "modern." By the 1920s and 1930s, advertisers, not scientists or even science popularizers, effectively asserted their claim to act in the maturing consumer culture as the heralds and instruments who introduced modern technology. The advertising innovation, planned obsolescence, was but the most obvious contribution of advertisers as they preempted the authority to identify innovation.[50]

But the authority of advertising, especially in the age of television, went, as I have suggested, far beyond depending upon the putative authority of science. Children learned to sing along with musical commercials and to think in terms of stereotypes, sentiments, and bits and pieces of isolated messages that carried substantial cultural authority—authority that, as has also been suggested, could and did override or replace both rational and naturalistic ways of thinking, whether directly, or as an aspect of the consumer culture.[51]

Advertising even fulfilled the function of superstition that Daniel Lawrence O'Keefe and others have identified as fundamental: defending the individual, the self, against fears of a changing world. In a culture in which people worried about loss of the self, traditional magical strategies became viable. Advertisers attempted to speak to "one person at a time." Kate Smith could sell World War II bonds because the typical consumer's reaction to her was "She was speaking straight to me." Friendly people sold friendly products, and copy writers indulged freely in animism: an automobile became a tiger. Altogether advertisers could deny the impersonality of both mass society and natural law with as much aplomb as a practitioner of a cargo cult.[52]

So it was that advertising came in via the mass media just as conventional superstition, combining isolated assertions, irrational authority, and self-interested purveyors, was fading out of most American families. Advertising constituted, then, a new but functionally identical force. It, too, involved isolated assertions, irrational authority, and pecuniary interest. Merely because the label was different, most people missed Malinowski's early insight that the way to identify superstition in a culture is precisely by function, and they did not see that advertising and superstition functioned identically. And of course in this case the identity was masked by people's familiarity with the bits-and-pieces approach, not to mention the sensationalizing tendencies, of journalism. Like conventional superstition, advertising relied upon authoritative assertions that were not only without context but defied religious and scientific views of the order of the universe and life. As with folk beliefs, common repetition gave life to commercials. Like primitive magical thinking, advertising, as many commentators noted, worked on fears and wishes. "A great deal of advertising," noted Federal Trade Commissioner Paul Rand Dixon in 1963, "is aimed at the optimism of the credulous rather than at the minds of the skeptical."[53]

This eerie resemblance between advertising and superstition did on occasion strike various commentators of the mid-and late twentieth century. One group of researchers, who were looking at science claims by advertisers late in the 1930s, observed, "The psychological reactions of the people concerned seem not unlike the reactions to common superstitions. Belief in the advertised product is deeply rooted in our American *mores* and most assiduously cultivated . . . by the sellers of commodities and the purveyors of advertising." When a group of Dallas teachers developed a "Science and Superstition Minicourse" in 1974, one of the tests of students' mastery was their ability to analyze ads, asking, were they reasonable, and were they ethical? But even observers who had seen the resemblance did not become fully aware of the significance of the parallels between superstition and advertising.[54]

In searching for a way of conceptualizing the place of advertising in twentieth-century American culture, Schudson has ingeniously described it as an art form. He rejects the suggestion of other commentators that advertising fulfills religious functions; after all, he points out, most adults find the gods of advertising ridiculous. Such an objection, however, does not apply to treating advertising as superstition, since ridiculousness does not necessarily impair superstitious belief. Moreover, advertising, unlike art, involves commercialism, if not cupidity. The consequences of art consumption are arguable; the impact of the forms and messages of advertising is not, although both, of course, operate in a nonrational world. The cognitive content of advertisements was not what was effective in changing behavior—even if one leaves to one side consumers' attitudes, which may be ineffective in determining actions. Researchers found, however, that repeated exposures to models of behavior did affect what people did—obviously creating a version of authority. Like superstition, advertising involves a personal authority, a special world view. What would happen, Joseph Agassi asks, if one were to remove superstition from superstitious people? They would be unable to think, he answers. A parallel question can be applied to consumers of advertising; without advertising, essential guidance would be missing from their lives. Furthermore, Agassi continues, superstitious people did not have to believe in the superstitions; purely attitudinal and behavioral bases sufficed. Physicist Niels Bohr, Agassi points out, enjoyed justifying his reliance on the lucky influence of horseshoes by saying that "he had it on good authority, it helps even when not believed in."[55]

It was in this functional sense, then, in attitude and behavior, that superstition won in the popular arena in the United States: through advertising, superstitious thinking and antirational authority to a substantial degree dominated the culture. Advertisers were engaged in remystifying the world, not demystifying it. Rationalists and skeptics were contained and diverted through specialization, and no serious public opposition appeared to challenge credulity of the most blatant kind. People who relied on the world of advertising did not need charms when they could obtain consumer goods that would protect them from various real and imaginary evils. Disdain for naturalistic thinking, by contrast, could not have been greater in the age of television commercials. And no naturalistic-positivistic view of the universe intruded upon people to suggest how to live their lives when the science that they did get came primarily from advertising and otherwise fragmented accounts, deprived of connections and rational context.

The Demise of the Man of Science

That superstition won tells, however, but part of the story of popularizing; the other part is how science lost—and particularly when popularization of science and health traditionally had consisted of a battle against superstition and error. What happened to the popularizers who for so long had fought against the forces of occultism and self-interested authority, indeed, who had even opposed their altruistic scientism to commercialism?

Science lost, as my narrative has shown, because the scientists left the field of popularization. The exceptions were an occasional surviving old-fashioned man or woman of science and some college-level teachers, especially the instructors in elementary psychology described in chapter 3. Harvard's E. G. Boring, for example, described the message of his World

War II popularization as "that man is a mechanism, that there are laws that govern his actions . . . that psychology is a great thing." But in general the mission to fight superstition brought out no conspicuous leaders; after all, most people, including professional scientists, did not perceive the extent to which superstitious thinking was flourishing in American society. Just at the beginning of the 1980s, especially, some specific concern about either error or anti-Darwinist legislation recruited a few eminent scientists into specifically corrective campaigns, along with the organized skeptics, but they seldom attempted popularization in the broader sense.[56]

The technically educated leaders who could have continued popularization in the traditional way in fact did not do so. Beyond their focus on "image," large numbers of researchers found their specialized worlds so far from even a high-class popular audience that it was easy to let other specialists, specialists in dealing with either adults or children, do the work and provide at least the guidance when a scientist did turn to a popular audience. As specialization, sophisticated quantification, uncertainty, and paradox alienated the popular level of understanding from that of the laboratory, the difficulties of filling the role of popularizer increased greatly for any investigator. By 1937, biologist Francis B. Sumner suggested that the job of informing the journalists about science should be left at least to the college teachers of elementary science who were used to translating. James R. Angell, the president of Yale, called the new popularized science not "unpopular science" but "non-popular science," noting, "Its significance is beyond the grasp of the average man."[57]

When such scientists stopped trying, and withdrew, popularization, as I have shown, fell into the hands of other kinds of translators, simplifiers, and nonscientific specialists. But beyond that, the cultural symbolism of popular science disintegrated—the idea that science stood for something: opposition to superstition, if not for a naturalistic "philosophy of life." Together the broader meaning of science and the spokespersons for science had both passed from the scene. "Who speaks for science?" asked Wallace Brode in 1966, as if it might be possible to do so. By then, he said, it could have been "not only the scientists, but also . . . the science writers, editors, review writers, abstractors, feature writers, science administrators, and popular science speakers." In fact, he said, people could not easily "identify the leader or authority, in broad areas of science, who [could] speak with the recognized support of the science community."[58]

Brode was not just voicing a nostalgia for a sense of community (a nostalgia not limited to scientists); he was reflecting the loss of the identity of science that earlier scientists had felt.

The retreat of the research elite from the arena of popularizing could be measured in many ways, as has been suggested by the foregoing chapters on health, psychology, and the natural sciences. Nor was the retreat always a willing one; the scientists' representatives struggled hard, for example, before commercialism overwhelmed their efforts at the New York World's Fair of 1939. But the direction of change was unmistakable. Perhaps the starkest index of cultural transformation was furnished by the American Medical Association when the leadership after the 1930s abandoned the effective and convincing fight against nostrums, quacks, and misleading advertising. By 1970, when a group surveying television content were looking for material for the public that was sponsored by organized medicine, the only items that showed up were four spot commercials dealing with socioeconomic aspects of medicine—commercials that the surveyors rated as "totally devoid of useful health information."[59]

It was, then, when the men of science left a vacuum in American society that journalists and educators proclaimed themselves the specialists who would carry out the function of popularizing science and health. By the mid-twentieth century, no significant body of bench or field scientists was willing to challenge the specialists. Where the primary- and secondary-level teachers often had the will to preach the religion of science, ultimately they had to make choices between it and the child-centered curriculum, choices that tempered the zeal that put science first. Just such a choice, for example, undermined the teaching of metrics, which were not "practical."[60] Even the family of curriculums associated with the new math, as I have suggested, made modifications only in material studied; enthusiasm was much harder to build in.

The influence of journalists, for their part, was altogether corrupting, turning high culture into trivial news items and reducing men of science to purveyors of bits and pieces of information. The founding director of Science Service, Slosson, was an excellent example, a truly transitional figure, as David J. Rhees has shown. While Slosson, a chemist before he was a writer and editor, was alarmed by the forces of occultism and superstition in American society, he chose to avoid direct attacks, for the most part, and instead tried to displace error from the media with sound science popularization. Although a person with ideals, passionately com-

mitted to uplifting the common man, Slosson thought that to be successful Science Service would have to compromise with the new mass media.
He personally believed in at least a conservative version of the religion of
science, but in his presentations he emphasized facts and utility at the expense of theory, fitting into the demands of journalism for short, concrete
items with snappy headlines. As he told the Science Service trustees in
1921, "We must go into the newspapers and their demand is for short
paragraphs ending in -*est*." In his collection *Chats on Science*, Slosson was
explicit in his intention to follow the journalistic format: "If the reader
finds a page dull he can skip over to another without fear of losing the
thread of the story," he wrote. "I have," he continued, "purposely mixed
up the pages lest the reader should be misled into thinking that he had got
engaged in a continuous treatise and so would be compelled by his conscience to read longer than he liked." By diluting urgent messages and
insights from the science he believed in, Slosson tragically helped move
popularization into the jurisdiction of journalism.[61]

Technicians Instead of Scientists

Especially after World War II, then, in science, health, and, slightly later,
psychology, as nonscientists preempted public forums, few practitioners
stood up to speak for science or the religion of science. All of this occurred in the face of a very great increase in the number of people in
clearly scientific occupations. As all observers noted at the time, Sumner
and Angell were correct: no one could speak up, because scientists had
become so specialized that each was limited to his or her own very narrow
area of expertise. As early as 1922 William Bateson described his fellow
geneticists in the United States as "pathetic in their simplicity, knowing
nothing whatever outside Genetics" and as nothing more than "machines
for grinding out genetics."[62]

Mere specialization and narrowness were not in themselves impene-
trable barriers to scientists' popularizing. In addition, the specialists suffered a failure of nerve. The combination of specialization with the lack of
zeal, however, was conclusive. Already in 1937, R. S. Mulliken of the
University of Chicago was complaining, "Even among scientists themselves, outside their own specialties, the scientific attitude is far too rare
and is never fully developed." A quarter of a century later, philosopher of

science Stephen Toulmin paralleled science to Babel: "an assemblage of skills—practical, technological skills, and theoretical, mathematic skills—rather than . . . 'natural philosophy.'"[63]

All of the signs came to point in the same direction: American scientists, as a whole, were behaving like mere technicians—competent in a narrow, technical field but without the vision or identity with a larger calling in society such as would move them to make a public profession of naturalism and skepticism. One of the older school in 1945 had suggested that scientists as scientists ought to take an oath: "I pledge that I will use my knowledge for the good of humanity and against the destructive forces of the world and the ruthless intent of men; and that I will work together with my fellow scientists of whatever nation, creed, or color, for these, our common ends." Despite the timely liberal preoccupations of the author, the oath suggests both mission and identity and contrasts with the new style of diploma that Conway Zirkle (a man of science) sarcastically suggested for the young scientist of 1955:

The Johns Hopkins University
certifies that
John Wentworth Doe
does *not* know anything but
Biochemistry.

Please pay no attention to any pronouncement he may make on any other subject, particularly when he joins with others of his kind to save the world from something or other.

However, he worked hard for this degree and is potentially a most valuable citizen. Please treat him kindly.[64]

One of the marks of the narrow technician was his or her unwillingness to go beyond facts—again reflective of the cultural regard for "information" as well as specialization. Because of specialization, complained a biologist in 1930, too many science courses perpetuated the worst of old-fashioned teaching and were still taught at the most primitive levels, that is, emphasizing the factual and authoritarian, without the enlightenment of what investigation meant. In succeeding decades, other commentators watched the population of scientists increase and their specialization intensify and remarked that the result was not only narrowness but mediocrity. In a highly fragmented, technical system, people flourished professionally who in another day would have been handicapped by insufficiency of breadth, to say nothing of their lacking the culture and calling of Victorian scientists who argued for science because it was culture. Some contemporary critics extended the critique to note the scholastic qualities of teachers and students alike in the era of narrow specialization. When institutionalized science, embodying the technical-technician element, came under attack for contributing to environmental irresponsibility, it was entirely appropriate to lament, as did one observer of his times, "Einstein is dead," meaning broad, culturally responsible representatives of science.[65]

Consequences of the Eclipse of the Men of Science

The traditional cultural role of the men and women of science, as I have tried to emphasize, had two aspects. One was positive: advocating and exemplifying naturalism and rationality. The other was reactive: campaigning against error, even taking the responsibility to correct every advocate of superstition and pseudoscience who received media attention. That the new scientist technicians did not work for "science as a way of life" was therefore but one aspect of the decline of popularization. As technicians they looked upon science as an isolated part of their lives, a part that did not impinge on other, obviously irrational aspects of their existence. As social psychologist Kimball Young was working to keep his colleagues in line in 1924, he noted a "disconcerting fact": "Very often among scientists themselves is found the most curious mixture of modernism in a specialized field coupled with an intense adherence to some medieval or primitive superstition which is unworthy of them." The narrower figures who came to dominate American science therefore did not even react to opportunities to take a stand that would involve enlightening members of the public. Inaction in the face of brazen challenge was hard to miss. Except in rare cases of personal interest such as the constantly recurring antivivisection campaign, people who in other ways passed for scientists stood silent or actually worked with the enemy, whether that enemy was in a new guise or an older one. No significant group of investigators objected when some of the American astronauts—real technicians whose feats media controllers believed represented science—while in space flagrantly and even defiantly carried out supposedly religious exercises in a superstitious manner, or when one of them in

1971 even attempted to carry out extrasensory perception "experiments" during the Apollo XIV flight. Another of the most illuminating, if not amusing, incidents of the 1980s was the confrontation among psychologists when the American Psychological Association acquired *Psychology Today* and yet continued to accept and publish cigarette and liquor ads—on the basis that it was necessary in order to finance sound popularization! The official statement of these psychologists explicitly renounced responsibility for deciding what should be presented to the public.[66]

Although the *Psychology Today* episode was so extreme that many psychologists did object strenuously and publicly, the point is not that intellectually limited technicians or writers, editors, and scientists entangled in journalistic goals were misrepresenting science and even serving as the dupes of the new superstition. The point is that usually no large numbers of the most able investigators stood up in the popular arena—or anywhere else—for a scientific attitude. The corrupt version of science that the commercial media portrayed, for example, was not challenged by scientist groups. They were organized and available and for decades could have brought the same effective pressures to bear as did various other minority and interest groups. But they did not. Their interests when public were political, and popularization therefore remained in other hands.[67]

The most obvious and flagrant failure of American scientists as a whole was their passivity in the face of the "creation science" challenge. To meet the offensive of the religious zealots of the 1920s, Maynard Shipley had mobilized a special group, the Science League of America, but, even more significant, all across the country scientists did not hesitate to speak out individually to try to popularize sound science. In mid-century and after, a more insidious—more insidious because deliberately mislabeled "science," like a patent medicine—form of antievolutionary influence arose. As these aggressive antievolutionists for years were winning local battles all over the country, the silence of professional scientists before unmistakable, old-fashioned obscurantism and irrationalism was remarkable. Only after very long delay did a few scientist groups finally mount an effort to oppose "creation science," but the ranks of tens of thousands of Americans who passed for scientists did not produce recruits to speak plainly in the language of popular science; rather what was noticeable was that a number of those who were occupationally "scientists" broke ranks and served the enemy. Once again, in the media world no one could tell what science was and what it stood for.[68]

With few restraints on what appeared as popularized science in any medium (with the partial exception of the *Scientific American* and the like, as will be noted again below), the condition of popular learning about science deteriorated in the United States. As sociologist Edward Shils pointed out, the incorporation of the masses into social institutions and the denigration of cultural authorities could not have any effect but dilution; the large numbers of scientists and technicians therefore really belonged in the mediocre, rather than the high, intelligentsia as they evolved in American society, and the tiers of popularization therefore tended also to become indistinguishable. Only such a conceptualization can encompass the results of surveys of the extent to which Americans, even those identified with science, were not sympathetic to rationalism, much less reductionism. Of the 20 percent of the public in the science-attentive group in 1981, for example, two-thirds believed that "creationist science" should receive equal time in the schools with real science, and the additional 19 percent in the interested public group (presumably sensitive to science) showed even more softness on this issue. The broad sci-tech community, in short, tended not to be remarkably different from the general adult population. Among all Americans, Daniel Yankelovich found that the 30 percent who in 1970 believed "everything has a scientific explanation" had shrunk to 27 percent a decade later, and the 42 percent who said that they had given up the belief that science would explain the mysteries of nature had increased to 48 percent.[69] Between advertising and all of this manifest irrationalism, it would be difficult to generate a more complete portrait of the victory of the forces of superstition.

Popularization as an Institutional Support

Such changes in popular science were neither trivial nor merely intellectual. Popularized science had served a number of important functions in American culture. For some groups, in the nineteenth century, learning about science had provided uplift, culture, and civilization, or at the least had opened up a route through which they could fulfill some of their aspirations. Cultural analysts from a later time viewed popularization and especially the rationalism and self-abnegation in health instruction and popular science as elements that helped many Americans mesh into the processes of modernization.[70] Even as late as the 1980s, researchers found evidence of the potential of contemporary popularization of science to help socialize members of the public and school children into supporting fluoridation or serving humanity in professional capacities.[71]

But popular science also had more specific institutional uses. Beyond the impact on the general public, sometimes understood as the better educated, sometimes as the masses needing guidance, popularized science was important to science as an organized activity. From the late nineteenth century, at least, scientists, both amateur and professional, were among the most avid consumers of popularization, and they depended upon it to encourage, define, and reinforce their scientific activities, whether at microscopists' soirees or in research laboratories. Propaganda for "the public" therefore turned out to have a profound effect not just on various parts of the public but also on scientists themselves. In important ways, popularized science helped confirm investigators in their choice of occupation and, for some of them for a time, at least, in their belief in the religion of science. By the twentieth century, as I have noted, what passed for popularized science was helping professionals keep up with science— if not one kind of biologist learning about an allied field in the *American Naturalist*, then physicians learning about medical and health advances from the mass media.[72]

It was in this context of bolstering the institutions of science that such publications as the *Scientific American*, not to mention the *American Scientist*, the *American Psychologist*, and similar professional publications, took on such importance in the mid-twentieth century and after. Publications that were popular but still addressed the technical rather than the mass audiences therefore acted as standard supports of science as an institution. Journalists could joke that even though the editors of the *Scientific American* did eliminate mathematical exposition from the articles, the technical content was still so difficult that the magazine had 700,000 subscribers but only 700 readers. Yet the material was more attractive than the journalists let on, and it helped define a world of science. The *American Scientist*, which did include mathematical formulas in the articles, performed a parallel service (and by 1960 had almost 100,000 circulation). This was the classic case of popularization that served a small part of the population but in an essential way, in this case also playing an institutional role in science.[73] Writers in such publications did not have to dip back as in Covert's spiral to catch the completely naive reader but could continually assume substantial background.

The most important function of popularizers, however, was to create and maintain the role of science through the impressions that they made upon younger Americans, explaining what it meant to join the ranks and serve science. Not only did popularization recruit students into science, but it shaped basic expectations of what their activities would consist of. Anne Roe's case histories of eminent scientists, for example, suggest the effect that one single book had in interesting young people in scientific careers: Slosson's *Creative Chemistry* (1919). Slosson's book showed the power of scientists to devise applied science solutions to human problems, from agriculture to metallurgy. He showed how discovery could be fun, exciting, and, at the same time, helpful to humankind, a combination that for some creative youngsters was very exciting.[74] Others who became scientists were inspired by other popularizations that conveyed the fascination of curiosity and discovery. Some, for example, were affected by the quest for intellectual purity and worldly power that John B. Watson stimulated in his popular expositions of behavioristic psychology. Still others were no doubt inspired by the Health Heroes series.[75] All of these recruits in turn helped shape the actual events in science a generation or two later.

Popularization as Optimistic Reassurance

While popularized science and health maintained and broadened American scientific endeavors, particularly through material aimed at better-educated or elite groups, nevertheless certain basic elements cut across elite and mass audience reactions. The underlying, persistent intellectual appeal of well-presented scientific exposition was an element that could never be ignored, from the fascination in the early nineteenth century that Rossiter and Greene documented (as I mentioned in chapter 4) to the glossy presentations of special-audience publications and even public television programs of a much more recent time. But beyond the intellectual fascination was an equally compelling appeal.

In the hopeful and expansive days of the nineteenth century and in the darker days of atomic terror, popularized science was optimistic in tone. The repeated theme of discovery and progress let the professional, amateur, and lay person alike share in one aspect of the world in which there was the excitement of the actual achievement of the new and the promise of more innovation—"new hope." The testimony of observers across the decades was consistent. The practical scientists of the early twentieth century, wrote philosopher G.T.W. Patrick in 1913, had a positive outlook: "The world is pretty good, and we will make it better." "Science news is *good* news," declared Watson Davis of Science Service in 1934. And in 1981, the publisher of *Science Digest* observed, "The new science magazines tell you that there is a future, that you can go on forever, that you're immortal. These new publications will be successful for the same reasons as the *National Enquirer*." Eventually the reassuring and pollyannish quality of popular science caught the attention of the editors of the *New Yorker*, who at midcentury reprinted with appropriate ironic comment a statement from *Science News-Letter*: "One reassuring feature of the nerve gas picture: While very dangerous to people, they are not destructive of property and facilities as atom bombs are."[76] Science fiction, too, originally embodied this same upbeat message. Altogether optimism was extremely appealing; one midcentury observer paralleled the popular science books of his day with *Peace of Mind* and *How to Stop Worrying*.[77]

The major changes in popularization in the twentieth century, then, were not in the appeal or attraction, for intellectual fascination and a sense of progress and discovery were always present. The changes lay in the elements that tended to drop out, and these elements tended to be absent from both mass media, general audience popularization, on the one hand, and internal, sci-tech community or professional materials, on the other.

The Loss of Passion and Skepticism

One of the characteristics of popularized science and health after it left the hands of the men of science was the disappearance of a critical amount of enthusiasm and passion. The goal of superficial objectivity, as in journalism, for instance, could subtly damage any presentation, but it was noticeably deadly when applied to textbooks. Textbook writers, complained the editor of the *American Journal of Physics*, were too pat and hid both error and adventuresomeness, in short the excitement of actually *doing* science; the result, he complained, "is that revolutionary ideas in physics simply do not appear to the student to be revolutionary." Even in the 1980s, an observer of the new science magazines noted that since journalists tried to avoid taking sides in scientific controversies, their writing was much less pungent and interesting than that of scientists who were not afraid to speak out.[78]

Another element that began to disappear in the mid-twentieth century was the identification of scientists with science (even though the identity "scientist" persisted in some of the popular materials; obviously that is why it is necessary to distinguish from that identity "men of science," who did identify with science). The psychologists, who still needed the "science" imprimatur, continued to talk about science and the scientific method. Writers in the *American Scientist* still sometimes discussed science as an entity, and even an ideal. But the list of such exceptions was very short. By contrast, articles in the midcentury *Scientific American*, for example, almost never included the word "science," and the scientists and other authors who published there identified all investigators by specialty (at most, general bacteriology, physics, and the like), and neither the person nor the activity described suggested any sense of science as an entity.[79] In general in the United States, the "scientific community" came to have political, not methodological or epistemological, meanings.[80]

For subject matter purposes, of course description of a person by specialty was more precise than identification with "science." The facts were well served. For evangelistic purposes, however, the religion of science was the loser and the technician identity the gainer. The problem was not just, as Brode (above) pointed out, that no one knew who spoke for science.[81] The problem was that for large parts of even the interested public, being a man or woman of science was no longer conceptually possible.

Beyond passion and identity, what was most critically missing from popularization, as the twentieth century wore on, was skepticism. And this casualty in the warfare between science and superstition was decisive in the outcome. Earlier popularizers had managed to connect progress in solving the mysteries of nature with traditional skepticism. Joseph Jastrow in 1902 described the scientific "habit of mind that makes one keen-scented for right beliefs and secure, not from error indeed, but from rash credulity." By contrast, the new hope science writers did not convey effectively even the routine doubts of the investigators; in practice, new hope from the products of science was antithetical to a skeptical way of thinking.[82]

At one time, skepticism had been the weapon with which science advocates had labeled belief in superstition (and in the claims of advertising) socially deviant, at least among well-educated people.[83] As the narrative above has shown, by the late twentieth century, those who attempted to speak for science no longer tried to mobilize the skepticism that existed in either scientific personnel or the population in general; only rarely, as in the consumer movement or some small element's outrage at various, usually traditional, credulities, did any individual scientist speak up in the name of science, or even of controlled experiments, to challenge the authorities of the media.[84] The unrelenting campaign of scientists to upgrade journalistic treatments of science had long since died out; the best that they could do was to improve the quality of information available for journalists to use, especially since media scientist personalities were reduced to mere undifferentiated authorities. What skepticism there was, was directed often against science and medicine and other institutions and professions, not against either folk or commercial error.[85]

In 1904, astronomer Edward S. Holden wrote, "The mass of men believe that religion has come out vanquished, humiliated, and discredited from a long warfare with triumphant science." Within the ranks of cultivated Americans early in the twentieth century, there was much truth in Holden's hyperbole: in popularized science and health, the men of science had self-serving mysticism and superstition on the run. Half a century later, the advocates of science were divided and in confusion, largely unaware that the forces of conflicting irrational authority and commercial interest largely determined the form and tendency of delivering popularized science. The journalistic-advertising mode of presenting disconnected news about the products of the laboratory confused everyone, but one development was clear: the proponents of science no longer occupied the moral high ground. How could they, when scientists no longer believed in the religion of science but sent public relations mercenaries to fight the battles? As early as 1938, the English popularizer, Lancelot Hogben, believed that the failure of nerve and lack of faith that he was seeing grew out of a pessimistic and elitist view of mankind: "In the Victorian age big men of science like Faraday, T. H. Huxley and Tyndall did not think it beneath their dignity to write about simple truths with the conviction that they could *instruct* their audiences. . . . The key to the eloquent literature which the pen of Faraday and Huxley produced is their firm faith in the educability of mankind."[86] It was that kind of faith that was lacking in mid- and late twentieth-century American researchers.

Defection of Allies

Beginning at the end of the days of the men of science, two stages in the disintegration of the great popularizing effort emerge from my narrative. The high point of the men and religion of science lasted into the twentieth century, despite the rise of the mass media. In the first phase of disintegration, the journalistic mode began to dominate popularization, but the crusade against superstition persisted, particularly in the hands of a number of educators who were in fact still holding the moral high ground.[87] In the second stage, even that legacy, and with it the struggle against superstition, was lost, and not only journalistic bits and pieces but advertising sensationalism set the tone for all of American culture, including science. Ultimately there was little opposition to these trends, either from scientific personnel or from other intellectual elements.

Indeed, many influential Americans of various cultural levels responded to cultural cues and actually attacked the self-denying discipline of scientific endeavors. Important intellectuals denied the validity of narrowly focused research. Other elements found the restrictive and controlled style of science repugnant, and they rejected it along with the ideal of civilization and civilized behavior that had traditionally been part of the advocacy of the religion of science. The prominence of these critics of science—whose opinions often appeared in both highbrow and mass media—of course affected workers in health and science and created an unfriendly environment for popularization that had any advocacy, much less reductionism, in it.[88]

Intellectuals of the last period, influenced especially by technically shrewd philosophers of science, tried to show how a crude or naive, or even not naive, scientism, by which they meant the religion of science (not merely forms and products, as in Whalen's definition of popular scientism), was defective on many grounds, not least those of epistemology and metaphysics. The intellectuals' demands for rigor of thinking were effective in a negative way, but their positive ideas did not reach investigators in other fields who were, or at least could have been, the descendants of the men of science. Particularly absent was the optimistic belief that scientific rationalism could replace magical thinking. Instead, the message of the best thinkers was that only in technical detail was science respectable—that the ideal of science was a delusion. "The term, 'The Scientific Method,' has . . . become taboo," complained R. R. Haun of Drake University in 1960, and he observed also that college-level liberal arts survey courses in science had died out. A generation later, two researchers who, contrary to custom, did speak out in the name of science to denounce occultism, concluded that there was at least one reason for the weakness of scientists in the face of an obvious challenge:

Many students have the impression that science is entirely subjective and unable to assess or predict the validity of ideas, apparently on the basis of limited exposure to philosophers such as Polanyi, Hanson, and Kuhn. In presenting perspectives on science in our classrooms, we have perhaps overdone the critical view of the validity of our knowledge. . . . Students attribute more empirical validity to philosophy than to science itself. . . . We do not read these philosophers as subscribing to the total subjectivity of science, and we do not believe they would subscribe to such a position. It would seem a service to speak more plainly and more assertively about science's track record.[89]

Some of the debunkers of the naive religion of science pulled back a little when they saw the direction of their efforts, saying that the ideal of objectivity and rationality should be preserved, even though everyone knows that scientists cannot fulfill the ideal.[90] But, as in the cases of the students just noted, this message of sophisticated enlightenment did not translate well. It did not furnish, on the popular level, a basis on which either a scientist or a nonscientist could address life and the universe. Instead, the philosophers made a major contribution to the failure of nerve, so that relatively well educated scientists in particular were afraid to believe in science enough to enter into warfare against error and superstition.[91]

What was particularly and vitally missing from the work of the philosophers was, again, the keen sense of the negative element that had always animated the popularizers of science. The chic intellectual critics turned their skepticism against the late nineteenth-century ideal of science, not against superstition, mysticism, and commercial exploitation.[92]

Even in the 1980s, there were still a few men and women of science who had a sense of identification with science as a way to truth, civilization, morality, and other constructive values—and a high contempt for commercialism of any kind, much less mysticism, irrationalism, or occultism. Many represented their generation's quota of irrepressible skeptics, hardheaded nay-sayers deviant enough to speak out in both the lab and a public forum to enlighten one part or another of the public. Some may even have retained, like Voltaire and the other Encyclopedists of the eighteenth century, a sense of the danger that superstition could overturn an empire and its culture.

But these surviving men and women of science were swamped numerically by other scientists who at most counted some sort of political or professional association work, that is, bureaucratic activity, as their service to science. More likely, these "scientists" were in fact narrow technicians who did a job without a calling. In either case, such professionals did not struggle with other population elements for possession of the public mantle of science. Nor did they feel personally the obligation to · pick a fight with superstition, pseudoscience, or advertising. The chances were that they did not even know what civilization was, or perhaps science as such. Few Americans of that era did, whether or not part of the science-attentive public. Nowhere had the technical training, the education, or the milieu of the technicians prepared them for an obligation to summarize, simplify, or translate science for any nonspecialist audiences. Indeed, in functional terms, science probably did not exist any longer on the popular level. Superstition did.

Notes

Chapter 1: Superstition and the Popularizing of Science

1. General introductions to the popularization of science in the United States include Matthew D. Whalen, "Science, the Public, and American Culture: A Preface to the Study of Popular Science," *Journal of American Culture*, 4 (1981), 14–26; Annette M. Woodlief, "Science," in M. Thomas Inge, ed., *Concise Histories of American Popular Culture* (Westport, CT: Greenwood Press, 1982), pp. 354–362. Comparative perspective is provided especially in B. Dixon, "Telling the People: Science in the Public Press Since the Second World War," in A. J. Meadows, ed., *Development of Science Publishing in Europe* (Amsterdam: Elsevier Science Publishers, 1980), pp. 215–235. See also Robert Fox, "The Scientist and His Public in Nineteenth-Century France," *Social Science Information*, 21 (1982), 697–718. J. L. Crammer, "Popularization of Science through Cheap Books," *Illinois Libraries*, 31 (1949), 390, notes that foreigners often saw American popularizations as propaganda or attempts to further economic penetration of other countries. In the chapters that follow, a more cultural point of view will be taken.

2. A late interesting example is a chapter, "A Workable Philosophy of Life," in a health textbook, Thurman Brooks Rice, *Living* (Chicago: Scott, Foresman and Company, 1940), chap. 27.

3. Eugene E. Levitt, "Superstitions: Twenty-Five Years Ago and Today," *American Journal of Psychology*, 65 (1952), 443–449; Levitt cites much of the earlier literature on this subject.

4. It may be that the phenomenon in a postindustrial society is not different from that found in developing countries in which two wildly incompatible belief systems do in fact coexist not only in the same cultures but in very large numbers of individuals; see, for example, the summary in Warren O. Hagstrom, "The Production of Culture in Science," in Richard A. Peterson, ed., *The Production of Culture* (Beverly Hills: Sage Publications, 1976), pp. 102–103.

5. Marcello Truzzi, "The Occult Revival as Popular Culture: Some Random Reflections on the Old and Noveau Witch," *Sociological Quarterly*, 13 (1972), 16–36, and the perceptive essays in Howard Kerr and Charles L. Crow, eds., *The*

Occult in America: New Historical Perspectives (Urbana: University of Illinois Press, 1983). Mervin Block, "Flapdoodle Writ Large: Astrology in Magazines," *Columbia Journalism Review* (Summer 1969), 51–54. The phenomenon of the 1960s and 1970s probably is best conceptualized as a social phenomenon rather than a direct comment on superstition per se; see, for example, Frederick R. Lynch, "Toward a Theory of Conversion and Commitment to the Occult," *American Behavioral Scientist*, 20 (1977), 887–908; Stuart H. Blum, "Some Aspects of Belief in Prevailing Superstitions," *Psychological Reports*, 38 (1976), 579–582. Daniel Lawrence O'Keefe, *Stolen Lightning, The Social Theory of Magic* (New York: Continuum, 1982), pp. 568–569, notes the growing financial base of the occult revival. He also (p. 566) notes that "magic is always in some measure a game of 'acting as if;' even the magician is skeptical."

6. C. June Gregory, "Changes in Superstitious Beliefs among College Women," *Psychological Reports*, 37 (1975), 939–944, which contains an extensive list of relevant references.

7. Beginning in the late 1970s, a running bibliography on various contemporary credulities appeared in the *Skeptical Inquirer*. O'Keefe, *Stolen Lightning*, comments on antiscientific aspects of the magical aspects of superstition throughout his encyclopedic analysis of magic.

8. Karl E. Scheibe and Theodore R. Sarbin, "Toward a Theoretical Conceptualisation of Superstition," *British Journal for the Philosophy of Science*, 16 (1965), 143–158.

9. Chester H. Rowell, "The Cancer of Ignorance," *Survey*, 55 (1925), 159. O'Keefe, *Stolen Lightning*, p. 475, makes a similar point in a different context.

10. E.g., James R. Moore, *The Post-Darwinian Controversies: A Study of the Protestant Struggle to Come to Terms with Darwin in Great Britain and America, 1870–1900* (Cambridge: Cambridge University Press, 1979); Frank M. Turner, "The Victorian Conflict between Science and Religion: A Professional Dimension," *Isis*, 69 (1978), 356–358; David B. Wilson, "Victorian Science and Religion," *History of Science*, 15 (1977), 52–67.

11. Compare, for example, these early instances, long before the Darwinian debates: "Warfare of Misguided Zeal upon Science," *Knickerbocker*, 8 (1836), 666–674; "G.W.M.," "Geology—Its Facts and Inferences," *Universalist Quarterly and General Review*, 2 (1845), 5–21. James Thompson Bixby, "Science and Religion as Allies," *Popular Science Monthly*, 9 (1876), 690; Bixby, Wundt's first American Ph.D., believed that one service of science to religion was to defeat superstition. "The Warfare of Science," *Popular Science Monthly*, 39 (1891), 695. R. M. Wenley, "Science and Philosophy," *Popular Science Monthly*, 59 (1901), 361–372. John J. O'Shea, "'New Theology,' Old Superstition, and Modern Science," *American Catholic Quarterly*, 32 (1907), 222. Horace B. English, "The Conflict between Science and Religion," *Scientific Monthly*, 23 (1926), 423–426; the latter was only one of a flurry of "warfare" comments inspired by the Scopes case

(1925). See Willard B. Gatewood, Jr., *Controversy in the Twenties—Fundamentalism, Modernism, and Evolution* (Nashville: Vanderbilt University Press, 1969), pp. 148–153. Donald F. Brod, "The Scopes Trial: A Look at Press Coverage after Forty Years," *Journalism Quarterly*, 42 (1965), 219–226. William Ernest Hocking, "Illicit Naturalizing of Religion," *Journal of Religion*, 3 (1923), 561–589. See also John C. Burnham, "The Encounter of Christian Theology with Deterministic Psychology and Psychoanalysis," *Bulletin of the Menninger Clinic*, 49 (1985), 321–352.

12. E.g., John Fiske, *Edward Livingston Youmans, Interpreter of Science for the People* (1894; repr. Freeport, NY: Books for Libraries Press, 1972), pp. 244, 246. Walter C. Kraatz, "Pseudoscience and Antiscience in an Age of Science," *Ohio Journal of Science*, 58 (1958), 263. The issue still was not dead in the 1970s; see Edward E. Daub, "Demythologizing White's *Warfare of Science and Theology*," *American Biology Teacher*, 40 (1978), 553–556; Morris H. Goran, *Science and Anti-Science* (Ann Arbor: Ann Arbor Science Publications, 1974), pp. 15–21.

13. John William Draper, *History of the Conflict between Religion and Science* (1874; repr. New York: D. Appleton and Company, 1890); Andrew Dickson White, *A History of the Warfare of Science with Theology in Christendom* (2 vols., New York: D. Appleton and Company, 1896). A contemporary protest against confusing religion with superstition in the warfare was "Superstition in Religion and Science," *Open Court*, 2 (1889), 837–839.

14. G.E.R. Lloyd, *Early Greek Science, Thales to Aristotle* (New York: W. W. Norton & Company, 1970), especially pp. 9–10; G.E.R. Lloyd, *Magic, Reason, and Experience* (New York: Cambridge University Press, 1979). Francis Adams, ed. and trans., *The Genuine Works of Hippocrates* (2 vols., London: The Sydenham Society, 1849), 2: 843.

15. See in general Keith Thomas, *Religion and the Decline of Magic* (New York: Charles Scribner's Sons, 1971). Bert Hansen, "The Complementarity of Science and Magic before the Scientific Revolution," *American Scientist*, 74 (1986), 128–136. A. D. Wright, "The People of Catholic Europe and the People of Anglican England," *Historical Journal*, 18 (1975), 451–456. Margaret J. Osler, "Certainty, Scepticism, and Scientific Optimism: The Roots of Eighteenth-Century Attitudes toward Scientific Knowledge," in Paula Backscheider, ed., *Probability, Time, and Space in Eighteenth-Century Literature* (New York: AMS Press, 1979), pp. 3–28.

16. Thomas, *Religion and the Decline of Magic*; the quotation from Stephen is on p. 69. Thomas goes on to point out that after the Reformation the emphasis on self-help, in which humans looked out for themselves, opened the way for technological means to substitute for magic. James Turner, *Without God, Without Creed: The Origins of Unbelief in America* (Baltimore: Johns Hopkins University Press, 1985), especially p. 79.

17. Herbert Leventhal, *In the Shadow of the Enlightenment: Occultism and Renais-*

sance Science in Eighteenth-Century America (New York: New York University Press, 1967). Jon Butler, "Magic, Astrology, and the Early American Religious Heritage, 1600–1760," *American Historical Review*, 84 (1979), 317–346. The way in which theology and science came together in natural theology is taken up in chapter 4.

18. William A. Hammond, *On Certain Conditions of Nervous Derangement, Somnambulism—Hypnotism—Hysteria & Hysterical Affections, Etc.* (1881; repr. New York: G. P. Putnam's Sons, 1883), p. 229.

19. Proscience skeptics, ironically, often propagandized with evangelical fervor and even used the religious forms with which they, and everyone else, were familiar; the resulting confusion is alluded to below.

20. Marcus Selden Goldman, "Sidney and Harrington as Opponents of Superstition," *Journal of English and Germanic Philology*, 54 (1955), 526–548. J. Bronowski, *Magic, Science, and Civilization* (New York: Columbia University Press, 1978), places this tradition in another version of the development of modern science.

21. Compare, for example, Paolo Rossi, *Francis Bacon: From Magic to Science*, trans. Sacha Rabinovitch (Chicago: University of Chicago Press, 1968), especially chaps. 1–2, with the American nineteenth century described in George H. Daniels, *American Science in the Age of Jackson* (New York: Columbia University Press, 1968). Kendrick Frazier, "Editor's Afterword," *Skeptical Inquirer* (Fall 1979), 80.

22. Elihu Palmer, *Principles of Nature; Or, A Development of the Moral Causes of Happiness and Misery among the Human Species* (New York: n.p., 1801), pp. iv–v. Turner, *Without God, Without Creed,* in general deals with the history of unbelief, which is only partly the history of skepticism.

23. Turner, *Without God, Without Creed.* Albert P. Mathews, "Science and Morality," *Popular Science Monthly*, 74 (1909), 284.

24. Both translation and context are from John Frederick Logan, "Superstition, Impiety, and an Enlightened Legal Order: The Theological Politics of the Abbé Mably," in W. Warren Wagar, ed., *The Secular Mind: Transformations of Faith in Modern Europe* (New York: Holmes & Meier, 1982), especially pp. 56–57. Italics in original (and in all other quotations unless otherwise noted).

25. Jerome Rosenthal, "Voltaire's Philosophy of History," *Journal of the History of Ideas*, 16 (1955), 151–178.

26. Gregory, "Changes in Superstitious Beliefs."

27. A partial exception might be satanism, but even there belief tended to consist of a series of related, but not systematic, authoritative assertions.

28. E.g., A. Lesser, "Superstition," *Journal of Philosophy*, 28 (1931), 617–628. Theodore Roszak, "On the Contemporary Hunger for Wonders," *Michigan Quarterly Review*, 19 (1980), 311–321. A. R. Kantor, "Logic and Superstition," *Journal of Philosophy*, 29 (1932), 234. By the 1970s it was clear that rebellion against au-

thority could include rejection of anything other than subjective feelings; see, for example, George Sheehan, *Running and Being: The Total Experience* (New York: Warner Books, 1978).

29. Lynn Thorndike, "Censorship by the Sorbonne of Science and Superstition in the First Half of the Seventeenth Century," *Journal of the History of Ideas*, 16 (1955), 119–125. John Immerwahr, "The Failure of Hume's Treatise," *Hume Studies*, 3 (1977), 57–71.

30. As will be noted in chapter 6, in the twentieth century a similar fate befell aggressive proponents of science.

31. Horatio Hackett Newman, *Outline of General Zoology* (New York: The Macmillan Company, 1924), pp. 11–12; other examples are Agnes Repplier, "On the Benefits of Superstition," *Atlantic Monthly*, 58 (1886), 177–186; A. W. Meyer, "Reflections on Credulity," *Scientific Monthly*, 24 (1927), 530–536. Robert S. Carroll, "Professional Contributions to Invalidism," *Scientific Monthly*, 2 (1916), 83. Fletcher Bascomb Dresslar, "Superstition and Education," *University of California Publications, Education*, 5 (1907), 1–239. Otis W. Caldwell and Gerhard E. Lundeen, "Students' Attitudes Regarding Unfounded Beliefs," *Science Education*, 15 (1931), 246–266. An excellent example tying psychopathology to other types of deviance is Iago Galdston, "The Psychodynamics of the Triad, Alcoholism, Gambling, and Superstition," *Mental Hygiene*, 35 (1951), 589–598. A more modern version was psychologists' labeling nonadaptive behavior in pigeons "superstition"; see, for example, John Oliver Cook, "'Superstition' in the Skinnerian," *American Psychologist*, 18 (1963), 516–518. L. J. Vance, "Superstition in American Life," *Open Court*, 3 (1889), 1823. Claudia de Lys, *A Treasury of American Superstition* (New York: The Philosophical Library, 1948), p. ix, offered readers a "mental flight into the past." Magical thinking was of course a standard category in psychopathology.

32. This phenomenon was noticed as early as the 1890s: Elizabeth Ferguson Seat, "The Survival of Superstition," *Lippincott's Monthly Magazine*, 56 (1895), 428–431. *New York Times*, December 6, 1930, p. 5.

33. Dresslar, "Superstition and Education," p. 231. Victor C. Smith, "Science Methods and Superstition," *School & Society*, 31 (1930), 66–68. John Dewey was of course already the most influential advocate of this general point of view. O. U. Vicklund, "The Elimination of Superstition in Junior High School Science," *Science Education*, 24 (1940), 93–99.

34. Edward Sutfin, "Bacon's Opinion of His Predecessors," *New Scholasticism*, 18 (1944), 147–184. Rossi, *Francis Bacon*, especially chap. 2. Robert G. Ingersoll, "Why Am I an Agnostic?" *North American Review*, 149 (1889), 744. Compare [Paul Carus], "Superstition in Religion and Science," *Open Court*, 2 (1888–1889), 837–839. Those opposed to religious authority in general tended not to recognize that traditional theology was reasonable.

35. Frederick Lewis Allen, *Only Yesterday: An Informal History of the Nineteen-*

268 Notes to Pages 22–23

Twenties (1931; repr. New York: Perennial Library, 1964), p. 166. This passage is often quoted in textbooks.

36. Emily C. Davis, "A Maze of Superstitions: The Age-Old Battle between Enlightened Medicine and Superstitious 'Cures' Is by No Means at an End," *Science News-Letter*, 35 (1939), 138–140.

37. Roger C. Smith, "Popular Misconceptions Concerning Natural History," *Scientific Monthly*, 10 (1920), 163. The magnitude of the partisan forces, or at least their cultural importance, is suggested to some extent in chapters 3–5, but in general the point here is the manifestation of popularization rather than the particular size of the groups involved.

38. Nathan Reingold, "Definitions and Speculations: The Professionalization of Science in America in the Nineteenth Century," in Alexandra Oleson and Sanborn C. Brown, eds., *The Pursuit of Knowledge in the Early American Republic* (Baltimore: Johns Hopkins University Press, 1976), pp. 33–69, attempts to define the scientific community and its adherents in terms appropriate for that day. See also Matthew D. Whalen and Mary F. Tobin, "Periodicals and the Popularization of Science in America, 1860–1910," *Journal of American Culture*, 3 (1980), 195–200.

39. Lincoln C. Blake, "The Concept and Development of Science at the University of Chicago, 1890–1905" (doctoral diss., University of Chicago, 1966). Statements from the full bloom of the movement included John Merle Coulter, "The Scientific Spirit," *Educational Bi-Monthly*, 1 (1907), 293–299, and William Graham Sumner, "The Scientific Attitude of Mind," in *Earth-Hunger and Other Essays* (New Haven: Yale University Press, 1913), pp. 17–28.

40. J. A. Cummings, *First Lessons in Geography and Astronomy, With Seven Plain Maps and a View of the Solar System, For the Use of Young Children as Preparatory to Ancient and Modern Geography* (Boston: Cummings and Hilliard, 1818), p. 82.

41. Donald Fleming, *John William Draper and the Religion of Science* (1950; repr. New York: Octagon Books, 1972), constitutes a revealing case history. This was substantially different from that described in Donald Harvey Meyer, "Paul Carus and the Religion of Science," *American Quarterly*, 14 (1962), 597–607; Carus, who had a European background, compromised more with religion than most American enthusiasts. David Tyack and Elisabeth Hansot, *Managers of Virtue: Public School Leadership in America, 1820–1980* (New York: Basic Books, 1982). Turner, *Without God, Without Creed*. A. Hunter Dupree, "Christianity and the Scientific Community in the Age of Darwin," in David C. Lindberg and Ronald L. Numbers, eds., *God and Nature: Historical Essays on the Encounter between Christianity and Science* (Berkeley: University of California Press, 1986), pp. 351–368. A strong characterization of the religious equivalent of science is in James Oliver Robertson, *American Myth, American Reality* (New York: Hill & Wang, 1980), p. 280.

42. Robertson, *American Myth, American Reality*. Dupree, "Christianity and the Scientific Community"; the term appears to have been dropped from the published version, but Dupree's discussion makes the point. A surprisingly frank example of the Nature cult was by a National Bureau of Standards scientist, Paul R. Heyl, in "The Solid Ground of Nature," *Scientific Monthly*, 25 (1927), 25–33. In the history of thought the separation of science and faith has a long history. Maurice Mandelbaum, *History, Man, and Reason: A Study in Nineteenth-Century Thought* (Baltimore: Johns Hopkins University Press, 1971), especially pp. 30–31, for example, traces this separation to Kant. But on the popular level such formal ideas were not of substantial importance.

43. Howard N. Brown, "Modern Superstition," *Unitarian Review*, 3 (1875), 50–51.

44. [C. W. Eliot], "Popularizing Science," *Nation*, 4 (1867), 34. Herbert N. Casson, *The Crime of Credulity* (New York: Peter Eckler, 1901), p. 89. Bromide of potassium was a standard treatment in mental diseases at that time.

45. William J. Wainwright, *Mysticism: A Study of Its Nature, Cognitive Value and Moral Implications* (Madison: University of Wisconsin Press, 1981), pp. 5–7, distinguishes between occult or magical aspects of mysticism and religious mysticism proper. The Victorian popularizers of science had in mind, of course, only commonplace mysticism.

46. This frequently cited example is explicated in I. Bernard Cohen, "The Fear and Distrust of Science in Historical Perspective: Some First Thoughts," in Andrei S. Markovits and Karl W. Deutsch, eds., *Fear of Science—Trust in Science: Conditions for Change in the Climate of Opinion* (Cambridge, MA: Oelge Schlager, Gunn & Hain, 1980), pp. 29–58. E. P. Evans, "Recent Recrudescence of Superstition," *Popular Science Monthly*, 48 (1895), 92.

47. J. W. Powell, "Certitudes and Illusions: Chuar's Illusion," *Science*, n.s. 3 (1896), 263–271. See especially Daniels, *American Science in the Age of Jackson*. In Americans' opposition to arid scholasticism and their devotion to facts lay also a bias in favor of practical results; see below. For example, Gerhard E. Lundeen and Otis W. Caldwell, "A Study of Unfounded Beliefs among High School Seniors," *Journal of Educational Research*, 22 (1930), 257n.

48. Edwin E. Slosson, *Chats on Science* (New York: The Century Co., 1924), pp. 190–191.

49. "From Superstition to Humbug," *Science*, 2 (1883), 637. "Clearing House," *Journal of Adult Education*, 6 (1934), 324. Cyril H. Hancock, "An Evaluation of Certain Popular Science Misconceptions," *Science Education*, 24 (1940), 208–213.

50. Asa Gray to R. W. Church, August 22, 1869, quoted in A. Hunter Dupree, *Asa Gray, 1810–1888* (1959; repr. New York: Atheneum, 1968), p. 340, and an 1860 commentator, "Darwin and His Reviewers," *Atlantic Monthly*, 6 (1860), 424, both noted that "the English mind is prone to positivism and kindred forms of materialistic philosophy . . . ," as the latter put it.

51. Charles A. McMurry and Lida B. McMurry, *Special Method in Natural Science for the First Four Grades of the Common School* (3rd ed., Bloomington, IL: Public-School Publishing Company, 1899), p. 28. Basic distinctions noted by Frederick Gregory, *Scientific Materialism in Nineteenth Century Germany* (Dordrecht: D. Reidel Publishing Company, 1977), especially pp. 1–10, were not well observed in American popularization, but connections to skepticism, optimism, and antiauthoritarianism were.

52. "The Domain of Science," *Popular Science Monthly*, 35 (1889), 842.

53. See especially the analysis of William E. Leverette, Jr., "Science and Values: A Study of Edward L. Youmans' *Popular Science Monthly*" (doctoral diss., Vanderbilt University, 1963), especially pp. 131–133; the points were mostly already explicit in "Purpose and Plan of Our Enterprise," *Popular Science Monthly*, 1 (1872), 113–115.

54. W. M. Davis, "The Reasonableness of Science," *Harvard Graduates' Magazine*, 31 (1922), 5. John Trowbridge, "The Study of Physics in the Secondary School," *Popular Science Monthly*, 15 (1879), 165. Jennie Mohr, *A Study of Popular Books in the Physical Sciences* (New York: [Columbia University dissertation], 1942), pp. 7–12.

55. Again, this emphasis on method was a viewpoint soon well known in education from the teachings of John Dewey. See especially David A. Hollinger, *Morris R. Cohen and the Scientific Ideal* (Cambridge, MA: The MIT Press, 1975). [E. L. Youmans], review of Helmholtz, *Popular Lectures on Scientific Subjects*, in *Popular Science Monthly*, 3 (1873), 514. S. B. Barnes and R.G.A. Dolby, authors of "The Scientific Ethos: A Deviant Viewpoint," *Archives Européannes Sociologiques*, 11 (1970), 3–25, note the credal nature of the "norms" of science and the fact that they flourished when the warfare between science and religion was particularly active.

56. Mohr, *A Study of Popular Books*.

57. For example, Stow Persons, *The Decline of American Gentility* (New York: Columbia University Press, 1973); Morton White, *Social Thought in America: The Revolt against Formalism* (2nd ed., Boston: Beacon Press, 1957).

58. William P. Atkinson, "Liberal Education of the Nineteenth Century," *Popular Science Monthly*, 4 (1873), 1–26. Turner, *Without God, Without Creed*, traces these general trends.

59. Whalen and Tobin, "Periodicals and the Popularization," p. 200. J. B. Maller and G. E. Lundeen, "Superstition and Emotional Maladjustment," *Journal of Educational Research*, 27 (1934), 592–617. David Starr Jordan, "Science and Sciosophy," *Science*, 59 (1924), 569. The early twentieth-century perspective is described from various points of view in Charles William Heywood, "Scientists and Society in the United States, 1900–1940: Changing Concepts of Social Responsibility" (doctoral diss., University of Pennsylvania, 1954); Ronald C. Tobey, *The*

American Ideology of National Science, 1919–1930 (Pittsburgh: University of Pittsburgh Press, 1971); and Hollinger, *Morris R. Cohen*. This theme is also explored further in chapter 5.

60. Michael Sokal, "James McKeen Cattell and the Failure of Anthropometric Mental Testing, 1890–1901," in William R. Woodward and Mitchell Ash, eds., *The Problematic Science: Psychology in Nineteenth-Century Thought* (New York: Praeger, 1982), p. 323, first alerted me to the importance of the category "man of science." The concept has a venerable history; see, for example, Moody E. Prior, "Bacon's Man of Science," *Journal of the History of Ideas*, 15 (1954), 348–370; Herbert Spencer, *Education: Intellectual, Moral, and Physical* (New York: D. Appleton and Company, [1860]), p. 82, puts the concept in the context that "true science is essentially religious." Ritchie Calder, "Common Understanding of Science," *Impact of Science on Society*, 14 (1964), 180.

61. See, for example, "Popular Psychology," *Science*, 7 (1886), 106; Truman Lee Kelly, "Mental Traits of Men of Science," in Leo E. Saidla and Warren E. Gibbs, eds., *Science and the Scientific Mind* (New York: McGraw-Hill Book Company, 1930), pp. 220–222.

62. "Narrowness among Men of Science," *Popular Science Monthly*, 12 (1877), 108. Years later T. C. Mendenhall, "The Relations of Men of Science to the General Public," *Popular Science Monthly*, 38 (1890), 19–31, was still urging participation.

63. C. E. Vail, "Our Duty to the Future," *Scientific Monthly*, 3 (1916), 585. In an introductory lecture at Johns Hopkins University, biologist Newell Martin, "The Study and Teaching of Biology," *Popular Science Monthly*, 10 (1876), 301, noted that the man of science need not be a great investigator, but could be only a humble worker (or soldier): "That an army may attain its best success, needs indeed that every man be brave and loyal, but it is by no means required that every soldier be a brigadier-general; so in the army of Science there is a place for soldiers of all ranks and capabilities."

64. E.g., Josiah P. Cook, Jr., "Scientific Culture," *Popular Science Monthly*, 7 (1875), 513–531.

65. John M. Coulter, "Nature Study and Intellectual Culture," *Science*, n.s. 4 (1896), 742; Wesley C. Mitchell, "The Public Relations of Science," *Science*, 90 (1939), 604–605. Turner, *Without God, Without Creed*, gives the background for the moralistic trend.

66. Quoted in Charles M. Haar, "E. L. Youmans: A Chapter in the Diffusion of Science in America," *Journal of the History of Ideas*, 9 (1948), 199. A good example is Mendenhall, "The Relation of Men of Science." Hollinger, *Morris R. Cohen*. The English background, always a model for American intellectuals, is summarized in Turner, "The Victorian Conflict."

67. Daniels, *American Science in the Age of Jackson*, p. 40. [Orville Dewey],

"Diffusion of Knowledge," *North American Review*, 30 (1830), 295, 297. See the interesting distinction between "diffusion of science," in which it is unchanged, as opposed to "transmission of science," in which ideas evolved as they passed from person to person, in R.G.A. Dolby, "The Transmission of Science," *History of Science*, 15 (1977), 1–43.

68. See the first part of this chapter. Owsei Temkin, "Health Education through the Ages," *American Journal of Public Health*, 30 (1940), 1091–1095, shows the long tradition, before the nineteenth century, of the connection between the fight against superstition and the development of health popularization to improve the condition of the masses.

69. Charles Sayle, ed., *The Works of Sir Thomas Browne* (2 vols., Edinburgh: John Grant, 1912), especially 1: 140. Toby Gelfand, "Demystification and Surgical Power in the French Enlightenment," *Bulletin of the History of Medicine*, 57 (1983), 216–217, gives an important early general example of the use of popularizing and publicizing to undermine superstition and establish the authority of science.

70. Thomas Dick, *On the Improvement of Society by the Diffusion of Knowledge; or, An Illustration of the Advantages which Would Result from a More General Dissemination of Rational and Scientific Information Among All Ranks* (Philadelphia: Edward C. Biddle, 1842 [the book had several American editions]), especially pp. 21, 28, 29; punctuation as in the original.

71. Franklin Henry Giddings, *The Mighty Medicine: Superstition and Its Antidote: A New Liberal Education* (New York: The Macmillan Company, 1929), p. 143.

72. Eliot, "Popularizing Science," p. 32. Much British background appears in Ian Inkster and Jack Morrell, eds., *Metropolis and Province: Science in British Culture, 1780–1850* (London: Hutchinson, 1983).

73. Daniels, *American Science in the Age of Jackson*. "The 'News,'" *Popular Science News and Boston Journal of Chemistry*, 17 (1883), 43. John Theodore Merz, *A History of European Thought in the Nineteenth Century* (4 vols., Edinburgh: William Blackwood & Son, 1904), 1: 44. Sally Gregory Kohlstedt, *The Formation of the American Scientific Community: The American Association for the Advancement of Science, 1848–60* (Urbana: University of Illinois Press, 1976). Ritchie Calder, "Common Understanding of Science," *Impact of Science on Society*, 14 (1964), 179–195.

74. E.g., Calder, "Common Understanding of Science." William A. Satariano, "Immigration and the Popularization of Social Science, 1920 to 1930," *Journal of the History of the Behavioral Sciences*, 15 (1979), 310–320, provides a specific twentieth-century example. Terry Shinn and Richard Whitley, eds., *Expository Science: Forms and Functions of Popularisation* (Dordrecht: D. Reidel Publishing Company, 1985), contains essays that attempt to conceptualize popularization as a

mere subset of scientific communication in general. Based largely upon current European materials, this interesting idea is not particularly appropriate for the present historical work.

75. George Basalla, "Pop Science: The Depiction of Science in Popular Culture," in Gerald Holton and William A. Blanpied, eds., *Science and Its Public: The Changing Relationship* (Dordrecht: D. Reidel Publishing Company, 1976), pp. 261–278. Pop science of course tended to contain traditional elements. This phenomenon is analyzed in detail from a modern viewpoint in C. E. Ashworth, "Flying Saucers, Spoon-Bending, and Atlantis: A Structural Analysis of New Mythologies," *Sociological Review*, 28 (1980), 353–376. "Du Bois-Reymond on Exercise," *Popular Science Monthly*, 21 (1882), 544.

76. Jerome R. Ravetz, *Scientific Knowledge and Its Social Problems* (Oxford: Clarendon Press, 1971), pp. 386–397.

77. No attempt is made here to deal systematically with the social function of popularization in terms of audience use, such as the teenager's using "popular" music or the 1920s conversationalist's using the "Five-Foot Shelf" of classics.

78. The literature on this subject is extensive; see especially Donald M. Scott, "The Popular Lecture and the Creation of a Public in Mid-Nineteenth-Century America," *Journal of American History*, 66 (1980), 791–809. Jean Pradal, *The Literature of Science Popularisation: A Study of the Present Situation in Member States of the Council for Cultural Cooperation* (Strasbourg: Council of Europe, [1969]), pp. 14–15. A recent summary of the early period is to be found in Kohlstedt, *The Formation*, and a particularly graceful one in A. Hunter Dupree, "Public Education for Science and Technology," *Science*, 134 (1961), 716–718. The rise of specialized popular science magazines of course had a magnified effect because it was still the custom frequently for both newspaper and other magazine editors to copy material from the leading periodicals, and the more popular science material was available from any source, therefore, the more it was available for copying. The subject comes up again especially in chapter 4.

79. Dupree, *Asa Gray*, p. 127. Whalen, "Science, The Public."

80. The aspirations of members of the intelligent public are suggested by the title of a European journal of the 1790s as quoted in Preserved Smith, *A History of Modern Culture* (2 vols., New York: Henry Holt, 1934), 2: 138: *News of the Learned and Curious World, in which is contained the Quintessence of manifold Learning, and remarkable things in History, Chronology, Genealogy, Geography, political intelligence, astronomy, the law of nature, the civil and administrative law, theology, political science, ethics, physics, medicine, philosophy, philology, military and civil matters; in which also many old and new books and authors are noticed and criticized; and not a few notices of persons important in station, in office, in the army, and in learning, are intermingled; faults and needs of all sorts are pointed out; good doctrines are taught; and the means of*

learning many sciences are given; and finally many pleasing stories and merry jests are added, and all is briefly treated by the collaboration of a curious and learned society and so gotten up that by this one may obtain a gentleman's Erudition. Published Monthly.

81. Carl Bode, *The Anatomy of American Popular Culture* (Berkeley: University of California Press, 1959), pp. 116–131. Franklin H. Giddings, "A Provisional Distribution of the Population of the United States into Psychological Classes," *Psychological Review*, 8 (1901), 349, found that of 4,759 books published in 1899, 176 were "Physical and Mathematical," and an additional 120 were "Medical and Hygiene."

82. Whalen and Tobin, "Periodicals and the Popularization." Tobey, *The American Ideology.* James Steel Smith, "The Day of the Popularizers: The 1920's," *South Atlantic Quarterly*, 62 (1963), 297–309. Benjamin C. Gruenberg, *Science and the Public Mind* (New York: McGraw-Hill Book Company, 1935). Hillier Krieghbaum, *Science and Mass Media* (New York: New York University Press, 1967). Stephen J. McDonough, "Covering the Science Beat," *Quill* (October 1936), 6. David J. Rhees, "A New Voice for Science: Science Service under Edwin E. Slosson, 1921–29" (master's thesis, University of North Carolina, 1979).

83. Following the Three Mile Island nuclear incident in 1980, press demands for information were so great that Scientists' Institute for Public Information, another scientist group, established an information service, Media Resource Service, comparable to Science Service.

84. "Professor Newcomb on American Science," *Popular Science Monthly*, 6 (1874), 243. William D. Carey, "Foreword," in June Goodfield, *Reflections on Science and the Media* (Washington: American Association for the Advancement of Science, 1981), p. vii. The general points listed here are covered in some detail in the chapters that follow.

85. See especially Pradal, *The Literature.* Peter Farago, *Science and the Media* (Oxford: Oxford University Press, 1976). The best practical description of popularization as such remains David S. Evans, "The Theory and Practice of Popular Science," *Pilot Papers*, 1 (1946), 27–41. Steven Shapin, "'Nibbling at the Teats of Science': Edinburgh and the Diffusion of Science in the 1830s," in Ian Inkster and Jack Morrell, eds., *Metropolis and Province: Science in British Culture, 1780–1850* (London: Hutchinson, 1983), p. 151, points out that the diffusion of science is an active, not a passive, procedure.

86. George Cotkin, "The Socialist Popularization of Science in America, 1901 to the First World War," *History of Education Quarterly*, 24 (1984), 201–214.

87. Catherine Covert, "Freud on the Front Page: Transmission of Freudian Ideas in the American Newspaper of the 1920's" (doctoral diss., Syracuse University, 1975).

88. See especially Mohr, *A Study of Popular Books*, p. 27. Helen Margaret Bar-

ton, "A Study of the Development of Textbooks in Physiology and Hygiene in the United States" (doctoral diss., University of Pittsburgh, 1942), p. 188.

89. [E. L. Youmans], "Scientific Lectures," *Popular Science Monthly*, 4 (1873), 242. See especially chapter 6.

90. See, for example, Irving S. Wright, "The Five Pillars of Science Writing," *Nieman Reports* (July 1953), 10. Researchers found most of the biology in 1920s newspapers "homocentric"; W. Edgar Martin, "A Chronological Survey of Research Studies Relating to Biological Materials in Newspapers and Magazines," *School Science and Mathematics*, 45 (1945), 549. Dale Marvin Herder, "Education for the Masses: The Haldeman-Julius Little Blue Books as Popular Culture during the Nineteen-Twenties" (doctoral diss., Michigan State University, 1975), especially pp. 207, 212. William R. Oates, "Social-Ethical Content in Science Coverage by Newsmagazines," *Journalism Quarterly*, 50 (1973), 681.

91. David L. MacKaye, "They Don't Want Dead Ones," *Adult Education Journal*, 4 (1945), 45.

92. "Science Stories Require Judgment Standard Same as Routine News," *Editor & Publisher*, April 25, 1931, p. 44. Vernon F. Wolthoff, "A Survey of Medical Writing in Leading American Magazines" (master's thesis, University of Missouri, 1949), p. 110. M. Amrine, "Space Filler," *American Psychologist*, 13 (1958), 185.

93. "Editorial," *American Naturalist*, 17 (1883), 58. Evart G. Routzahn, "Education and Publicity," *American Journal of Public Health*, 16 (1926), 1070. Hadley Cantril and Gordon W. Allport, *The Psychology of Radio* (New York: Harper & Brothers, 1935), pp. 90–95. Benjamin J. Novak, "Science in the Newspaper," *Science Education*, 26 (1942), 140–141. Marvin Howard Alisky, "A Study of the Sunday Science Reporting in the New York *Times* and the New York *Herald-Tribune*, From September 8, 1946, to June 1, 1947" (master's thesis, University of Texas, 1947), p. 42; the *Herald-Tribune* was 30 percent medicine and health. E. G. Sherburne, Jr., "Science on Television: A Challenge to Creativity," *Journalism Quarterly*, 40 (1963), 300–305 (commentators have criticized the basis of this sample). "Media Resource Service, 1983–1984" (New York: Scientists' Institute for Public Information, [1984?]), p. [5].

94. Thomas Hardy Leahey and Grace Evans Leahey, *Psychology's Occult Doubles: Psychology and the Problem of Pseudoscience* (Chicago: Nelson-Hall, 1983), especially pp. 242–243. Sayle, *The Works of Sir Thomas Browne*.

Chapter 2: The Popularizing of Health

1. Guenter B. Risse, Ronald L. Numbers, and Judith Walzer Leavitt, eds., *Medicine Without Doctors, Home Health Care in American History* (New York: Science History Publications, 1977); Judith Ward-Steinem Karst, "Newspaper Medicine: A Cultural Study of the Colonial South, 1730–1770" (doctoral diss., Tulane University, 1971).

2. The great collection (well known in the United States) was Sir John Sinclair, *The Code of Health and Longevity; or, A Concise View of the Principles Calculated for the Preservation of Health, And the Attainment of Long Life. Being an Attempt to Prove the Practicability of Condensing, Within a Narrow Compass, The Most Material Information Hitherto Accumulated, Regarding the Most Useful Arts and Sciences, Or Any Particular Branch Thereof* (2nd ed., 4 vols., Edinburgh: Arch. Constable & Co., 1807). Sinclair reprinted as one of his appendices in this edition an 1805 lecture on health advice for young people by the Boston physician Benjamin Waterhouse, cited in note 15. Robley Dunglison, *On the Influence of Atmosphere and Locality; Change of Air and Climate; Seasons; Food; Clothing; Bathing; Exercise; Sleep; Corporeal and Intellectual Pursuits, &c &c on Human Health; Constituting Elements of Hygiene* (Philadelphia: Carey, Lea & Blanchard, 1835), pp. iii–v. William B. Walker, "The Health Reform Movement in the United States, 1830–1870" (doctoral diss., Johns Hopkins University, 1955), especially pp. iii, 4.

3. For example, Sinclair, *The Code of Health*, 1: 10. William Coleman, "Health and Hygiene in the *Encyclopédie*: A Medical Doctrine for the Bourgeoisie," *Journal of the History of Medicine and Allied Sciences*, 29 (1974), 399–421; Saul Jarcho, "Galen's Six Non-Naturals: A Bibliographic Note and Translation," *Bulletin of the History of Medicine*, 44 (1970), 372–377; Jerome J. Bylebyl, "Galen on the Non-Natural Causes of Variation in the Pulse," *Bulletin of the History of Medicine*, 45 (1971), 482–485; Peter H. Niebyl, "The Non-Naturals," *Bulletin of the History of Medicine*, 45 (1971), 486–492; and Chester R. Burns, "The Nonnaturals: A Paradox in the Western Concept of Health," *Journal of Medicine and Philosophy*, 1 (1976), 202–211. The most recent and explicit discussion is James C. Whorton, *Crusaders for Fitness: The History of American Health Reformers* (Princeton, NJ: Princeton University Press, 1982), especially p. 14.

4. William A. Alcott, "On the Construction of School-Rooms," in *The Introductory Discourse and the Lectures Delivered Before the American Institute of Instruction Annual Meeting, 1831* (Boston: Hilliard, Gray, Little and Wilkins, 1832), p. 273.

5. See especially Walker, "The Health Reform Movement;" Whorton, *Crusaders for Fitness*, especially p. 5; and Stephen Nissenbaum, *Sex, Diet, and Debility in Jacksonian America: Sylvester Graham and Health Reform* (Westport, CT: Greenwood Press, 1980). Still another factor is explored in Regina Markell Morantz,

"Making Women Modern: Middle Class Women and Health Reform in 19th Century America," *Journal of Social History,* 10 (1977), 490–503.

6. Nissenbaum, *Sex, Diet, and Debility*; Whorton, *Crusaders for Fitness.*

7. Walker, "The Health Reform Movement," especially pp. 29–30. Caleb Ticknor, *The Philosophy of Living; or, The Way to Enjoy Life and Its Comforts* (New York: Harper & Brothers, 1836), p. 21. Compare, for example, Thomas Joseph Pettigrew, *On Superstitions Connected with the History and Practice of Medicine and Surgery* (London: John Churchill, 1844), who (p. 24) quoted Bacon: "Witches and imposters have always held a competition with physicians." Worthington Hooker, *Human Physiology: Designed for Colleges and The Higher Classes in Schools, and For General Reading* (New York: Pratt, Oakley, & Company, 1859), p. viii.

8. John Harley Warner, "The Nature-Trusting Heresy: American Physicians and the Concept of the Healing Power of Nature in the 1850's and 1860's," *Perspectives in American History,* 11 (1977–1978), 291–324. J. R. Black, *The Laws of Health; or, How Diseases Are Produced and Prevented: And Family Guide* (1872; 2nd ed., Baltimore: The Author, 1885), especially pp. 28–29.

9. The only work of a general nature is Helen Margaret Barton, "A Study of Textbooks in Physiology and Hygiene in the United States" (doctoral diss., University of Pittsburgh, 1942), which can be supplemented by Whorton, *Crusaders for Fitness,* and Walker, "The Health Reform Movement." Anita Clair Fellman and Michael Fellman, *Making Sense of Self: Medical Advice Literature in Late Nineteenth-Century America* (Philadelphia: University of Pennsylvania Press, 1981), focus on the ideological point of view.

10. The present work will not deal in detail with the intellectual history of the content of health popularization, although some attempt will be made to convey general approaches.

11. Walker, "The Health Reform Movement," especially pp. 132–133; Whorton, *Crusaders for Fitness,* especially p. 140. Frank Luther Mott, *A History of American Magazines, 1850–1865* (Cambridge, MA: Harvard University Press, 1938), p. 87.

12. Walker, "The Health Reform Movement," especially p. 180, takes up one side of this relationship; many authors survey the medical side, including John Duffy, *The Healers: The Rise of the Medical Establishment* (New York: McGraw-Hill Book Company, 1976); Joseph F. Kett, *The Formation of the American Medical Profession: The Role of Institutions, 1780–1860* (New Haven: Yale University Press, 1968); William G. Rothstein, *American Physicians in the Nineteenth Century: From Sects to Science* (Baltimore: Johns Hopkins University Press, 1972).

13. Hattie Hopeful, "Exercise," *Lady's Home Magazine,* 12 (1858), 233–234. Elizabeth Blackwell, *The Laws of Life, With Special Reference to the Physical Education of Girls* (New York: George P. Putnam, 1852).

14. William F. Mavor, *The Catechism of Health, Containing Simple and Easy*

Rules and Directions for the Management of Children, and Observations on the Conduct of Health in General. For the Use of Schools and Families . . . with Alterations and Improvements (New York: Samuel Wood & Sons, 1819), especially pp. 60–61, 3. Mavor was of course himself English.

15. Benjamin Waterhouse, *Cautions to Young Persons Concerning Health, In a Public Lecture Dedicated at the Close of the Medical Course in the Chapel at Cambridge, Nov. 20, 1804* (Cambridge, MA: University Press by W. Hilliard, 1805), pp. 12–13. See, in general, Walker, "The Health Reform Movement," and Whorton, *Crusaders for Fitness*; Charles E. Rosenberg and Carroll Smith-Rosenberg, "Pietism and the Origins of the American Public Health Movement: A Note on John H. Griscom and Robert M. Hartley," *Journal of the History of Medicine and Allied Sciences*, 23 (1968), 16–35. Elisha Bartlett, *Obedience to the Laws of Health: A Moral Duty; A Lecture Delivered Before the American Physiological Society, January 30, 1838* (Boston: J.A. Noble, 1838). Catharine Esther Beecher, *Physiology and Calisthenics for Schools and Families* (New York: Harper, 1856), p. 78. Ronald L. Numbers, *Prophetess of Health: A Study of Ellen G. White* (New York: Harper & Row, 1976).

16. Whorton, *Crusaders for Fitness*, especially p. 134. Morantz, "Making Women Modern." John B. Blake, "Mary Gove Nichols, Prophetess of Health," *Proceedings of the American Philosophical Society*, 106 (1962), 219–234.

17. See especially Walker, "The Health Reform Movement," pp. 97–98, 118–123, 229–230.

18. "Health and the Love of Nature," *Lady's Home Magazine*, 11 (1858), 294.

19. John W. Draper, *Human Physiology, Statical and Dynamical; or, The Conditions and Course of the Life of Man* (New York: Harper & Bros., 1856), p. v.

20. [Galen E. Bishop], "Medicine and Medical Humbuggery," *Journal of Popular Medicine and Collateral Sciences*, 1 (1853), 34.

21. Walker, "The Health Reform Movement." Whorton, *Crusaders for Fitness*. Richard Cole Newton, "The Re-Awakening of the Physical Conscience," *Popular Science Monthly*, 71 (1907), 156–164. Clifford J. Waugh, "Bernarr Macfadden: The Muscular Prophet" (doctoral diss., State University of New York at Buffalo, 1979). Macfadden was of course preceded by Dio Lewis and other figures.

22. Numbers, *Prophetess of Health*; Richard W. Schwarz, *John Harvey Kellogg, M.D.* (Nashville: Southern Publishing Association, 1970); Whorton, *Crusaders for Fitness*.

23. See, for example, Frederick A. P. Barnard, "The Germ Theory of Disease and Its Relations to Hygiene," *Reports and Papers, American Public Health Association*, 1 (1873), 70–87; "The 'Celebrated Physician,'" *Popular Science News*, 28 (1894), 14. Phyllis Allen Richmond, "American Attitudes toward the Germ Theory of Disease (1860–1880)," *Journal of the History of Medicine and Allied Sciences*, 9 (1954), 428–454. There is an extensive specialized literature on the history of American public health; see, for example, James H. Cassedy, *Charles V. Chapin*

and the Public Health Movement (Cambridge, MA: Harvard University Press, 1962).

24. George H. Perkins, "The Physician of the Future," *Popular Science Monthly*, 21 (1882), 638–639. Frank Overton, *Applied Physiology, Including the Effects of Alcohol and Narcotics* (New York: American Book Company, 1897), p. 30. Characterization of the body as a machine was not new, but later Victorians tended to be literal and reductionistic in their characterization. A late example is R. Bache, "Efficiency of the Human Machine," *Scientific American*, 98 (1908), 130.

25. "A Sober Reality," *Health Magazine*, 5 (1898), 208. "Sanitary Warnings," *Health Magazine*, 5 (1898), 322. Andrew Dickson White, in his "New Chapters in the Warfare of Science. XIII. From Fetich to Hygiene," *Popular Science Monthly*, 39 (1891), 434–435, blamed simple lack of sanitation for visitations of disease that earlier ignorant churchmen had attributed to religious causes.

26. No public seemed immune; see, for example, one of many informative health articles in a children's magazine: W. S. Harwood, "The Pulse and the Temperature," *St. Nicholas*, 20 (1893), 855. Frank Luther Mott, *A History of American Magazines, 1865–1885* (Cambridge, MA: Harvard University Press, 1938), pp. 138–139.

27. *Popular Science News*, 25 (1891), 41. See, for example, F. L. Oswald, "Sanitary Superstitions," *Chautauquan*, 32 (1901), 489–492. Distortions in ads are cogently summarized in James Harvey Young, "The Regulation of Health Quackery," *Pharmacy in History*, 26 (1984), 3–12.

28. See, in general, Richard K. Means, *A History of Health Education in the United States* (Philadelphia: Lea & Febiger, 1962); Barton, "A Study of Textbooks." While the WCTU-approved texts embodied some of the moralizing typical of an earlier period, it was now in a more secular, not to mention scientific, context. Albert Mordell, quoted in Mark Sullivan, *Our Times: The United States, 1900–1925* (6 vols., New York: Charles Scribner's Sons, 1931–1935), 2: 192. James Johonnot and Eugene Bolton, *Lessons in Hygiene; or, The Human Body and How to Take Care of It. The Elements of Anatomy, Physiology, and Hygiene* (New York: D. Appleton and Company, 1889), p. 74. See, for example, the notice of pirating of the *American Health Primers, Boston Journal of Chemistry*, 15 (1881), 21.

29. William Gilman Thompson, "The Present Aspect of Medical Education," *Popular Science Monthly*, 27 (1885), 590. Sanitation and health—and in the early years, the ideal of science—also entered educational curriculums by way of the developing home economics programs; Virginia Bramble Vincenti, "A History of the Philosophy of Home Economics" (doctoral diss., Pennsylvania State University, 1981), pp. 126–128; Marie Negri Carver, "Home Economics as an Academic Discipline," University of Arizona College of Education, Center for the Study of Higher Education, *Topical Paper* no. 15 (1979).

30. Whorton, *Crusaders for Fitness*, especially chap. 6. "Editorial Note," *Cos-*

mopolitan, 49 (1910), 326. Frank Luther Mott, *A History of American Magazines, 1885–1905* (Cambridge, MA: Harvard University Press, 1957), pp. 310–311. No attempt is made here to describe the eugenics movement, which is now the focus of a large and substantially irrelevant literature; the basic historical work is Mark H. Haller, *Eugenics: Hereditarian Attitudes in American Thought* (New Brunswick: Rutgers University Press, 1963).

31. According to an editorial, "Sanitary Lapses," *Modern Medicine*, 2 (1920), 581, "No sanitary campaign has ever had such immediate and complete success as this one," against the public drinking cup. See the certainties listed in D. B. Armstrong, "Can It Now Be Told?" *Journal of Health and Physical Education* (June 1935), 7.

32. Frederick G. Kilgour, "Scientific Ideas of Atomicity in the Nineteenth Century," *Proceedings of the Tenth International Congress of the History of Science*, (2 vols., Paris: Hermann, 1964), 1: 329–331; Garland E. Allen, *Life Science in the Twentieth Century* (New York: Wiley, 1975). Emma E. Walker, "When to Be Afraid: A Common-Sense Talk about Children's Diseases," *Good Housekeeping* (March 1909), 341. W.R.C. Latsom, "Wonders of the Human Body," *Health-Culture*, 9 (1903), 417–418. Andrew McClary, "Germs are Everywhere: The Germ Threat as Seen in Magazine Articles, 1890–1920," *Journal of American Culture*, 3 (1980), 33–46. John C. Burnham, "The Fragmenting of the Soul: Intellectual Prerequisites for Ideas of Dissociation in the United States," in Jacques Quen, ed., *Split Minds and Split Brains* (New York: New York University Press, 1986), pp. 63–83, develops this point even more generally.

33. "Food and Health," *American Journal of Public Health*, 11 (1921), 159–161. C.-E.A. Winslow, review of Putnam, *School Janitors, Mothers, and Health*, in *American Journal of Public Health*, 3 (1913), 827, quoted H. W. Hill: "The old sanitation was concerned with the environment, the new is concerned with the individual, and finds the sources of infectious disease in man himself rather than in his surroundings."

34. Iago Galdston, "The Problem of Motivation in Health Education," in *Motivation in Health Education; The 1947 Health Education Conference of the New York Academy of Medicine* (New York: Columbia University Press, 1948), pp. 16–18. Whorton, *Crusaders for Fitness*; Ruth E. Grout, "Health Education Today in the Light of Yesterday," *Yale Journal of Biology and Medicine*, 19 (1947), 573–580; C. E. Turner, "Present Trends in Health Education," *Public Health Nursing*, 29 (1937), 499; Charles M. De Forest, "The Crusade Method of Training for Right Living," *Nation's Health*, 6 (1924), 75–76. Lee K. Frankel, "Insurance Companies and Public Health Activities," *American Journal of Public Health*, 4 (1914), 1–6. James N. Giglio, "Voluntarism and Public Policy between World War I and the New Deal: Herbert Hoover and the American Child Health Association," *Presidential Studies Quarterly*, 13 (1983), 430–452. In New York at one point the state health depart-

ment was sending out boilerplate copy to newspapers in the state; Edward A. Moore, "Public Health Publicity: The Art of Stimulating and Focussing Public Opinion," *American Journal of Public Health*, 6 (1916), 278.

35. B. L. Arns, "Public Health News and Notes," *Journal of the American Public Health Association*, 1 (1911), 669–670. Surgeon General, Public Health Service, *Annual Report*, 1923, pp. 205–207; "Too Much Health Propaganda?" *American Journal of Public Health*, 21 (1931), 543–545; Benjamin C. Gruenberg, "Motivation in Health Education," *American Journal of Public Health*, 23 (1933), 116.

36. The *American Journal of Public Health* from time to time ran inventories of health columns in American newspapers. Typical discussions included Thomas D. Wood, "The Health Crisis in Education," *Addresses and Proceedings*, National Education Association, 1921, pp. 306–308; Eugene Lyman Fisk, *Health Building and Life Extension: A Discussion of the Means by Which the Health Span, the Work Span, and the Life Span of Man Can Be Extended* (New York: The Macmillan Company, 1923). Douglas Waples and Ralph W. Tyler, *What People Want to Read About* (Chicago: University of Chicago Press, 1931), pp. 70–73. The nature of the interest was suggested by a survey, J. R. Gergerich and J. A. Thalheimer, "Reader Interests in Various Types of Newspaper Content," *Journal of Applied Psychology*, 20 (1936), 471–480, in which medicine scored low but self-improvement was the highest category.

37. Means, *History of Health Education*, pp. 77–237; the quotation is from p. 138. See, for example, "The Swing of the Pendulum in Health Education," *Nation's Health*, 4 (1922), 482.

38. Means, *History of Health Education: Reorganization of Science in Secondary Schools* (Washington: Government Printing Office, 1920, U.S. Bureau of Education Bulletin no. 26), pp. 12–15. Lois Meier, *Health Material in Science Textbooks* (New York: Lincoln School of Teachers College, 1927). Maitland P. Simmons, "Changing Conceptions of Major Topics in General Science Textbooks (1911–1934)," *Journal of Educational Research*, 31 (1937), 199–204.

39. The rules are quoted in Means, *History of Health Education*, p. 129. Irving Fisher and Eugene Lyman Fisk, *How to Live: Rules for Healthful Living Based on Modern Science* (New York: Funk & Wagnalls Company, 1915), pp. 119–120. The influence of contemporary psychological belief and educational theory is evident, for example, Thomas D. Wood, ed., in *Health Education: A Program for Public Schools and Teacher Training Institutions* (New York: [The Joint Committee of the National Education Association and the American Medical Association], 1924).

40. Means, *History of Health Education*. William Walter Patty, "The Teaching of Health Education in Elementary Schools," *Journal of Health and Physical Education* (January 1934), 3–7, 60. Louise Franklin Bache, *Health Education in an American City: An Account of a Five-Year Program in Syracuse, New York* (Garden City, NY: Doubleday, Doran & Company, 1934). Benjamin C. Gruenberg, "Motivation in

Health Education," *American Journal of Public Health*, 23 (1933), 116. "Problems of Health Education," *Nation's Health*, 6 (1924), 108. Charles M. De Forest, "The Crusade Method of Training for Right Living," *Nation's Health*, 6 (1924), 75–76.

41. Herman N. Bundesen, "Selling Health—A Vital Duty," *American Journal of Public Health*, 18 (1928), 1454. Barbara Melosh, *"The Physician's Hand": Work Culture and Conflict in American Nursing* (Philadelphia: Temple University Press, 1982), especially pp. 115–143, shows how public health nurses translated the "gospel of health" into behavior. See, for example, John C. Burnham, "The Progressive Era Revolution in American Attitudes Toward Sex," *Journal of American History*, 59 (1973), 885–908; and "For Longer and Healthier Lives," *Literary Digest*, January 28, 1928, p. 15.

42. George A. Walker and Eleanor Saltzman, "False Health Notions," *Hygeia*, 20 (1942), 34. Julius Stieglitz, "Chemistry and Recent Medical Progress," *Scientific Monthly*, 37 (1933), 453, spoke approvingly of "medical control of life and health." G. B. Affleck, review of Rogers, *Life and Health*, in *American Journal of Physical Education*, 15 (1910), 486.

43. J. Mace Andress, *The Teaching of Hygiene in the Grades* (2nd ed., Boston: Houghton Mifflin Company, 1926), is an exemplary transition document in which behavior is emphasized. The advertising examples are from M. P. Ravenel, review of Osborne, *Health: What Everyone Ought to Know*, in *American Journal of Public Health*, 20 (1930), 229; Iago Galdston, "Hazards of Commercial Health Advertising," *American Journal of Public Health*, 21 (1931), 248.

44. Armstrong, "Can It Now Be Told?"

45. Irving Fisher, *National Vitality: Its Wastes and Conservation* (Washington: Government Printing Office, 1909, Committee of One Hundred on National Health, National Conservation Committee, Bulletin no. 30).

46. Vernon F. Wolthoff, "A Survey of Medical Writing in Leading American Magazines" (master's thesis, University of Missouri, 1949), p. 51. "Today's Health Revamps Format, Seeks More Ads," *Advertising Age*, May 5, 1948, p. 156.

47. See, for example, "God's Own Narcotic," *Time*, July 29, 1946, pp. 82–83. Carolyn Keith Cramp, "Popular Magazines as Medical Advisors: A Comparison of Medical Reports in Popular and Professional Journals" (master's thesis, Syracuse University, 1953), pp. 147–148, 174–180.

48. Robert Fuoss, quoted in Wolthoff, "A Survey of Medical Writing," p. 49.

49. See, for example, Wood, *Health Education*. Means, *History of Health Education*, especially pp. 250–255. The specialized literature is voluminous, but the main trends appeared in *Journal of Health, Physical Education, Recreation* [title varies].

50. Homer N. Calver, "Health Information, Please," *JAMA*, 115 (1940), 1251, for example, and *Hygeia* and other medically-sponsored publicity, but this confusion was carried over into many health educators' and journalists' work

also. As early as 1945, George M. Wheatley of Metropolitan Life questioned the wisdom of emphasizing the authority of the physician: "Have we oversold professional talents to young people? Have we so surrounded the subject of health with instruments and sera and textbooks that it became an unfathomable mystery, an esoteric body of knowledge forbidden to all but a small group?" ("Youth Talks Back," *Channels* [March 1945], 2). The educational impact of the physical examination by a physician is explored in Angela Nugent, "Fit for Work: The Introduction of Physical Examinations in Industry," *Bulletin of the History of Medicine*, 57 (1983), 578–595. As Herbert R. Edwards, in *Transactions of the Association of Life Insurance Medical Directors of America*, 1942, p. 9, observed, chest x rays may not have detected much tuberculosis but they did teach people that they could not have a health examination with their overcoats on. Means, *A History of Health Education*, p. 242.

51. Fisher and Fisk, *How to Live*. Wood, *Health Education*, pp. 21–22. Frank Ernest Hill, *Educating for Health: A Study of Programs for Adults* (New York: American Association for Adult Education, 1939), p. 207. Ernest I. Stewart, Jr., *Attention to Your Health* (New York: Teachers College, 1941).

52. Jean V. Latimer, "Is Specificity of Health Instruction Desirable?" *Journal of Health and Physical Education*, 10 (1939), 384.

53. J. Clarence Funk, *Stay Young and Live: Common Sense about Health in Wartime* (Richmond: Dietz Press, 1943), pp. 89–90.

54. See, for example, C. V. Akin, "The Present Status of Public Health Education," *American Journal of Public Health*, 30 (1940), 1438–1439; Robert M. Yoder, "Vitamania," *Hygeia*, 20 (1942), 264; Arthur H. Steinhaus, "Too Much Health," *Journal of the National Education Association*, 32 (1943), 43–44; Forrest E. Conner, "Focus on Health," *Journal of School Health*, 37 (1967), 3–4. John Tebbel, *Your Body: How to Keep It Healthy* (New York: Harper & Brothers, 1951), pp. 223–229. A description of the low state of affairs is in Hollis S. Ingraham, "Something Else That Johnny Doesn't Know," *Journal of School Health*, 36 (1966), 331–336.

55. Walter McQuade, "Why Are They Running, Stretching, Starving?" *Fortune* (August 1970), 132–135, 161. Means, *History of Health Education*, pp. 324–327. John F. Kennedy, "A Presidential Message to the Schools on the Physical Fitness of Youth," *School Life* (September 1961), 33. The concern for "youth" of course reflected more universal concern for the body. Sam S. Blanc, John W. Low, and George E. Mathes, "Trends in Science Education," *Science Education*, 42 (1958), 173.

56. Examples include Iago Galdston, ed., *Beyond the Germ Theory* (New York: Health Education Council, 1954); Lawrence K. Frank, "Health Education," *American Journal of Public Health*, 36 (1946), 357–366; and Justus J. Schifferes, *How to Live Longer* (New York: E. P. Dutton & Company, 1949). Philip G. Johnson, *The Teaching of Science in Public High Schools* (Washington: Government

Printing Office, 1950, Federal Security Agency, Office of Education Bulletin no. 9), p. 6.

57. Irwin M. Rosenstock, "What Research in Motivation Suggests for Public Health," *American Journal of Public Health*, 50 (1960), 295–302. A later version of this trend is found in the President's Committee on Health Education, *The Report of the President's Committee on Health Education* (New York: [The Committee, 1971]), especially p. 17; and, similarly, Earl Ubell, "Health Behavior Change: A Political Model," *Preventive Medicine*, 1 (1972), 209–221. New York Academy of Medicine, *Motivation in Health Education* (New York: Columbia University Press, 1948), contains much description of the context in which this trend developed. Elianne Riska and Peter Vinten-Johansen, "The Involvement of the Behavioral Sciences in American Medicine: Historical Perspective," *International Journal of Health Sciences*, 11 (1981), 583–596.

58. See, for example, Charles Kaiser, "A Bouncing Year-Old Baby," *Newsweek*, February 21, 1983, p. 76.

59. See the summary, Scott K. Simonds, "Health Education in the Mid-70's—State of the Art," in Anne R. Somers, ed., *Promoting Health, Consumer Education, and National Health* (Germantown, MD: Aspen Systems, 1976), pp. 105–108. A. R. Somers, "Priorities in Educating the Public about Health," *Bulletin of the New York Academy of Medicine*, 54 (1978), 39.

60. See, for example, Savel Zimand, "Tips and Tricks for the Practice," *American Journal of Public Health*, 35 (1945), especially 631–633; Lee W. Frederiksen, Laura J. Solomon, and Kathleen A. Brehony, eds., *Marketing Health Behavior: Principles, Techniques, and Applications* (New York: Plenum Press, 1984); John W. Farquhar et al., "Community Education for Cardiovascular Health," *Lancet*, June 4, 1977, pp. 1192–1195.

61. The pioneer popular statement, Public Health Service, Federal Security Agency, *Environment and Health: Problems of Environmental Health in the United States and the Public Health Service Programs Which Aid States and Communities in Their Efforts to Solve Such Problems* (Washington: [Government Printing Office], 1951), emphasized contamination but also pollution. Compare, for example, the summary, Michael G. Marmot and Warren Winkelstein, Jr., "Health and Technology," *Science*, 181 (1973), 1204.

62. See, for example, *The Report of the President's Committee on Health Education* (Washington: Department of Health, Education, and Welfare, Public Health Service, 1971); *Healthy People: The Surgeon General's Report on Health Promotion and Disease Prevention* (Washington: Government Printing Office, 1979, DHEW (PHS) Publication no. 79–55071); David A. Hamburg, Glen R. Elliott, and Delores L. Parron, eds., *Health and Behavior: Frontiers of Research in the Biobehavioral Sciences* (Washington: National Academy Press, 1982), p. 33; Paul I. Ahmed and George V. Coelho, eds., *Toward a New Definition of Health: Psychosocial Dimensions*

(New York: Plenum Press, 1979); Daniel I. Wikler, "Persuasion and Coercion for Health, Ethical Issues in Government Efforts to Change Life-Styles," *Milbank Memorial Fund Quarterly*, 56 (1978), 303–309. S. J. Kunitz, "The Historical Roots and Ideological Functions of Disease Concepts in Three Primary Care Specialities," *Bulletin of the History of Medicine*, 57 (1983), 412–432, elucidates the antireductionistic tendencies in holism and other streams of both popular and professional medicine.

63. Whorton, *Crusaders for Fitness*, pp. 331–349. In the magazines for the elderly, for example, *Lifetime Living*, health material diminished greatly and was by 1954 classified under "Art of Living." One general treatment is Julius A. Roth, *Health Purifiers and Their Enemies: A Study of the Natural Health Movement in the United States with a Comparison to its Counterpart in Germany* (New York: Prodist, 1977). See also Dennis Brisset and Lionel S. Lewis, "The Natural Health Food Movement: A Study of Revitalization and Conversion," *Journal of American Culture*, 1 (1978), 61–76; Christopher Lasch, *The Culture of Narcissism: American Life in an Age of Diminishing Expectations* (New York: W. W. Norton, 1979). Selskar M. Gunn and Philip S. Platt, *Voluntary Health Agencies: An Interpretive Study* (New York: The Ronald Press, 1945). Richard Carter, *The Gentle Legions* (Garden City, NY: Doubleday, 1961). Sally Guttmacher, "Whole in Body, Mind, and Spirit: Holistic Health and the Limits of Medicine," *Hastings Center Report* (April 1979), 15–21. *Report of the President's Committee*, p. 18, and, for example, "Proposed Report on the Educational Qualifications of Community Health Educators," *American Journal of Public Health*, 38 (1948), 843–850. Diane Starr Petryk, "A Content Analysis of Medical News in Four Metropolitan Dailies" (master's thesis, Michigan State University, 1979), pp. 40–41, found an absolute increase in medical stories in newspapers from 1967 to 1978.

64. For example, Elizabeth G. Pritchard, "Workers' Health Education," *American Journal of Public Health*, 32 (1942), 395. C.-E. A. Winslow, "Health Education Grows Up," *Channels*, 20 (1942–1943), 10. The change was very general; see, for example, Robert Olesen, "What People Ask about Health," *Public Health Reports*, 54 (1939), 765–779.

65. Daniel Fox, *Organizing Health Policy in Britain and the United States, 1911–1965* (Princeton University Press, 1986). The confusion appears clearly in Homer N. Calver, "Health Information, Please," *JAMA*, 115 (1940), 1251–1253, for example. John B. Morrison, "Periodic Conferences of Officers of Societies in Adjoining States," *American Medical Association Bulletin*, 23 (1928), 8. *Hygeia* for years embodied this program of health plus social advantages for physicians. John C. Burnham, "American Medicine's Golden Age: What Happened to It?" *Science*, 215 (1982), 1474–1482.

66. See, for example, a book with a significant title, J. D. Ratcliff, *Modern Miracle Men* (New York: Dodd, Mead & Company, 1940). Means, *History of Health*

Education, pp. 184–185. Clarence C. Little, quoted in *American Journal of Public Health*, 30 (1940), 1233, measured success of cancer education by the extent to which people came to see physicians at the cancer clinic.

67. Thurman B. Rice, *Living* (Chicago: Scott, Foresman and Company, 1940), p. v.

68. Examples include P. M. Hall, "Publicity and the Public Health," *American Journal of Public Health*, 4 (1914), 106; "Popular Medical Information," *JAMA*, 88 (1927), 324–325; Veterans Administration, Medical & General Reference Library, *Popular Medical Books Written by Physicians, 1940–1952: An Annotated Bibliography* (Washington: Veterans Administration, 1952); Jonathan Forman, "Education of the Public by Radio in Matters of Health," *Education on the Air*, 19 (1949), 339–343; M. Pinson Neal, "Health Education for the Public," *Southern Medical Journal*, 33 (1940), 763–768.

69. The best concrete account of advocacy groups' actual influence is Corinda Stewart Waters, "A Century of Health Instruction in the Public Schools of Maryland, 1872–1972" (doctoral diss., University of Maryland, 1972). Means, *History of Health Education*, pp. 181–184, 314–316. Specific group descriptions include Richard H. Shryock, *National Tuberculosis Association, 1904–1954: A Study of the Voluntary Health Movement in the United States* (New York: National Tuberculosis Association, 1957); *Twenty-Five Years of Life Conservation* (New York: Metropolitan Life Insurance Company, [1935]); Bruce V. Lewenstein, "Industrial Life Insurance Companies and Health Education in the Early 20th Century" (unpublished paper kindly furnished by the author); Richard A. Rettig, *Cancer Crusade: The Story of the National Cancer Act of 1971* (Princeton: Princeton University Press, 1977).

70. Carter, *The Gentle Legions*. John A. Ferrell, "America's Contributions and Problems in Public Health," *American Journal of Public Health*, 23 (1933), 1117.

71. See in general James Harvey Young, *The Medical Messiahs: A Social History of Health Quackery in Twentieth-Century America* (Princeton: Princeton University Press, 1967). Victor Herbert and Stephen Barrett, *Vitamins and 'Health' Foods: The Great American Hustle* (Philadelphia: George F. Stickley Company, 1982).

72. John E. Drewry, "Doctors and the Public," *Nieman Reports*, July, 1953, p. 12.

73. Edward Hitchcock, *Dyspepsy Forestalled and Resisted; or, Lectures on Diet, Regimen, and Employment; Delivered to the Students of Amherst College, Spring Term, 1830*, (2nd ed., Amherst, MA: J. S. & C. Adams, 1831).

74. Paul D. Stolley, "Cultural Lag in Health Care," *Inquiry*, 8 (1971), 71–76. Social class differentiation is summarized in Jacob J. Feldman, *The Dissemination of Health Information: A Case Study in Adult Learning* (Chicago: Aldine Publishing, 1966). Ralph A. Beals and Leon Brody, *The Literature of Adult Education* (New York: American Association for Adult Education, 1941), p. 177.

75. Tom Lee, "Cancer's Front-Page Treatment," *Nation*, September 18, 1976, p. 239.

76. See in general Feldman, *The Dissemination of Health Information*, and Charles F. Cannell and James C. MacDonald, "The Impact of Health News on Attitudes and Behavior," *Journalism Quarterly*, 33 (1956), 315–323. Edith M. Stern, "Medical Journalism—With and without Upbeat," *Saturday Review*, January 9, 1954, p. 10.

77. Stern, "Medical Journalism," pp. 9–10, 36. David Hellerstein, "Cures That Kill," Harper's (December 1980), 22. David Dietz, "Science, Newspapers, and the Future," *Quill* (July 1966), 14–15. Fred Jerome, "Gee Whiz! Is That All There Is?" in Sharon M. Friedman, Sharon Dunwoody, and Carol L. Rogers, eds., *Scientists and Journalists: Reporting Science as News* (New York: The Free Press, 1986), p. 148. The problem of the breakthrough story is taken up in Petryk, "A Content Analysis." A defense of the new hope school is Lois R. Chevalier, "Do Science Writers Raise False Hopes?" *Medical Economics* (April 1959), 69–71, 288, 290, 292, 296, in which the author claimed that pressure from the public, stimulated by the science writers' suggestions, actually led physicians to improve the medical care they were delivering. A late classic example is Charles Panati, *Breakthroughs—Astonishing Advances in Your Lifetime in Medicine, Science, and Technology* (Boston: Houghton Mifflin Company, 1980).

78. Martin S. Pernick, "Thomas Edison's Tuberculosis Films: Mass Media and Health Propaganda," *Hastings Center Report* (June 1978), 21–27. Allan M. Brandt, *No Magic Bullet: A Social History of Venereal Disease in the United States Since 1880* (New York: Oxford University Press, 1985), especially pp. 68–69. H. E. Kleinschmidt, "What of the Future of the Health Movie?" *American Journal of Public Health*, 35 (1945), 55–56. Ralph P. Creer, "Movies That Teach Health," *Today's Health* (October 1954), 36–37, 50–51, claimed that some movies were very successful and hoped to use them as a basis for television programming.

79. See, for example, Evart G. Routzahn, "Public Health Education," *American Journal of Public Health*, 27 (1937), 930; "Old Nostrum Rides Again," *American Journal of Public Health*, 34 (1944), 182–183; Fred V. Hein, "Health Information, Please," *Education on the Air*, 21 (1951), 450–451. See, in general, Erik Barnouw, *The Sponsor: Notes on a Modern Potentate* (New York: Oxford University Press, 1978).

80. Barnouw, *The Sponsor*. Anne Hudson Jones, "Medicine and the Physician," in M. Thomas Inge, ed., *Concise Histories of American Popular Culture* (Westport, CT: Greenwood Press, 1982), pp. 312–315. Frank A. Smith et al., "Health Information During a Week of Television," *New England Journal of Medicine*, 286 (1972), 516–520. George Gerbner et al., "Health and Medicine on Television," *New England Journal of Medicine*, 305 (1981), 901–904. Bibliography is in ibid. and Somers, *Promoting Health*, pp. 32–37.

81. *Cincinnati Chronicle*, June 1, 1840, p. 1.

82. Examples include Effie F. Knowlton, "Using Scientific Sources," *Hygeia*, 18 (1940), 566; Gertrude I. Duncan and Frederick H. Lund, "The Validity of Health Information Gained through Radio Advertising," *Research Quarterly*, 16 (1945), 102–105. Ingraham, "Something Else That Johnny Doesn't Know," p. 331. Details are in James Harvey Young, *The Toadstool Millionaires, A Social History of Patent Medicines in America before Federal Regulation* (Princeton: Princeton University Press, 1961), and Young, *The Medical Messiahs.*

83. Rita S. Rosenberg, "An Investigation of the Nature, Utilization, and Accuracy of Nutritional Claims in Magazine Food Advertisements, An Analysis and Evaluation of the Nutritional Statements Made in Food Advertisements Over a Fifty Year Period" (doctoral diss., New York University, 1955); copy generously lent by the author. Christie Jelen, "The Application of Marketing Techniques to Social Advertising: Dental Health Case Study" (master's thesis, University of Texas, 1975), pp. 61–62.

84. Young, *Toadstool Millionaires.* "Smoking and News, Coverage of a Decade of Controversy," *Columbia Journalism Review* (Summer 1963), 6–12, is a good example because it was in itself censored in the name of journalism. *The Report of the President's Committee*, p. 11.

85. Cramp, "Popular Magazines as Medical Advisors." A later example is in Herbert and Barrett, *Vitamins and "Health" Foods*, pp. 139–147. Cramp's findings tend to cast doubt on the editors' claims, reported in Wolthoff, "A Survey of Medical Writing," that they often checked stories with medical authorities.

86. Waters, "A Century of Health Instruction," pp. 415–420. James Frederick Rogers, quoted in Means, *History of Health Education*, p. 285.

87. Charles H. Keene, review of Kreuger, *The Fundamentals of Personal Hygiene*, in *American Journal of Public Health*, 23 (1933), 401. An excellent example of mechanical translation is Laura Cairns, "A Scientific Basis for Health Instruction in Public Schools," *University of California Publications in Education*, 2 (1929), 339–434. A good example of regret is Delbert Oberteuffer, "Two Problems in Health Education," *Journal of Health and Physical Education* (February 1931), 3, 5.

88. Howard M. Parshley, *Biology* (New York: John Wiley & Sons, 1940), pp. 3–4.

89. An anonymous quote in Hillier Krieghbaum, ed., *When Doctors Meet Reporters* (New York: New York University Press, 1957), p. 3.

90. "The Public Interest in Science," *Modern Medicine*, 2 (1920), 710. "The Swing of the Pendulum in Health Education," p. 482.

91. For example, John J. Burt, Linda Brower Meeks, and Sharon Mitchell Pottebaum, *Toward a Healthy Lifestyle through Elementary Health Education* (Belmont, CA: Wadsworth Publishing, 1980); Marion C. Chafetz, *Health Education: An Annotated Bibliography on Lifestyle, Behavior, and Health* (New York: Plenum

Press, 1981). Gwendolyn D. Scott and Mona W. Carlo, *On Becoming a Health Educator* (Dubuque, IA: Wm. C. Brown Company, 1974). John S. Sinacore, *Health: A Quality of Life* (New York: The Macmillan Company, 1968), p. 3. Michael S. Haro, "An Editorial: A Philosophy 'For the Health of It,'" *Journal of School Health*, 43 (1973), 7; Barton, "Study of Textbooks," p. 173.

92. Steven Polgar, "Health and Human Behavior: Areas of Interest Common to the Social and Medical Sciences," *Current Anthropology*, 3 (1962) 170. Peter Morell, *Poisons, Potions, and Profits: The Antidote to Radio Advertising* (New York: Knight Publishers, 1937), p. 137. "Problems of Health Education," *Nation's Health*, 6 (1924), 108. See, for example, Duncan and Lund, "The Validity of Health Information"; Smith et al., "Health Information during a Week of Television"; and Gerbner et al., "Health and Medicine on Television."

93. See, for example, Aubrey D. Gates, "Health Education and Community Responsibility," *JAMA*, 139 (1949), 933. Two important midcentury popularizations suggest the shift underway: Justus J. Schifferes, *How to Live Longer* (New York: E. P. Dutton, 1949), still took up prevention and cure of killing diseases, but E. Patricia Hagman, ed., *Good Health for You and Your Family* (New York: A. S. Barnes, 1951), emphasized health, not disease. Jonathan E. Fielding, "Successes of Prevention," *Milbank Memorial Fund Quarterly*, 56 (1978), 274–302, offers a number of examples of complexity, such as the decline of cholesterol-fostering foods and fluoridation that involve different levels of science and authority and can require or not require active participation by the citizen.

94. Treffie Cox, J. S. McCollum, and Ralph K. Watkins, "Science Claims in Magazine Advertising," *Science Education*, 22 (1938), 14.

95. See chapter 6 for explicit discussion of other aspects of cultural change.

Chapter 3: The Popularizing of Psychology

1. "Professor" Babcock, "The Power of Mind," *Knickerbocker*, 11 (1838), 297. I have not been able to identify Babcock from standard sources.

2. O. S. Fowler, L. N. Fowler, and Samuel Kirkham, *Phrenology Proved, Illustrated, and Applied, Accompanied by a Chart; Embracing an Analysis of the Primary, Mental Powers in Their Various Degrees of Development; The Phenomena Produced by Their Combined Activity; And the Location of the Phrenological Organs in the Head. Together with a View of the Moral and Theological Bearing of the Science* (New York: Fowlers and Wells, 1849), pp. iii–vi. John D. Davies, *Phrenology: Fad and Science—A 19th-Century American Crusade* (New Haven: Yale University Press, 1955). Madeline B. Stern, *Heads and Headlines: The Phrenological Fowlers* (Norman: University of Oklahoma Press, 1971). The Fowlers of course were for some years publishers of the *Water-Cure Journal* and were stalwarts in health and other re-

forms. Roger Cooter, *The Cultural Meaning of Popular Science: Phrenology and the Organization of Consent in Nineteenth-Century Britain* (Cambridge: Cambridge University Press, 1984), provides background and comparison.

3. See especially R. Laurence Moore, *In Search of White Crows: Spiritualism, Parapsychology, and American Culture* (New York: Oxford University Press, 1977). General summaries include Merle Curti, *Human Nature in American Thought: A History* (Madison: University of Wisconsin Press, 1980), especially chaps. 5–6, and Nathan G. Hale, Jr., *Freud and the Americans: The Beginnings of Psychoanalysis in the United States, 1876–1917* (New York: Oxford University Press, 1971), especially chap. 9.

4. See previous note and Robert C. Fuller, *Mesmerism and the American Cure of Souls* (Philadelphia: University of Pennsylvania Press, 1982). Richard Weiss, *The American Myth of Success: From Horatio Alger to Norman Vincent Peale* (New York: Basic Books, 1969), and Donald Meyer, *The Positive Thinkers: Religion as Pop Psychology from Mary Baker Eddy to Oral Roberts* (2nd ed., New York: Pantheon Books, 1980), especially explore the secularization process often involved. Another perspective is offered in Thomas Hardy Leahey and Grace Evans Leahey, *Psychology's Occult Doubles: Psychology and the Problem of Pseudoscience* (Chicago: Nelson-Hall, 1983).

5. *Southern Literary Messenger*, quoted in Davies, *Phrenology*, pp. 41–42. John Bigham, "The New Psychology," *Methodist Review*, 78 (1896), 345.

6. See, for example, S. Osgood, "The Practical Study of the Human Soul," *Christian Examiner*, 63 (1857), 335: "The Human Soul in its Essential Life is the Human Personality." J. P. Gordy, *Lessons in Psychology, Designed Especially as an Introduction to the Subject for Private Students, and as a Text-Book in Normal and Secondary Schools* (Athens, OH: Ohio Publishing Company, 1890), pp. 4, 45. Joseph Haven, "Mental Science as a Branch of Education," *American Journal of Education*, 3 (1857), 137. No attempt is made here to cite the extensive literature on philosophical psychology.

7. Joseph Jastrow, "Popular Psychology," *Science*, 7 (1886), 106. The discipline of psychology as such is treated insightfully in John M. O'Donnell, *The Origins of Behaviorism: American Psychology, 1870–1920* (New York: New York University Press, 1985).

8. Compare, for example, the lack of enthusiasm in John E. Bradlee, "Application of the Principles of Psychology to the Work of Teaching," *Education*, 4 (1884), 346–359, with the fervor of proponents of the new psychology. John Dewey, "The New Psychology," *Andover Review*, 2 (1884), 282. E. W. Scripture, *Thinking, Feeling, Doing* (Meadville, PA: Flood and Vincent, 1895), especially p. 282; ibid. (2nd ed., New York: G. P. Putnam's Sons, 1907), especially p. iii. Scripture was teaching at Yale in 1895.

9. G. Stanley Hall, "The New Psychology," *Harper's Monthly Magazine*, 103

(1901), 727–732. Hall even incorporated a rat maze into the devices he used to illustrate the article. Not all of the consumers of popularization were convinced of the ability of psychologists to carry out their program. As a Delaware teacher, W. L. Gooding, "Psychology and Pedagogy," *School Review*, 3 (1895), 560, observed, in a restrained way, about the resources of psychologists and the applications of psychology, "The output of this psychologic mine is altogether uncertain." Even the philosopher Josiah Royce, who was sympathetic, noted that "neither theoretical development nor novelty is as marked a feature of the New Psychology as some hopeful accounts would imply." ("The New Psychology and the Consulting Psychologist," *Forum*, 26 [1898], 87). R. M. Wenley, "The Movement towards Physiological Psychology," *Popular Science Monthly*, 73 (1908), 143. O'Donnell, *Origins of Behaviorism*, especially pp. 122–123.

10. Isaac Cook, "Psychology *versus* Metaphysics," *Methodist Review*, 77 (1895), 223. J. H. Hyslop, "The New Psychology," *New Princeton Review*, 6 (1888), 155. Walter Hayle Walshe, "Physiology *versus* Metaphysics," *Popular Science Monthly*, 25 (1884), 249. The materialist platform was laid out (disapprovingly) by John W. Draper, "Mental Physiology," *International Review*, 2 (1875), 277–279. Virtually none of the men of science was a materialist, but they emphasized naturalism with the result that their tendencies, at least, were clear. See, more generally, John C. Burnham, "The Encounter of Christian Theology with Deterministic Psychology and Psychoanalysis," *Bulletin of the Menninger Clinic*, 49 (1985), 321–352.

11. William James, *The Principles of Psychology* (2 vols., New York: Henry Holt and Company, 1890).

12. James Rowland Angell, "Contemporary Psychology," *Chautauquan*, 40 (1905), 453. Historical surveys of the image of psychology have just appeared: Michael S. Pallak and Richard Kilburg, "Psychology, Public Affairs, and Public Policy: A Strategy and Review," *American Psychologist*, 41 (1986), 933–940; Ludy T. Benjamin, Jr., "Why Don't They Understand Us? A History of Psychology's Public Image," *American Psychologist*, 41 (1986), 941–946; Wendy Wood, Melinda Jones, and Ludy T. Benjamin, Jr., "Surveying Psychology's Public Image," *American Psychologist*, 41 (1986), 947–953.

13. See, for example, the cartoon in *Life*, November 9, 1916, p. 820.

14. Warner Fite, "The Human Soul and the Scientific Prepossession," *Atlantic Monthly*, 122 (1918), 796–804. Hugo Münsterberg, "Psychology and Mysticism," Atlantic Monthly, 83 (1899), 67–85. Leahey and Leahey, *Psychology's Occult Doubles*.

15. Joseph Jastrow, "The Versatility of Psychology," *The Dial*, 45 (1908), 38–41. The fools were of course the religiously or mystically inclined thinkers whom popularizers dared not attack too openly, as Jastrow indicated.

16. Edward A. Ayres, "Measuring Thought with a Machine," *Harper's Weekly*, May 9, 1908, p. 27. "Physiological Discovery That Explains the Forma-

tion of Bad Habits," *Current Opinion*, 58 (1915), 101–102. George Stuart Fuller-ton, "Is Man an Automaton?" *Popular Science Monthly*, 70 (1907), 149–156. These are random examples.

17. Mandel Sherman, "Book Selection and Self-Therapy," in Louis R. Wilson, ed., *The Practice of Book Selection* (Chicago: University of Chicago Press, 1940), pp. 172–174. Garry Robert Austin, "An Analysis of Certain Characteristics of Recent Widely Distributed Psychology Books for the Lay Reader" (doctoral diss., Northwestern University, 1950), especially pp. 32–35.

18. See especially Wayne Viney, Tom Michaels, and Alan Ganong, "A Note on the History of Psychology in Magazines," *Journal of the History of the Behavioral Sciences*, 17 (1981), 270–272, and Marcel Evelyn Chotkowski La Follette, "Authority, Promise, and Expectation: The Images of Science and Scientists in American Popular Magazines, 1910–1955" (doctoral diss., Indiana University, 1979), p. 77.

19. E. B. Titchener, "Recent Advances in Psychology," *International Monthly*, 2 (1900), 154–168.

20. Details are in Matthew Hale, Jr., *Human Science and Social Order, Hugo Münsterberg and the Origins of Applied Psychology* (Philadelphia: Temple University Press, 1980). See, for example, Fabian Franklin, "Should Psychology Supervise Testimony?" *Popular Science Monthly*, 72 (1908), 465–474.

21. Hale, *Human Science*. "Soothing Syrup of Psychology," *Living Age*, 283 (1914), 573–575. In general on this period see Thomas M. Camfield, "The Professionalization of American Psychology, 1870–1917," *Journal of the History of the Behavioral Sciences*, 9 (1973), 66–75.

22. See, for example, Daniel J. Kevles, "Testing the Army's Intelligence: Psychologists and the Military in World War I," *Journal of American History*, 55 (1968), 565–581. Charles William Heywood, "Scientists and Society in the United States, 1900–1940: Changing Concepts of Social Responsibility" (doctoral diss., University of Pennsylvania, 1954). Such a book from an earlier period as Henry Smith Williams, *Miracles of Science* (New York: Harper & Brothers, 1913), did not include psychology, whereas after World War I most popular surveys of science did. John C. Burnham, "The New Psychology: From Narcissism to Social Control," in Braeman, Bremner, and Brody, eds., *Change and Continuity in Twentieth-Century America: The 1920's* (Columbus: The Ohio State University Press, 1968), 351–398. The standard work is Thomas M. Camfield, "Psychologists at War: The History of American Psychology and the First World War" (doctoral diss., University of Texas, 1969). A survey in 1927 showed that psychology stories were the most popular among all of those issued by Science Service; David J. Rhees, "A New Voice for Science: Science Service under Edwin E. Slosson, 1921–29" (master's. thesis, Univerity of North Carolina, 1979), p. 62.

23. See La Follette, "Authority, Promise, and Expectation," especially p. 79.

Sherman, "Book Selection." Stephen Leacock, "A Manual of the New Mentality," *Harper's Monthly Magazine*, 148 (1924), 472. Madison Bentley, in *Science*, 58 (1923), 70, correctly perceived that professional psychologists had lost control of the definition of their own discipline. An excellent general treatment of psychology in this period is Michael M. Sokal, "James McKeen Cattell and American Psychology in the 1920s," in Josef Brozek, ed., *Explorations in the History of Psychology in the United States* (Lewisburg, PA: Bucknell University Press, 1984), pp. 273–323.

24. See, for example, Paul M. Dennis, "The Edison Questionnaire," *Journal of the History of the Behavioral Sciences*, 20 (1984), 23–37. Burnham, "The New Psychology." Dorothy Hazeltine Yates, *Psychological Racketeers* (Boston: R. G. Badger, 1932). B. Crider, "Who Is a Psychologist? Pseudo-Psychologies," *School and Society*, 43 (1936), 370–371. See the estimate in *Psychological Exchange* (August 1932), 3.

25. A contemporary account is "Psychology as a Business," *Scientific American*, 127 (1922), 112–113, 142. Loren Baritz, *The Servants of Power, A History of the Use of Social Science in American Industry* (Middletown, CT: Wesleyan University Press, 1960). Michael M. Sokal, "The Origins of the Psychological Corporation," *Journal of the History of the Behavioral Sciences*, 17 (1981), 54–67.

26. A well-known literary piece using the humorous potential in the psychological expert was James Thurber, *Let Your Mind Alone, and Other More or Less Inspirational Pieces* (New York: Harper & Brothers, 1937).

27. See, for example, Edward S. Robinson, "A Little German Band: The Solemnities of Gestalt Psychology," *The New Republic*, November 27, 1929, pp. 10–14. William P. King, ed., *Behaviorism: A Battle Line* (Nashville: Cokesbury Press, 1930).

28. See, for example, John C. Burnham, "Psychiatry, Psychology and the Progressive Movement," *American Quarterly*, 12 (1960), 457–465; Hamilton Cravens, *The Triumph of Evolution: American Scientists and the Heredity-Environment Controversy, 1900–1941* (Philadelphia: University of Pennsylvania Press, 1978); H. A. Overstreet, "A Quarter-Century of Psychology, a Science That Has Only Just Been Born," *Century*, 113 (1927), 526–535; and note 4.

29. A contemporary account is J.v.D. Latimer, "Putting the Psyche to Work," *American Mercury* (June 1928), 142–150.

30. Philip R. Jenkins, "The Success Book: Phony Guidance?" *The Clearing House*, 13 (1939), 336–339. Austin, "An Analysis." Sherman, "Book Selection." Burnham, "The New Psychology." Dale Carnegie, *How to Win Friends and Influence People* (New York: Simon and Schuster, 1936). Henry C. Link, "Man in Chains," *Saturday Evening Post*, May 7, 1938, pp. 25, 72, 75–76, is a late example

by an important figure. A good example of conventional psychology not only popularized but pitched to the success market was H. Clay Skinner, *Psychology for the Average Man* (Boston: Richard G. Badger, 1927).

31. An excellent early example is Knight Dunlap, "The Social Need for Scientific Psychology," *Scientific Monthly*, 10 (1920), 502–517. The program of the psychologists is summarized in H. K. Nixon, "Popular Answers to Some Psychological Questions," *American Journal of Psychology*, 36 (1925), 418–423. *Recent Social Trends in the United States: Report of the President's Research Committee on Social Trends* (2 vols., New York: McGraw-Hill Book Company, 1933), 1: 411–412, suggests that the campaign to make the occult unrespectable had some success. See, for example, Morris A. Copeland, "Psychology and the Natural-Science Point of View, *Psychological Review*, 37 (1930), 461–487. A. P. Weiss, "Bridgman's New Vision of Science," *Scientific Monthly*, 29 (1929), 514, pointed out that psychologists were better able to adjust to rapid change in science—i.e., in fact had a better grasp on the scientific outlook—than physicists.

32. Suggestions of a substantial decline in media attention are in Austin, "An Analysis," p. 36, and, in kindred material, in George Gerbner, "Psychology, Psychiatry, and Mental Illness in the Mass Media: A Study of Trends, 1900–1959," *Mental Hygiene*, 45 (1961), 89–93. La Follette, "Authority, Promise, and Expectation," does not confirm any dramatic decline until 1940. For radio, see, for example, "Broadcasting Table of Information," *Library Journal*, January 1, 1932, pp. 40–41, and the pamphlet out of the program, Henry E. Garrett and Walter V. Bingham, *Psychology Today* (Chicago: University of Chicago Press, 1931); Morris S. Vitales, "Psychology and Reemployment," *Scientific Monthly*, 39 (1934), 271.

33. Benjamin R. Simpson, "A Pragmatist Examines the Discard of Mechanistic Psychology," *Scientific Monthly*, 44 (1937), 453–463. John Wright Buckham, "What Has Psychology Done to Us?" *Christian Century*, 57 (1940), 1171–1172.

34. Among accounts of the hard times of psychology was Grace Adams, "The Rise and Fall of Psychology," *Atlantic Monthly* (January 1934), 82–92. Ben Harris, "Psychology at the 1939 World's Fair," unpublished. On world's fair publicity in general, Robert Perloff and Linda S. Perloff, "The Fair—An Opportunity for Depicting Psychology and Conducting Behavioral Research," *American Psychologist*, 32 (1977), 220–229.

35. A contemporary survey is Robert J. Lewinski and Daniel D. Feder, "Science versus Sensationalism in Psychology for the Layman," *Journal of Applied Psychology*, 23 (1939), 429–435. Austin, "An Analysis."

36. See Burnham, "The New Psychology," pp. 368–369.

37. Edgar James Swift, *The Jungle of the Mind* (New York: Charles Scribner's Sons, 1933), pp. 4–5.

38. Among contemporary accounts is "Psychologists Organize in National Emergency," *Science News Letter*, January 18, 1941, p. 38. John G. Darley and Dael Wolfle, "Can We Meet the Formidable Demand for Psychological Services?" *American Psychologist*, 1 (1946), 179–180. Robert P. Fischer and Robert P. Hinshaw, "The Growth of Student Interest in Psychology," *American Psychologist*, 1 (1946), 117, suggest that student interest had risen dramatically already in 1940–1941. The growth of psychological interest in medicine and health was noted in chapter 2.

39. Fillmore Sanford, "The Growth of APA," *American Psychologist*, 9 (1954), 125. Fillmore Sanford, "Notes on the Future of Psychology as a Profession," *American Psychologist*, 6 (1951), 75. Samples of the intraprofessional discussion are Karl E. Pottharst, "Comment," *American Psychologist*, 23 (1968), 284–286, and C. W. Crannell, "Are Rat Psychologists Responsible for Fission?" *American Psychologist*, 2 (1947), 22–23. APA Education and Training Board, "Anticipations of Developments During the Next Decade Which Will Influence Psychology," *American Psychologist*, 11 (1956), 686–688. Dael Wolfle, "The Reorganized American Psychological Association," *American Psychologist*, 1 (1946), 3–4. Roy Schafer, quoted in Eugene D. Fleming, "Tests That Tell All About You," *Cosmopolitan* (September 1957), 40. A general treatment is Albert R. Gilgen, *American Psychology Since World War II: A Profile of the Discipline* (Westport, CT: Greenwood Press, 1982).

40. Franklin Fearing, "Psychology and the Films," *Hollywood Quarterly*, 2 (1947), 119. Alfred H. Fuchs, George R. Klare, and Maxwell S. Pullen, "Student Reactions to Topics in General Psychology," *American Psychologist*, 12 (1957), 219–221.

41. Alton L. Blakeslee, "Psychology and the Newspaper Man," *American Psychologist*, 7 (1952), 91–94. M. Amrine, "Psychology in the News," *American Psychologist*, 13 (1958), 659.

42. See La Follette, "Authority, Promise, and Expectation," *Reader's Guide*; R. R. Blake, "Some Quantitative Aspects of *Time* Magazine's Presentation of Psychology," *American Psychologist*, 3 (1948), 124–126, 132; and Austin, "An Analysis." M. Amrine, "A Report on APA's Press Room," *American Psychologist*, 12 (1957), 585. Kary K. Wolfe and Gary K. Wolfe, "Metaphors of Madness: Popular Psychological Narratives," *Journal of Popular Culture*, 9 (1976), 895–907. And, for example, Gordon Kahn, "One Psychological Moment, Please," *Atlantic Monthly* (October 1946), 135–137; Cecile Starr, "Psychiatry without Jargon," *Saturday Review*, July 10, 1954, pp. 32, 34.

43. For example, George J. Dudycha, "Recent Literature on Careers in Psychology," *Occupations*, 28 (1950), 455–461; Ross Stagner, "Attitudes of Corporate Executives Regarding Psychological Methods in Personnel Work," *American Psychologist*, 1 (1946), 540–541; Ronald Taft, "The Staff Psychologist in Industry,"

American Psychologist, 55–61. Robert F. Creegan, "Psychologist, Know Thyself!" *American Psychologist*, 8 (1953), 52. Elizabeth Ogg, "Psychologists in Action," *Public Affairs Pamphlet*, no. 229 (Washington: Public Affairs Committee, 1955).

44. Blake, "Some Quantitative Aspects."

45. Frederic Wertham, "The Cult of Contentment," *New Republic*, March 29, 1948, pp. 22–24. Christopher Lasch, *The Culture of Narcissism: American Life in an Age of Diminishing Expectations* (New York: Warner Books, 1979).

46. Lester Guest, "The Public's Attitude toward Psychologists," *American Psychologist*, 3 (1948), 135–139. Elton B. McNeil, "The Public Image of Psychology," *American Psychologist*, 14 (1959), 520. Jacques Bacal, E. J. Shoben, Jr., and Isabella Taves, "Beware of the Psycho-Quacks," *Look*, September 25, 1951, pp. 54–61, is a good example. See the general comments of Leahey and Leahey, *Psychology's Occult Double*, especially pp. 242–243.

47. For example, Jim Nunnally and John M. Kittross, "Public Attitudes Toward Mental Health Professions," *American Psychologist*, 13 (1958), 589–594; Jacob Cohen and G. D. Wiebe, "Who Are These People?" *American Psychologist*, 10 (1955), 54–55; Harry C. Aichner, "Bravo, Dr. Brothers!" *American Psychologist*, 11 (1956), 53; M. Amrine, "Psychology in the News," *American Psychologist*, 13 (1958), 609. Ernest Havemann, *The Age of Psychology* (New York: Simon and Schuster, 1957); the series ran in *Life* from January 7 to February 4, 1957, and included illustrations not in the book.

48. Blake, "Some Quantitative Aspects," confirms the impression conveyed by surveying *Science News-Letter*.

49. Vance Packard, *The Hidden Persuaders* (New York: D. McKay Co., 1957). The literature on this general subject is vast; see, for example, James V. McConnell, Richard L. Cutler, and Elton B. McNeil, "Subliminal Stimulation: An Overview," *American Psychologist*, 13 (1958), 229–242; Peter Watson, *War on the Mind: The Military Uses and Abuses of Psychology* (London: Hutchinson, 1978). Emerson Coyle, "Psychology and Slycology," *American Psychologist*, 10 (1955), 87. Carl R. Rogers and B. F. Skinner, "Some Issues Concerning the Control of Human Behavior," *Science*, 124 (1956), 1057–1066. Wilson L. Taylor, "Gauging the Mental Health Content of the Mass Media," *Journalism Quarterly*, 34 (1957), described the simplistic level of psychological thinking purveyed in the mass media, especially the lowest levels of the mass media.

50. The public relations discussions can be followed beginning in 1946 in *American Psychologist*, which contained committee reports that from one year to the next turned out to be very similar, regardless of committee compostion; for example, Dael Wolfle, "Publicity for Psychology," *American Psychologist*, 3 (1948), 35–36; Daniel Katz, "Public Relations Activities of the American Psychological Association," *American Psychologist*, 5 (1950), 627–633; "Report of the Committee on Public Relations, 1952–1953," *American Psychologist*, 8 (1953), 676–681;

Roger W. Russell, "Annual Report of the Executive Secretary: 1959," *American Psychologist*, 14 (1959), 738. Robert Tyson, "Is It Respectable to Publish Interesting Material for Popular Consumption?" *American Psychologist*, 4 (1949), 535–536.

51. For example, Edwin B. Newman, "Public Relations—For What?" *American Psychologist*, 12 (1957), 509–514; Fillmore H. Sanford, "Summary Report on the 1954 Annual Meeting," *American Psychologist*, 9 (1954), 715.

52. For example, "Highlights in Recent Psychology," *Science Digest* (June 1940), 81–84. Clark Newlon, "How Do You Feel About Your Boss?" *Cosmopolitan* (January 1953), 103; Robert Wernick, "Modern-Style Mind Reader," *Life*, September 12, 1955, pp. 97–102. A random example is "Rivalry and Reward Speed Accomplishment in School," *Science News-Letter*, 23 (1933), 216.

53. A cartoon in the *APA Monitor* (April 1972), 3, has one psychologist say to the other: "You say you *know* when psychology will have it made? Yes. When there is a Nobel Prize for psychology? No. When we are included in National Health Insurance? No. When? When we get our own TV hero."

54. For example, Arthur H. Brayfield, "Report of the Executive Officer: 1963," *American Psychologist*, 18 (1963), 753; Charles A. Kiesler, "Report of the Executive Officer: 1976," *American Psychologist*, 32 (1977), 398; "Town Meetin' Tonight!" *American Psychologist*, 16 (1961), 208; James Gaffney, "Who's OK, What's OK?" *New Catholic World*, 216 (1973), 273. Robert T. Lewis and Hugh M. Petersen, *Human Behavior: An Introduction to Psychology* (New York: The Ronald Press, 1974), p. 9. Robert Sklar, "Prime-Time Psychology," *American Film* (March 1979), 59–63. On another level, book clubs specializing in psychology sprang up.

55. Irwin Spector, "Publisher's Page," *Popular Psychology* (July 1973), 4.

56. Later, of course, changes in ownership and staff did result in a substantial lowering of quality.

57. Nicolas H. Charney, "What Is Psychology?" *Psychology Today* (June 1968), 36–37. Public discussions included "Psyched Out," *Time*, May 17, 1976, p. 78.

58. An evaluation of one part of the intellectual context is Jan Zimmerman, "Transcendent Psychology: Erik H. Erikson, Erich Fromm, Karen Horney, Abraham H. Maslow, and Harry Stack Sullivan and the Quest for a Healthy Humanity" (doctoral diss., Northwestern University, 1982).

59. For example, Erwin M. Segal and Roy Lachman, "Complex Behavior or Higher Mental Process: Is There a Paradigm Shift?" *American Psychologist*, 27 (1972), 46–55; David Bakan, "Psychology Can Now Kick the Science Habit," *Psychology Today* (March 1972), 26, 28, 86–87. One discussion was Georgine M. Pion and Mark W. Lipsey, "The Challenge of Change," *American Psychologist*, 39 (1984), 739–754.

60. An authoritative example is Mona Marie Olean, "Communicating with

the Public about Psychology" (Washington: American Psychological Association, 1977), especially p. 2. The public relations model for popularizing psychology was widely, perhaps pervasively, assumed; see, for example, Earl Ubell, "Should There Be a Behavioral Science Beat?" in Frederick T. C. Yu, ed., *Behavioral Sciences and the Mass Media* (New York: Russell Sage Foundation, 1968), pp. 240–241.

61. Leona Tyler, "An Approach to Public Affairs: Report of the Ad Hoc Committee on Public Affairs," *American Psychologist*, 24 (1969), 1–4. Arthur H. Brayfield, "Introduction," *American Psychologist*, 22 (1967), 179. Richard H. Blum and Mary Lou Funkhouser, "A Lobby for People?" *American Psychologist*, 20 (1965), 209–210. George A. Miller, "Psychology as a Means of Promoting Human Welfare," *American Psychologist*, 24 (1969), 1063, 1067–1069. Patrick H. DeLeon, Gary R. VandenBos, and Alan G. Kraut, "Federal Legislation Recognizing Psychology," *American Psychologist*, 39 (1984), 933–946. As the citations indicate, the *American Psychologist* documents the changes, which also appear in the *APA Monitor*, especially after it changed from a Washington newsletter, alerting members to grants and programs, into a public affairs journal. (Background is in Jeffrey Mervis, "Up Through the Years with the *Monitor*," *APA Monitor* [January 1986], 38, 42, 44.) One ad for an action group, run repeatedly in the *APA Monitor* in the early 1970s, read: "Help Harness Psychology's Political Power."

62. An example would be Roger W. McIntire, "Parenthood Training or Mandatory Birth Control," *Psychology Today* (October 1973), 33–39, 132–133, 143. Leona E. Tyler, "Design for a Hopeful Psychology," *American Psychologist*, 28 (1973), 1021. Helen B. Shaffer, "Human Engineering," in *Editorial Research Reports on the Scientific Society*, 1971. A good example was a program that took psychologists to inner city facilities as consultants; see, for example, *APA Monitor* (December 1970), 8.

63. Eli A. Rubenstein, "A View on the TV Violence Report: Turning Social Science Research into Public Policy," *APA Monitor* (June 1972), 3.

64. Douglas G. Mook, "In Defense of External Invalidity," *American Psychologist*, 38 (1983), 379.

65. M. Amrine, "Report on APA's Press Room," *American Psychologist*, 13 (1958), 659. Victor Cohn, quoted in *American Psychologist*, 20 (1965), 371. James Grunig, in Norman Metzger, ed., *Science in the Newspaper* (Washington: American Association for the Advancement of Science, 1974), p. 12. See, for example, James W. Tankard, Jr., and Rachael Adelson, "Mental Health and Marital Information in Three Newspaper Advice Columns," *Journalism Quarterly*, 59 (1982), 592–596.

66. Dunlap, "The Social Need," p. 511. "Menace of the Intellectual Underworld," *Current Opinion*, 56 (1914), 44.

67. Dunlap, "The Social Need." Fite, "The Human Soul." Gilbert Love, "De-

bunking Our Superstitions," *Scholastic*, October 26, 1935, pp. 7–8, is a good example of a general article based largely on the work of psychologists.

68. Dalmas A. Taylor and Sidney A. Manning, *Psychology: A New Perspective* (Cambridge, MA: Winthrop Publishers, 1975). Similar findings are reported in Amedeo Giorgi, *Psychology as a Human Science: A Phenomenologically Based Approach* (New York: Harper & Row, 1970), pp. 12–20. It is a common observation among schematic historians of the sciences that concern with method is a defensive posture in an immature science, whether in the eighteenth century or in the twentieth.

69. Edward John Hamilton, *The Human Mind: A Treatise in Mental Philosophy* (New York: Robert Carter & Brothers, 1883). Floyd C. Dockeray, *General Psychology* (New York: Prentice-Hall, 1932), p. 19. Howard H. Kendler, *Basic Psychology* (New York: Appleton-Century-Crofts, 1963), p. xi. In the course of surveying psychology textbooks, I ultimately stopped my sampling because I had found not a single one in which the author had omitted the exhortatory scientific methods section. These texts were almost all designed for college freshmen, although by the middle of the twentieth century many high schools were offering some instruction in the subject, often using whatever textbooks were available. T. L. Engle, *Psychology, Principles, and Applications* (Yonkers-on-Hudson, NY: World Book Company, 1945), p. v, for example, spoke of a "growing demand for instruction in psychology at high school and junior college levels."

70. O'Donnell, *Origins of Behaviorism*, p. 23, notes that from the beginning, laboratory work even in elementary psychology served to indoctrinate students into the culture of science. Much post-World War II oral tradition confirms the role of the methods training in psychology; when suddenly many people—typically physicians—were drawn into supported research, the only training that they had had in scientific methods had been in a psychology class, even though every physician, for example, had had years of premedical courses in the natural sciences.

71. See, for example, "The Big Promises of Pop Psych," *Psychology Today* (October 1975), 52. Kathleen Fisher, "Self-Help Authors Lack 'How-To' Manual," *APA Monitor* (April 1984), 20–21. Harold B. Clemenko, "What Do You Know about You?" *Look*, May 9, 1950, p. 108.

72. Edward S. Robinson, "Psychology and Public Policy," *School and Society*, 37 (1933), 537–543. Ross Stagner and T. F. Karwoski, *Psychology* (New York: McGraw-Hill Book Company, 1952), especially pp. 21–24.

73. Gertrude Schmeidler, "Following Up on Cultural Lag (and How to Give It a Push)," *American Psychologist*, 19 (1964), 137–138. See, for example, James Randi, *Flim Flam* (Buffalo, NY: Prometheus Books, 1982). Clifford T. Morgan published in 1966 a series of statements that he found most beginning psychology

students would mark as true but that psychological research had shown false; the statements included "Slow learners remember better than fast learners," "If a person is honest with you, he can usually tell you what his motives are," "Only human beings, not animals, have the capacity to think," and "When one is working for several hours, it is better to take a few long rests than several short ones." Morgan was able to show that many erroneous ideas were commonplace in the student population and that the study of psychology was needed to correct them. See Robert T. Lewis and Hugh M. Petersen, *Human Behavior: An Introduction to Psychology* (New York: The Ronald Press, 1974), pp. 10–11.

74. Sigmund Koch, "Psychology Cannot Be a Coherent Science," *Psychology Today* (September 1969), 14. Gregory A. Kimble, "Psychology's Two Cultures," *American Psychologist*, 39 (1984), 833–850.

75. See, for example, "What is Psychology?" *Psychology Today* (June 1968), 36–37. Michael S. Pallak, "Report of the Executive Officer: 1984," *American Psychologist*, 40 (1985), 611.

76. An example is David Bakan, "Political Factors in the Development of American Psychology," *Annals of the New York Academy of Sciences*, 291 (1977), 222–232. It is ironic that one survey of a middle class population found more favorable public attitudes toward psychologists than toward scientists; Anita Rosario Webb and James Ramsey Speer, "The Public Image of Psychologists," *American Psychologist*, 40 (1985), 1063–1064.

77. See, for example, "Robert M. Gagné," *American Psychologist*, 38 (1983), 24: "Influenced by his reading of popular works, Robert Gagné decided in high school that he wanted to study psychology and perhaps become a psychologist." See also chapter 6.

Chapter 4: Popularizing the Natural Sciences in the Nineteenth Century

1. Standard works are Brooke Hindle, *The Pursuit of Science in Revolutionary America, 1735–1789* (Chapel Hill: The University of North Carolina Press, 1956); John C. Greene, "Science and the Public in the Age of Jefferson," *Isis*, 49 (1958), 13–25; and John C. Greene, *American Science in the Age of Jefferson* (Ames: Iowa State University Press, 1984), especially chap. 1.

2. Greene, *American Science in the Age of Jefferson*, passim; John C. Greene, "The Founding of Peale's Museum," in Thomas R. Buckman, ed., *Bibliography & Natural History* (Lawrence: University of Kansas Libraries, 1966), pp. 66–72. Charles Coleman Sellers, *Mr. Peale's Museum; Charles Willson Peale and the First Popular Museum of Natural Science and Art* (New York: W. W. Norton & Company, 1980).

3. See, for example, besides general intellectual histories, David D. Hall, "The Victorian Connection," *American Quarterly*, 27 (1975), 561–574. An excellent sampling of popular science materials showing the dominance of English material in a wide-ranging selection is in Tyrus Hillway, "Melville's Education in Science," *Texas Studies in Literature and Language*, 16 (1974), 411–425.

4. Full-time scientists were of course rare not just in the United States but everywhere in the world outside of France until well into the nineteenth century. George H. Daniels, *American Science in the Age of Jackson* (New York: Columbia University Press, 1968), especially p. 34. William Martin Smallwood and Mabel Sarah Coon Smallwood, *Natural History and the American Mind* (New York: Columbia University Press, 1941), make little distinction (except for children's and educational material) between popularized and other science, and they explicitly close off their treatment at the point at which professional scientists appeared and natural explanations became more dominant.

5. Alexandra Oleson and Sanborn C. Brown, eds., *The Pursuit of Knowledge in the Early American Republic* (Baltimore: Johns Hopkins University Press, 1976); Merle Curti, *The Growth of American Thought* (3rd ed., New York: Harper & Row, 1964), 205–413. Historical commentators tend to believe that Americans took a special interest in science because frontier conditions brought a substantial part of the population into close contact with nature even beyond the rural life that was for so long a part of common experience; see, for example, Donald Zochert, "The Natural Science of an American Pioneer: A Case Study," *Transactions of the Wisconsin Academy of Sciences, Arts, and Letters*, 60 (1972), 7–15; James Oliver Robertson, *American Myth, American Reality* (New York: Hill & Wang, 1980), especially pp. 113–123.

6. There were other popular science books, such as the chapbooks, but their number and importance is uncertain; see, e.g., Emanuel D. Rudolph, "Botany in American and British Chapbooks before 1860," *Plant Science Bulletin*, 19 (1973), 34–36. Smallwood and Smallwood, *Natural History*, describe many examples and types of the various types of publications.

7. R. E. Peterson, ed., *Peterson's Familiar Science; or, The Scientific Explanation of Common Things* (1851; repr. Philadelphia: J. B. Lippincott & Co., 1860), p. iv. Paul Leonard Shank, "The Evolution of Natural Philosophy (Physics) Textbooks Used in American Secondary Schools before 1880" (doctoral diss., University of Pittsburgh, 1951), pp. 13, 16.

8. Michael Borut, "The *Scientific American* in Nineteenth Century America" (doctoral diss., New York University, 1977), pp. 27–33.

9. See in general Frank Luther Mott, *A History of American Magazines, 1850–1865* (Cambridge, MA: Harvard University Press, 1938); Matthew D. Whalen and Mary F. Tobin, "Periodicals and the Popularization of Science in America, 1860–1910," *Journal of American Culture*, 3 (1980), 195–203; John C.

Nerone, "The Press and Popular Culture in the Early Republic: Cincinnati, 1793–1848" (doctoral diss., University of Notre Dame, 1982), especially chap. 6; Donald deB. Beaver, "Altruism, Patriotism and Science: Scientific Journals in the Early Republic," *American Studies*, 12 (1971), 5–19. Smallwood and Smallwood, *Natural History*, pp. 224–225, take special note of children's magazines with substantial science content. "Our Hopes and Aims," *American Journal of Microscopy and Popular Science*, 1 (1875), 6.

10. [Benjamin Silliman], "Introductory Remarks," *American Journal of Science*, 1 (1818), 1–8; "Plan of the Work," *American Journal of Science*, 1 (1818), pp. v–vi.

11. "Preface," *Boston Journal of Philosophy and the Arts*, 1 (1823), iii. The articles in fact tended to be reprinted English material.

12. The proportion varied widely. In *Godey's Lady's Book*, for example, in 1840–1841 science and medicine came to less than four percent of the contents (Margaret F. Sommer, "Science in *Godey's Lady's Book*, 1840–1841" [unpublished paper]). Although of course the mortality rate for all types of magazines was high, the popular science ventures were notable not only in their brief duration but the fact that not one of them persisted.

13. Stanley M. Guralnick, *Science and the Ante-Bellum American College* (Philadelphia: The American Philosophical Society, 1975). Deborah Jean Warner, "Science Education for Women in Antebellum America," *Isis*, 69 (1978), 58–67.

14. Guralnick, *Science and the Ante-Bellum American College*, p. 22. Paul Johnson Fay, "The History of Science Teaching in American High Schools" (doctoral diss., The Ohio State University, 1930), especially pp. 89–124. Sidney Rosen, "The Rise of High-School Chemistry in America (to 1920)," *Journal of Chemical Education*, 33 (1956), 627–633. Sidney Rosen, "A History of the Physics Laboratory in the American Public High School (to 1910)," *American Journal of Physics*, 22 (1954), 194–204.

15. Rosen, "A History of the Physics Laboratory," pp. 195–196. Orra E. Underhill, *The Origins and Development of Elementary-School Science* (Chicago: Scott, Foresman and Company, 1941), pp. 13–74. Heber Eliot Rumble, "*More* Science Instruction?" *Science Education*, 33 (1949), 32–40, which describes especially efforts of educators to increase and improve science instruction in the nineteenth century.

16. "Nursery Rhymes for Little Scientists," reprinted from *Open Hand*, in *American Educational Monthly*, 10 (1873), 123. Barbara Joan Finkelstein, "Governing the Young: Teacher Behavior in American Primary Schools, 1820–1880—A Documentary History" (doctoral diss., Columbia University, 1970), especially pp. 92–96, found that even when textbook writers suggested illustrative materials and exercises, teachers tended to stick to simple recitation and memorization.

17. Emanuel D. Rudolph, "Learning Botany by Rote: The Way of the Nine-

teenth Century Catechisms," *Plant Science Bulletin*, 24 (1978), 39–40. C. Irving, *A Catechism of Botany, Containing a Description of the Most Familiar and Interesting Plants, Arranged According to the Linneaean System. With an Appendix on the Formation of An Herbarium. Adopted to the Use of Schools in the United States* (3rd American ed., New York: Collins and Hannay, 1829), pp. 6–7 (examined through the generosity of Emanuel D. Rudolph). [Jane Kilby Welch], *Botanical Catechism: Containing Introductory Lessons for Students in Botany* (Northampton: T. W. Shepard and Co., 1819), p. 31. Welch was the niece of the early American scientist Amos Eaton.

18. Bruno A. Casile, "An Analysis of Zoology Textbooks Available for American Secondary Schools before 1920" (doctoral diss., University of Pittsburgh, 1953). *The Rose Bud or Youths Gazette*, quoted in Thomas Cary Johnson, Jr., *Scientific Interests in the Old South* (New York: D. Appleton-Century Company, 1936), p. 113. A pioneer science educator recalled that in 1847 "in science, the instruction was wholly by catechism" (Elbridge Smith, quoted in Rosen, "A History of the Physics Laboratory," p. 194). As late as 1883 a series of parodies, "Popular Science Catechism," appeared in *Life*, 2 (1883).

19. William Mavor, quoted in Rudolph, "Learning Botany by Rote," p. 39. Underhill, *The Origins and Development*, especially pp. 74–92. E. M. Brigham, "Object Teaching," *American Educational Monthly*, 9 (1872), 212. Dora Otis Mitchell, "A History of Nature-Study," *Nature-Study Review*, 19 (1923), 261–269. The influence of the object lesson was evident in William T. Harris's *How to Teach Natural Science in Public Schools* (2nd ed., Syracuse: C. W. Bardeen, 1895), which was first issued in 1871 and was reprinted many times afterward. Harris advocated one hour a week, and object lessons were subordinated to a prescribed set of subject matters that could have had the effect of graded, progressive instruction had so much leeway not been given to what individual teachers thought they could carry out successfully.

20. See especially Fay, "The History of Science Teaching," p. 123. No attempt is made here to assemble a complete list of the secondary works dealing with the history of science education. See, for example, Alan M. Voelker and Charles A. Wall, "Historical Documents of Significance to Science Educators," *Science Education*, 57 (1973), 111–119. Ruth Miller Elson, *Guardians of Tradition: American Schoolbooks of the Nineteenth Century* (Lincoln: University of Nebraska Press, 1964), especially pp. 15–25, 35–40, analyzes the content of the textbooks.

21. Wyndham D. Miles, "Public Lectures on Chemistry in the United States," *Ambix*, 15 (1968), 129–153; the Eaton quotation is from pp. 141–142.

22. Fay, "The History of Science Teaching," pp. 29–30. Donald M. Scott, "The Popular Lecture and the Creation of a Public in Mid-Nineteenth Century America," *Journal of American History*, 66 (1980), 791–809, estimates that in the

1850s four hundred thousand people in the North and West alone heard public lectures each week. Margaret W. Rossiter, "Benjamin Silliman and the Lowell Institute: The Popularization of Science in Nineteenth-Century America," *New England Quarterly*, 44 (1971), 602–626. Oleson and Brown, *The Pursuit of Knowledge*, passim. Carl Bode, *The American Lyceum: Town Meeting of the Mind* (New York: Oxford University Press, 1956). Johnson, *Scientific Interests*, especially p. 49. Charles Upham Shepard, quoted in John C. Greene, "Prostestantism, Science, and American Enterprise: Benjamin Silliman's Moral Universe," in Leonard G. Wilson, ed., *Benjamin Silliman and His Circle: Studies on the Influence of Benjamin Silliman on Science in America, Prepared in Honor of Elizabeth H. Thomson* (New York: Science History Publications, 1979), p. 22. Ian Inkster, "Robert Goodacre's Astronomy Lectures (1823–1825) and the Structure of Scientific Culture in Philadelphia," *Annals of Science*, 35 (1978), 353–363.

23. Oleson and Brown, *The Pursuit of Knowledge*, passim. Johnson, *Scientific Interests*, especially pp. 54–61.

24. John Richards Betts, "P. T. Barnum and the Popularization of Natural History," *Journal of the History of Ideas*, 20 (1959), 353–368. Neil Harris, *Humbug: The Art of P. T. Barnum* (Boston: Little, Brown and Company, 1973), traces the way in which Barnum's educational work changed in context to the increasingly spectacular at the end of the nineteenth century. M. H. Dunlop, "Curiosities Too Numerous to Mention: Early Regionalism and Cincinnati's Western Museum," *American Quarterly*, 36 (1984), 524–548.

25. Scott, "The Popular Lecture"; Granville Sharp Pattison, *Syllabus of a Popular Course of Lectures on General Anatomy and Physiology, As Illustrative of the Natural History of Man* (Philadelphia: n.p., 1819), p. 3.

26. Robb Sagendorph, *America and Her Almanacs* (Dublin, NH: Yankee, Inc., 1970), especially pp. 125, 246. Charles E. Jorgenson, "The New Science in the Almanacs of Ames and Franklin," *New England Quarterly*, 8 (1935), 555–561. Phineas Raymond Stearns, *Science in the British Colonies of America* (Urbana: University of Illinois Press, 1970), p. 506. Marion Baker Stowell, *Early American Almanacs: The Colonial Weekday Bible* (New York: Burt Franklin, 1977). Lemuel H. Parsons, "Espy's Theory of Storms," *American Almanac and Repository of Useful Knowledge*, 1843, pp. 79–86.

27. The standard work is Richard A. Overfield, "Science in the *Virginia Gazette*, 1736–1780," *Emporia State Research Studies*, 16 (1968), 1–53.

28. Scott, "The Popular Lecture," pp. 798–799. Hillier Krieghbaum, "American Newspaper Reporting of Science News," *Kansas State College Bulletin*, 25 (1941), 17–18.

29. This account is based largely and freely on Donald Zochert, whose findings on Milwaukee in the 1830s and 1840s, "Science and the Common Man in

Ante-Bellum America," *Isis*, 65 (1974), 448–473, can be replicated for the rest of the country and for decades after his sample stops. See, for example, the discussion in Nerome, "The Press and Popular Culture." *Providence Gazette*, January 12, 1825, p. 1. The Boston *Transcript*, for example, while not dissimilar, did emphasize the many local lectures. William Peirce Randel, "Huxley in America," *Proceedings of the American Philosophical Society*, 114 (1970), 73–99. *Constitutionalist & Republic* [Augusta], January 28, 1855, [p. 2].

30. Zochert, "Science and the Common Man."

31. Amateurs in the nineteenth century did tend to work in the natural history areas; full-timers, as Daniels, *American Science in the Age of Jackson*, points out, were not so lopsidedly distributed in their interests. Some of the pains of separation of the two viewpoints, with the added issue of practicality, are explored in Robert Post, "Science, Public Policy, and Popular Precepts: Alexander Dallas Bache and Alfred Beach as Symbolic Adversaries," in Nathan Reingold, ed., *The Sciences in the American Context: New Perspectives* (Washington: Smithsonian Institution Press, 1979), pp. 77–98.

32. Substantial accounts of this movement include the articles of Walter B. Hendrickson, summarized in "Science and Culture in the American Middle West," *Isis*, 52 (1961), 357–371; Ralph W. Dexter has done comparable work on the Northeast; for example, see his "History of the Pottsville (Pa.) Scientific Association, 1854–1862," *Science Education*, 53 (1969), 29–32, and "The Essex County Natural History Society, 1833–1848," *Essex Institute Historical Collections*, 113 (1977), 38–53; and Oleson and Brown, *The Pursuit of Knowledge*, especially Henry D. Shapiro, "The Western Academy of Natural Sciences of Cincinnati and the Structure of Science in the Ohio Valley, 1810–1850." John Harley Warner, "'Exploring the Inner Labyrinths of Creation': Popular Microscopy in Nineteenth-Century America," *Journal of the History of Medicine and Allied Sciences*, 37 (1982), 7–33.

33. David Meredith Reese, *Humbugs of New York: Being a Remonstrance Against Popular Delusion; Whether in Science, Philosophy, or Religion* (New York: John S. Taylor, 1838). Tom Telescope, *The Newtonian System of Philosophy, Explained by Familiar Objects in an Entertaining Manner, For the Use of Young Ladies and Gentlemen* (Philadephia: Jacob Johnson, 1803), p. 6; this book was originally published in England, and the authorship has been attributed to Oliver Goldsmith.

34. Borut, "The *Scientific American*," especially p. 160.

35. Oleson and Brown, *The Pursuit of Knowledge*. Johnson, *Scientific Interests*. James D. Teller, "Louis Agassiz and Men of Letters," *Scientific Monthly*, 65 (1947), 428–432. Ian F. A. Bell, "Divine Patterns: Louis Agassiz and American Men of Letters," *Journal of American Studies*, 4 (1976), 349–381. The latter two are mere examples; the subject of the influence of science on American literature is a special

subfield with its own literature. Literary figures were, however, consumers rather than producers of popular science. See, for example, Joseph Beaver, *Walt Whitman—Poet of Science* (1951; repr. New York: Octagon Books, 1974).

36. *Lynchburg Press*, quoted in *National Register*, October 12, 1816, p. 106. Rosen, "Rise of High-School Chemistry," p. 628.

37. Rossiter, "Benjamin Silliman." Greene, *American Science in the Age of Jefferson*, makes a similar point more indirectly.

38. See especially Fay, "History of Science Teaching," p. 21.

39. James Turner, *Without God, Without Creed: The Origins of Unbelief in America* (Baltimore: Johns Hopkins University Press, 1985). The English background is explored particularly in Robert M. Young, *Darwin's Metaphor: Nature's Place in Victorian Culture* (Cambridge: Cambridge University Press, 1985), chap. 5.

40. Pattison, *Syllabus of a Popular Course*, p. 4. The argument from design could serve merely religious purposes, but it could also reinforce a Deistic point of view; from the point of view of popularizing, the ultimate goal is not important at the initial level.

41. The basic works are Daniels, *American Science in the Age of Jackson*; Theodore Dwight Bozeman, *Protestants in an Age of Science: The Baconian Ideal and Antebellum American Religious Thought* (Chapel Hill: University of North Carolina Press, 1977); Herbert Hovenkamp, *Science and Religion in America, 1800–1860* (Philadelphia: University of Pennsylvania Press, 1978); Turner, *Without God, Without Creed*. Underhill, *Origins and Development*, 51–56. Elson, *Guardians of Tradition*, provides many examples. [Orville Dewey], review of *Library of Useful Knowledge*, in *North American Review*, 30 (1830), 293–313.

42. "My Aquarium," *Atlantic Monthly*, 1 (1858), 431. "Astronomy," *American Quarterly Review*, 3 (1828), 320. See especially Bozeman, *Protestants*, pp. 84–85; Turner, *Without God, Without Creed*. Edward Hitchcock, *Religious Truth, Illustrated from Science, In Addresses and Sermons on Special Occasions* (Boston: Phillips, Sampson and Company, 1856), pp. 36–37.

43. "Superstition and Knowledge," *The Quarterly Review*, 29 (1823), 474–475. Anonymous review of Wiseman, *Twelve Lectures on the Connexion Between Science and Revealed Religion*, in *North American Review*, 45 (1837), 247. Wilson Smith, "William Paley's Theological Utilitarianism in America," *William and Mary Quarterly*, 11 (1954), 402–424.

44. Benjamin Silliman, Jr., *First Principles of Chemistry, For the Use of Colleges and Schools* (1852; 44th ed., Philadelphia: H. C. Peck & Theo. Bliss, 1858), pp. 13–14.

45. Hyman Kuritz, "The Popularization of Science in Nineteenth-Century America," *History of Education Quarterly*, 21 (1981), 259–274, emphasizes the ideology in popularization that connected science to technology.

46. Zochert, "Science and the Common Man," pp. 464–466. Daniels, *American Science in the Age of Jackson.* P. T. Barnum, quoted in Betts, "P. T. Barnum," p. 358.

47. The classic secular document spelling out this general attitude is Timothy Walker, "Defence of Mechanical Philosophy," *North American Review*, 33 (1831), 122–136. Turner, *Without God, Without Creed*, especially pp. 116–121, 132–137. See, for example, Alex Inkeles et al., *Exploring Individual Modernity* (New York: Columbia University Press, 1983), especially p. 14.

48. See, for example, [J. Lovering], "Skepticism in Science," *Christian Examiner*, 51 (1851), 209–250. Turner, *Without God, Without Creed*, treats this intellectual theme in detail.

49. Chauncy Wright, "Natural Theology as Positive Science," *North American Review*, 100 (1865), 177–185, especially 184. D. H. Meyer, *The Instructed Conscience: The Shaping of the American National Ethic* (Philadelphia: University of Pennsylvania Press, 1972), pp. 126–129, describes the "secularization of scientific thought."

50. *The Young Florist's Companion, Being Concise Explanations of Botanical Terms Used in Describing Flowers; Together with Illustrations of the Classes and Orders, By Familiar Examples* (Hartford: S. G. Goodrich, 1819), p. 12 and passim.

51. A good example of bad science early in the century can be found in the *Columbian Almanac*—in which the attempt is nevertheless to use naturalistic explanation. See, for example, Edgar Allan Poe's ironically titled "Sonnet—To Science," in James A. Harrison, ed., *The Complete Works of Edgar Allan Poe* (17 vols., 1902; repr. New York: AMS Press, 1965), 7: 22. Obviously even the functional or teleological explanations were immediately secular and rational. Turner, *Without God, Without Creed.*

52. [Denison Olmsted], *Outlines of the Lectures on Chemistry, Mineralogy, & Geology, Delivered at the University of North-Carolina—For the Use of Students* (Raleigh: J. Gales, 1819), p. 3. W. H. C. Bartlett, *Elements of Natural Philosophy, Section 1: Mechanics* (New York: A. S. Barnes & Co., 1850), p. 9.

53. Daniels, *American Science in the Age of Jackson*, chap. 3, notes the parallel between unsystematic fact gathering and religious belief without a rational theology, which would be chiefly interpretations of the Bible without context—not uncommon then.

54. J. G. Holland, "The Popular Lecture," *Atlantic Monthly*, 15 (1865), 367.

55. See Rossiter, "Benjamin Silliman," pp. 623–624. Taylor Stoehr, *Hawthorne's Mad Scientists: Pseudoscience and Social Science in Nineteenth-Century Life and Letters* (Hampden, CT: Archon Books, 1978), especially pp. 21–29, contains an up-to-date summary of the literature as well as original insights.

56. There were at first not many of them. There were 759 members of the American Association for the Advancement of Science in 1851, and 4,000 names

appeared in the first comprehensive American directory of scientists in 1906. Edward Lurie, "Science in American Thought," *Journal of World History*, 8 (1965), 641, notes that the scientific outlook had great influence even though the culture did not produce many great scientists.

57. Oliver Wendell Holmes, quoted in Edward Lurie, *Nature and the American Mind: Louis Agassiz and the Culture of Science* (New York: Science History Publications, 1974), p. 51. *Atlantic Monthly*, 29 (1872), 382. Matthew D. Whalen, "Science, the Public, and American Culture: A Preface to the Study of Popular Science," *Journal of American Culture*, 4 (1981), 19–20.

58. F. W. Clarke, "Scientific Dabblers," *Popular Science Monthly*, 1 (1872), 594–601, especially p. 600.

59. John C. Branner, "The Education of a Naturalist," *School Review*, 3 (1895), 134–143. See, for example, anonymous review of *Natural Science*, in *Popular Science Monthly*, 41 (1892), 418. At one point, an editor—presumably Youmans—of the *Popular Science Monthly*, 5 (1874), 741–744, complained that the American Association for the Advancement of Science was not doing enough popularizing and suggested that the name be changed to An Association for the Promotion of Science by Original Research. Perspective on late nineteenth-century amateur movements is found in Douglas Sloan, "Science in New York City, 1867–1907," *Isis*, 71 (1980), 35–76, and an important additional aspect is described in Emanuel D. Rudolph, "Women in Nineteenth Century Botany: A Generally Unrecognized Constituency," *American Journal of Botany*, 69 (1982), 1346–1355.

60. Krieghbaum, "American Newspaper Reporting," pp. 38–39.

61. "Newspaper Science," *Dial*, 26 (1899), 233–235. "Newspaper Science," *Current Literature*, 33 (1902), 677–678. *Popular Science News*, 29 (1895), 73. *Popular Science News*, 27 (1893), 9. Italics in original *Popular Science News* article to indicate obviously ridiculous material. John Trowbridge, "South Sea Bubbles in Science," *Popular Science Monthly*, 56 (1900), 401–408.

62. *Chicago Tribune*, January 2, 1898, p. 1; January 3, 1898, p. 4. For a whole hodgepodge of correction, including errors about the moon's appearance found in American novels of the day, see *Popular Science News*, 21 (1887), 57; or, on another occasion, 21 (1888), 137.

63. "Physicist," "Science and Fiction," *Popular Science Monthly*, 57 (1900), 326. "Mr. Tesla's Science," *Popular Science Monthly*, 58 (1901), 436–437. *Popular Science News*, 26 (1892), 153. At one point accurate and constructive reporting was unusual enough to elicit comment: "Brooklyn's Feast of Science," *Popular Science News*, 28 (1894), 149.

64. Details are in Whalen and Tobin, "Periodicals and the Popularization."

65. For example, see the "Chautauqua Edition" of Dorman Steele and J. W. P. Jenks, *Popular Zoology* (New York: Chautauqua Press, [1887?]).

66. Specifically relevant general background is in Geraldine Joncich, "Scientists and the Schools of the Nineteenth Century: The Case of American Physicists," *American Quarterly*, 18 (1966), 667–685.

67. The classic, not necessarily disinterested, observation is Daniel C. Gilman, "On the Growth of American Colleges and Their Present Tendency to the Study of Science," *Papers Read Before the American Institute of Instruction*, 1871, pp. 96–115. The standard discussion of science in higher education is Laurence R. Veysey, *The Emergence of the American University* (Chicago: University of Chicago Press, 1965), chap. 3. See also Stanley M. Guralnick, "The American Scientist in Higher Education, 1820–1910," in Nathan Reingold, ed., *The Sciences in the American Context: New Perspectives* (Washington: Smithsonian Institution Press, 1979), pp. 99–141.

68. *Boston Journal of Chemistry*, 15 (1881), 12. Rosen, "A History of the Physics Laboratory," especially p. 202, where Conant is quoted. Casile, "An Analysis of Zoology Textbooks," p. 182. E. J. Hallock, "Experiments for Young Chemists," *Boston Journal of Chemistry*, 15 (1881), 110. The revulsion against mere textbook instruction and the sentiment to let students confront nature, particularly by experiment, is documented in exquisite detail in Charles K. Wead, "Aims and Methods of the Teaching of Physics," Bureau of Education, *Circulars of Information*, 7 (1884), and, to a lesser extent, in John P. Campbell, "Biological Teaching in the Colleges of the United States," Bureau of Education, *Circulars of Information*, 9 (1891), in which the gaps and limitations are displayed, also. Of course as T. C. Mendenhall observed, in "Physics in General Education," *Popular Science Monthly*, 23 (1883), 24, the experiments were not always successful, for if they were not done skillfully, "The result of the crude experiments of the student was often to disprove the law which he was expected to establish."

69. Wilbur S. Jackman, quoted in Underhill, *The Origins and Development*, p. 121, which see in general. Rodger W. Bybee, "The New Transformation of Science Education," *Science Education*, 61 (1977), 87–88.

70. Tyree G. Minton, "The History of the Nature-Study Movement and Its Role in the Development of Environmental Education" (doctoral diss., University of Massachusetts, 1980). Mitchell, "A History of Nature Study," pp. 295–311. Louis I. Kuslan, "Science in the 19th Century Normal School," *Science Education*, 40 (1956), 138–144. Nature study is discussed further in the next chapter.

71. Elson, *Guardians of Tradition*, emphasizes the conservative nature of common school books. William G. Farlow, "Biological Teaching in Colleges," *Popular Science Monthly*, 28 (1886), 578. See especially Casile, "An Analysis of Zoology Textbooks." S. S. Cornell, *Cornell's Physical Geography: Accompanied with Nineteen Pages of Maps, A Great Variety of Map-Questions, and One Hundred and Thirty Diagrams and Pictorial Illustrations: And Embracing a Detailed Description of the*

Physical Features of the United States (New York: D. Appleton and Company, 1870), p. 3. Around 1900 the subject tended to become less general science and naturalism and more like the modern geography.

72. See especially Fay, "The History of Science Teaching."

73. Rumble, "*More* Science Instruction?" Whitelaw Reid, quoted in Frank Luther Mott, "*A History of American Magazines, 1865–1885* (Cambridge, MA: Harvard University Press, 1938), p. 105.

74. Simon Newcomb, "Exact Science in America," *North American Review*, 119 (1874), 306–307; Newcomb listed the major signs but found much of the activity wanting in quality. *Boston Journal of Chemistry*, 15 (1881), 7. Compare the later survey of readers, "The Eighteenth Volume," *Popular Science News*, 18 (1884), 9. "James Robinson Nichols," *Popular Science News*, 22 (1888), 25. Edwin G. Conklin, "The Early History of the American Naturalist," *American Naturalist*, 78 (1944), 29–37.

75. Charles M. Haar, "E. L. Youmans: A Chapter in the Diffusion of Science in America," *Journal of the History of Ideas*, 9 (1948), 199–200. Frank Luther Mott, *A History of American Magazines, 1865–1885* (Cambridge, MA: Harvard University Press, 1938), pp. 104–107. E. A. Washburn, "Address to Medical Students," *Popular Science Monthly*, 7 (1875), 63.

76. Mott, *A History of American Magazines*, pp. 495–499. Whalen and Tobin, "Periodicals and the Popularization of Science." "The Progress of Science," *Popular Science Monthly*, 58 (1901), 555. "Science in American Journals," *Popular Science Monthly*, 61 (1902), 474–475. Aline Gorren, "The New Criticism of Genius," *Atlantic Monthly*, 74 (1894). Frank L. Mott, "The Magazine Revolution and Popular Ideas in the Nineties," *Proceedings of the American Antiquarian Society*, 64 (1954), 195–214, notes that the new magazines were aimed at the upwardly mobile, as opposed to the genteel audience of the earlier periodicals. See, for example, Elmer F. Suderman, "Popular Fiction (1870–1900) Looks at Darwin and the Nature of God," in Ray B. Browne, ed., *Challenges in American Culture* (Bowling Green: Bowling Green University Popular Press, 1970), pp. 142–149. Sally Gregory Kohlstedt, "From Learned Society to Public Museum: The Boston Society of Natural History," in Alexandra Oleson and John Voss, eds., *The Organization of Knowledge in Modern America, 1860–1920* (Baltimore: Johns Hopkins University Press, 1979), pp. 400–401.

77. Harlan H. Ballard, *Three Kingdoms: A Hand-Book of the Agassiz Association* (New York: The Writers Publishing Company, 1888), pp. 18–19 and passim; and a somewhat different account, Harlan H. Ballard, "History of the Agassiz Association," *Swiss Cross*, 1 (1887), 4–7. *Popular Science News*, 24 (1890), 169, 9, and passim for the 1890s, when the *News* was serving in lieu of the *Swiss Cross* (which see) and other independent publications that before and after served the association. The "Editorial Notes," *Swiss Cross*, 1 (1887), 195–196, provide insight into

how this and other amateur groups worked, with the usual difficulties about cycles of interest, devising tasks to maintain active membership, etc.

78. Over the years innumerable editorials in the *Popular Science Monthly* spelled out this idea; see similarly Josiah Parsons Cooke, *Scientific Culture and Other Essays* (2nd ed., New York: D. Appleton and Company, 1885). Just at the end of the century scientists appeared in as much as 5 percent of the inspirational biography published in the better magazines (in contrast to none of it three-quarters of a century earlier); Theodore P. Greene, *America's Heroes: The Changing Models of Success in American Magazines* (New York: Oxford University Press, 1970), especially p. 153.

79. *Popular Science News*, 29 (1895), 69.

80. Frank Sargent Hoffman, *The Sphere of Science: A Study of the Nature and Method of Scientific Investigation* (New York: G. P. Putnam's Sons, 1898), pp. 18–19.

81. All of these attitudes were, of course, in addition to the specifically naturalistic views described in chapter 1, above. Mark Sullivan, *Our Times: The United States, 1900–1925* (6 vols., New York: 1927–1935), 2: 195. The *Boston Journal of Chemistry and Popular Science* in 1882 had editorial headings that suggested the emphasis of a practical point of view: "Familiar Science," "Practical Chemistry and the Arts," "Agriculture," and "Medicine and Pharmacy."

82. "'The Conflict of Ages,'" *Popular Science Monthly*, 8 (1876), 494; "Who Are the Propagators of Atheism?" *Popular Science Monthly*, 5 (1874), 367. William E. Leverette, Jr., "Science and Values: A Study of Edward L. Youmans' *Popular Science Monthly*" (doctoral diss., Vanderbilt University, 1963). William E. Leverette, Jr., "E. L. Youmans' Crusade for Scientific Autonomy and Respectability," *American Quarterly*, 17 (1965), 12–32. A perceptive contemporary example of reconciliation was H. W. Conn, "Study of Science and the Christian Faith," *Methodist Review*, 72 (1890), 79–92.

83. Horace Bushnell, quoted on p. 591 in D. H. Meyer, "American Intellectuals and the Victorian Crisis of Faith," *American Quarterly*, 27 (1975), 585–603. N. P. Gilman, "'The Creed of Science,'" *Unitarian Review and Religious Magazine*, 19 (1883), 507–508. It was a question, noted an author in "The Carboniferous Era," *Popular Science News*, 2 (1887), 19, whether one attributed processes to "nature" or to the "Author of nature." In the early history of the nature study movement, some workers voiced concern that Nature was set up as an infallible guide— especially when mankind was included as part of Nature; Minton, "History of the Nature-Study Movement," pp. 90–91. While nature worship was perhaps romantic, people at the time saw that it was quite different from superstition.

84. See, for example, M. J. Gorton, "Hysteria and Its Allies—Ghosts and Superstitions," *Popular Science News*, 25 (1891), 139–140, and other issues of this journal in the 1880s and 1890s. "The Mysteries of Plant-Growth," *Popular Science News*, 21 (1887), 39.

85. Lewis Swift, "A Mystery of the Skies," *Cosmopolitan*, 1 (1886), 22. "The Reason Why," *Popular Science News*, 23 (1889), 71–72. Ibid., 25 (1891), 135.

86. E. A. Washburn, "The Conflict of Religion and Science," *International Review*, 3 (1876), 36. George H. Williams, "Some Modern Aspects of Geology," *Popular Science Monthly*, 35 (1889), 640. A recent discussion of the concept emphasizes the element of analysis as distinct from complexity; Keith Stewart Thomson, "Reductionism and Other Isms in Biology," *American Scientist*, 72 (1984), 388–390. Nineteenth-century popularizers did not usually make such fine distinctions and sometimes confused analogy with explanation, although the direction of their efforts was clear enough.

87. Anonymous review of Bastian, *The Brain as an Organ of Mind*, in *Popular Science Monthly*, 17 (1880), 846. E. B. Rosa, "The Human Body as an Engine," *Popular Science Monthly*, 57 (1900), 491–499. For examples of this kind of discussion, see John Bascom, *Science, Philosophy and Religion* (New York: G. P. Putnam & Sons, 1871), p. 20; J. M. Stillman, "The Source of Muscular Energy," *Popular Science Monthly*, 24 (1884), 377–387; William James, "Are We Automata?" *Mind*, 4 (1879), 1–22; and Milic Capek, "James's Early Criticism of the Automaton Theory," *Journal of the History of Ideas*, 15 (1954), 260–279.

88. John Trowbridge, "What is Electricity?" *Popular Science Monthly*, 26 (1884), 76–78. "The Unity of Nature," *Boston Journal of Chemistry*, 15 (1881), 25–26.

89. John W. Dickinson, "Elementary and Scientific Knowledge," *Addresses and Journal of Proceedings of the National Education Association*, 1873, p. 178. "Easy Chemical Experiments," *Popular Science News*, 19 (1885), 17. Stanley Coulter, "The Contribution of Nature Study to the Future of the Child Who Must Leave School at the End of the Eighth Grade," *Educational Bi-Monthly*, 1 (1907), 306–311. William G. Peck, *Elementary Treatise on Mechanics, For the Use of Colleges and Schools of Science* (New York: A. S. Barnes & Company, 1870); the quote is on p. 4. [Mary Mapes Dodge], "The Giant Watabore," *St. Nicholas*, 1 (1873), 56–57, for example, explicitly contrasted for children the chaos of undigested fact and opinion with the orderly knowledge of science checked through one's own microscope.

90. "Supernatural Stories," *Eclectic Magazine of Foreign Literature, Science, and Art*, 15 (1850), 105–118. See in general Ronald E. Martin, *American Literature and the Universe of Force* (Durham: Duke University Press, 1981).

91. E. L. Youmans et al., "Science Teaching in the Public Schools," *Popular Science Monthly*, 23 (1883), 207–214. Diana Postlethwaite, *Making it Whole: A Victorian Circle and the Shape of Their World* (Columbus: The Ohio State University Press, 1984), emphasizes the Victorians' sense that the world was changing rapidly.

92. John M. Coulter, "The Mission of Science in Education," *Science*, n.s. 12 (1900), 283. Turner, *Without God, Without Creed*. [E. L. Youmans], "Our First

Year's Work," *Popular Science Monthly*, 2 (1873), 745. [Brother Azarias], "Literary and Scientific Habits of Thought," *American Catholic Quarterly Review*, 10 (1885), 217–239. One classic statement was William Graham Sumner, "The Scientific Attitude of Mind," in *Earth-Hunger and Other Essays* (New Haven: Yale University Press, 1913), pp. 17–28. John Brisben Walker, "What is Education? The Studies Most Important for the Modern Man. Who Should Study Science," *Cosmopolitan*, 37 (1904) 401–403. Commentators have pointed out that literature showed that cultivated people did learn the lesson of the ideal of the scientific attitude; see, for example, Harry Hayden Clark, "The Influence of Science on American Literary Criticism, 1860–1910, Including the Vogue of Taine," *Transactions of the Wisconsin Academy of Sciences, Arts, and Letters*, 41 (1952), 109–138; Donald Pizer, "Evolutionary Ideas in Late Nineteenth-Century English and American Literary Criticism," *Journal of Aesthetics and Art Criticism*, 19 (1961), 305–310. The pessimistic, sometimes antiscientific "bankruptcy of science" discussion in Europe did not find a sympathetic audience in the United States, where traditional views and a growing interest in pure research dominated the scientific community. See Harry W. Paul, "The Debate Over the Bankruptcy of Science in 1895," *French Historical Studies*, 5 (1968), 299–327; Roy MacLeod, "The 'Bankruptcy of Science' Debate: The Creed of Science and Its Critics, 1885–1900," *Science, Technology, and Human Values* (Fall 1982), 2–15. Compare D. C. Gilman, "The Bankruptcy of Science," *Cosmopolitan*, 23 (1897), 338–339.

93. W J McGee, "50 Years of American Science," *Atlantic Monthly*, 82 (1898), 307. Michael D. Stephens and Gordon W. Roderick, "American and English Attitudes to Scientific Education During the Nineteenth Century," *Annals of Science*, 30 (1973), 435–456, show that Americans had industrial advance in mind relatively more frequently than the British. John Joseph Zernel, "John Wesley Powell: Science and Reform in a Positive Context" (doctoral diss., Oregon State University, 1983), especially pp. 231ff. *Popular Science News*, 18 (1894), 9. David A. Hollinger, "Inquiry and Uplift: Late Nineteenth-Century American Academics and the Moral Efficacy of Scientific Practice," in Thomas L. Haskell, ed., *The Authority of Experts: Studies in History and Theory* (Bloomington: Indiana University Press, 1984), pp. 142–156, emphasizes the moral aspects of the religion of science in his incisive summary.

94. See, for example, Robert C. Bannister, *Social Darwinism: Science and Myth in Anglo-American Social Thought* (Philadelphia: Temple University Press, 1979); and the summary of recent scholarship included in John R. Reed, *Victorian Conventions* (Athens, OH: Ohio University Press, 1975), especially pp. 451–453. Another type of popular science in the service of civilization is described in Lisa Mighetto, "Science, Sentiment, and Anxiety: American Nature Writing at the Turn of the Century," *Pacific Historical Review*, 54 (1985), 33–50.

95. The influence of Karl Pearson was transparent and eagerly accepted; see, for example, "The Scientific Mind," *Popular Science News*, 26 (1892), 181.

96. "The Mysteries of Chemistry," *Popular Science News*, 23 (1889), 10.

97. John Trowbridge, "Science from the Pulpit," *Popular Science Monthly*, 6 (1875), 735.

Chapter 5: Popularizing the Natural Sciences in the Twentieth Century

1. Marcel Evelyn Chotkowski La Follette, "Authority, Promise, and Expectation: The Images of Science and Scientists in American Popular Magazines, 1910–1955" (doctoral diss., Indiana University, 1979). Bernhard M. Auer, "A Letter from the Publisher," *Time*, January 2, 1961, p. 1. See especially Normand Parent DuBeau, "Some Social Aspects of Science News" (master's thesis, University of Missouri, 1941), pp. 70, 88–94, etc.; J. S. Sorenson and D. D. Sorenson, "A Comparison of Science Content in Magazines in 1964–65 and 1969–70," *Journalism Quarterly*, 50 (1973), 97–101; George Comstock and Heather Tully, "Innovation in the Movies, 1939–1976," *Journal of Communication* (Spring 1981), 97–105; Louise Nathe, in Norman Metzger, ed., *Science in the Newspaper* (Washington: American Association for the Advancement of Science, 1974), pp. 14–18. "The Science Boom," *Newsweek*, September 17, 1979, pp. 104–107.

2. It is of course true that quantitative indicators can be misleading; see, for example, Jonathon T. Rich, "A Measure of Comprehensiveness in Newsmagazine Science Coverage," *Journalism Quarterly*, 58 (1981), 248–253, and below in this chapter. Nevertheless the proper point to begin a narrative is with the quantitative profile.

3. John M. Coulter, "Public Interest in Research," *Popular Science Monthly*, 67 (1905), 306. "The Popularization of Science," *Popular Science Monthly*, 72 (1908), 382–384. "The Scientific Monthly and the Popular Science Monthly," *Popular Science Monthly*, 87 (1915), 307–309; "Scientific Journals and the Public," *Popular Science Monthly*, 87 (1915), 309–310.

4. Will Irwin, *Propaganda and the News; or, What Makes You Think So?* (New York: Whittlesey House, 1936), pp. 89–94. Hillier Krieghbaum, "American Newspaper Reporting of Science News," *Kansas State College Bulletin*, 25 (1941), 38–40. J. O'H. Cosgrave of the *World* presented an early defense in *Science*, 55 (1922), 594–595. La Follette, "Authority, Promise, and Expectation," p. 88. A convenient sample of the better coverage is Walter Sullivan, ed., *Science in the Twentieth Century* (New York: Arno Press, 1976).

5. John D. Buenker, John C. Burnham, and Robert M. Crunden, *Progressivism* (Cambridge, MA: Schenkman Publishing Company, 1977), pp. 19–20; Russel B. Nye, "The Juvenile Approach to American Culture, 1870–1930," in Ray B. Browne et al., eds., *New Voices in American Studies* (West Lafayette: Purdue University Studies, 1966), pp. 79–81. E.g., Fred D. Barber, "Fundamental Considerations in the Reorganization of High School Science," *General Science Quar-*

terly, 1 (1917), 102–111; and see below in this chapter. It is possible that existing sources on the level of popularizing are misleading—that, for example, the magazines that La Follette sampled were not representative. Or it may be true that English popularization, too, may have declined in this period, and, as will be noted below, English writings were still very important in U.S. popularized science. All such possibilities have yet to be explored in systematic scholarship that is not yet in sight; for the time being the paradox must stand.

6. Lawrence Badash, "Radium, Radioactivity, and the Popularity of Scientific Discovery," *Proceedings of the American Philosophical Society*, 122 (1978), 147–149.

7. See below in this chapter. "Announcement," *Scientific American Monthly*, 4 (1921), 291. The sources may, of course, not be accurate, but at this point no scholar has shown in the popularizing of technology a configuration different from that described here.

8. DuBeau, "Some Social Aspects," p. 34. See especially Charles William Heywood, "Scientists and Society in the United States, 1900–1940: Changing Concepts of Social Responsibility" (doctoral diss., University of Pennsylvania, 1954), chap. 2; and Ronald C. Tobey, *The American Ideology of National Science, 1919–1930* (Pittsburgh: University of Pittsburgh Press, 1971). I shall not attempt here to explore the effects of the attenuation of certain kinds of reform after World War I. Warren I. Susman, *Culture as History: The Transformation of American Society in the Twentieth Century* (New York: Pantheon Books, 1984), pp. 107–108, points out that popularization of other areas of high culture—besides science—also reached a high point during the 1920s.

9. See Krieghbaum, "American Newspaper Reporting," pp. 42–46; Tobey, *The American Ideology*, especially chap. 4; James Walter Weslowski, "Before Canon 35: WGN Broadcasts the Monkey Trial," *Journalism History*, 2 (1975), 76–79, 86. Sidney Ratner, "Evolution and the Rise of the Scientific Spirit in America," *Philosophy of Science*, 3 (1936), 104. Paul A. Carter, *Another Part of the Twenties* (New York: Columbia University Press, 1977), chap. 4. Marshall Missner, "Why Einstein Became Famous in America," *Social Studies of Science*, 15 (1985), 267–292. *Life*, April 6, 1922, p. 14.

10. DuBeau, "Some Social Aspects," pp. 36, 41. Krieghbaum, "American Newspaper Reporting," pp. 41, 46–47; Hillier, Krieghbaum, "A Pioneer in Plain English," *Kansas Magazine*, 8 (1940), 91–94. The best treatment is David J. Rhees, "A New Voice for Science: Science Service under Edwin E. Slosson, 1921–29" (master's thesis, University of North Carolina, 1979). See Tobey, *The American Ideology*, chap. 3 and passim for the more general context; Heywood, "Scientists and Society," pp. 97–101.

11. E. T. Bell, "Mathematics and Speculation," *Scientific Monthly*, 32 (1931), 193. Rhees, "A New Voice."

12. See, for example, "The Ninth Planet," *Nation*, 130 (1930), 386; "The

Latest News from Pluto," *Literary Digest*, September 6, 1930, p. 18. Ralph O. Nafziger, "A Reader-Interest Survey of Madison, Wisconsin," *Journalism Quarterly*, 7 (1930), 137: "Popularized science is eagerly read by both men and women, as is also news of scientific discoveries."

13. DuBeau, "Some Social Aspects," pp. 5, 46–49, in which John J. O'Neill's letter is quoted. Emma Behnke, "Cultural Trends in Radio" (master's thesis, University of Iowa, 1941). The war had a similar effect on motion picture newsreels; Robert C. Davis, "The Public Impact of Science in the Mass Media: A Report on a Nation-Wide Survey for the National Association of Science Writers" (Ann Arbor: University of Michigan Survey Research Center, 1958), p. 3n. The classic 1930s survey is Benjamin C. Gruenberg, *Science and the Public Mind* (New York: McGraw-Hill Book Company, 1935).

14. See especially Heywood, "Scientists and Society," pp. 139–160. Jack Schuyler, "Science and Society," *Journal of Adult Education*, 9 (1937), 69–73. Gerald Wendt, *Science for the World of Tomorrow* (New York: W. W. Norton & Company, 1939). John Allen Harmon, "Scientists in the United States During the 1930's: Image and Status" (master's thesis, The Ohio State University, 1970). The amount of hostile comment about science was quite remarkable. In the *New Yorker*, May 11, 1935, p. 33, appeared a poem entitled "Science," by "C. D.," in which the author described how scientists throughout the Depression swapped stories "in expensive laboratories" and messed with protoplasms and "jars of jelly." "C. D." concluded sarcastically that "science is a grand profession!"

15. Hillier Krieghbaum, "Science News Doubled in a Decade, Editors Say," *Editor and Publisher*, April 7, 1951, p. 22.

16. *Impact of Science on Society*, 8 (1957), 55. Hillier Krieghbaum, "At Sputnik Plus 8: More Science News," *Editor and Publisher*, October 30, 1965, pp. 14, 47, and Hillier Krieghbaum, *Science and the Mass Media* (New York: New York University Press, 1967), which summarizes the numerous detailed studies on this whole period. Robert W. Hayden, "A History of the 'New Math' Movement in the United States" (doctoral diss., Iowa State University, 1981), p. 211. Ray Erwin, "Press Urged to Help U.S. Beat U.S.S.R. in Science," *Editor and Publisher*, November 30, 1957, p. 9. Victor Cohn, "Are We Really Telling the People about Science?" *Quill* (December 1965), 12.

17. See John Tebbel, "Newspapers and the Culture Beat," *Saturday Review*, April 13, 1963, p. 61; and in general Krieghbaum, *Science and the Mass Media*, especially p. 30. In 1963 a prize of $10,000 for a popular science book was not awarded because no suitable candidate could be found (Alan D. Williams, "$10,000 Going Begging?" *NASW Newsletter* [December 1963], 14).

18. Sharon M. Friedman, in Metzger, *Science in the Newspaper*, pp. 19–20. A. Clay Schoenfeld, "The Environmental Movement as Reflected in the American Magazine," *Journalism Quarterly*, 60 (1983), 470–475; James S. Bowman and

Kathryn Hanaford, "Mass Media and the Environment since Earth Day," *Journalism Quarterly*, 54 (1977), 160–165; James S. Bowman, "American Daily Newspapers and the Environment," *Journal of Environmental Education* (Fall 1978), 1–11. One chapter in what happened to environmentalist popularization of science is summarized in John Walsh, "Science Information: SIPI Expands, Puts New Emphasis on the Economy," *Science*, 192 (1976), 122–124.

19. See especially John Lear, "The Trouble with Science Writing," *Columbia Journalism Review* (Summer 1970), 30–34. "Science Newspaper under Consideration," *Editor and Publisher*, October 30, 1965, p. 14. Warren Burkett, "There's More Going on in Science Than Some Would Tell," *Quill* (May 1970), 19. Mary Bubb, "Nostalgic Look Back into Space," *Quill* (September 1974), 22–27. Carla Marie Rupp, "Breast Cancer Stories Have News Interest," *Editor and Publisher*, October 26, 1974, pp. 22, 24. Bruce J. Cole, "Trends in Science and Conflict Coverage in Four Metropolitan Newspapers," *Journalism Quarterly*, 52 (1975), 467. The failure of the *Saturday Review* in 1973 to sustain a separate science publication appeared at the time to symbolize lack of a market. An assessment at the low point was Philip C. Ritterbush, "The Public Side of Science," *Change* (September 1977), 26–33, 64. The finding of Wilbur Schramm and Serena Wade, "Knowledge and the Public Mind" (Stanford: Stanford University Institute for Communications Research, 1967), that print media were of major importance for science information, in contrast to television for public affairs, suggests that the media balance would be unusually important in determining the fate of popularized science.

20. E.g., William Bennett, "Science Hits the Newsstand," *Columbia Journalism Review* (January-February 1981), 53–56; William J. Broad, "Science Magazines: The Second Wave Rolls In," *Science*, 215 (1982), 272–273; La Follette, "Authority, Promise, and Expectation." Joye Patterson, "A Q Study of Attitudes of Young Adults about Science and Science News," *Journalism Quarterly*, 59 (1982), 406–413. Jack Weyland, "You Too Can Write the Science Version of Ann Landers," *Journal of College Science Teaching*, 13 (1984), 414–416. Bill Meyers, "The Advance of Science," *Washington Journalism Review* (November 1981), 36–37. "Science 84 Celebrates Fifth Anniversary," *Science*, 226 (1984), 530–531. Fred Jerome, "Gee Whiz! Is That All There Is?" in Sharon M. Friedman, Sharon Dunwoody, and Carol L. Rogers, eds., *Scientists and Journalists: Reporting Science as News* (New York: The Free Press, 1986), pp. 147–154. Josephine Gladstone, "Commentary: Remarks on the Portrayal of Scientists," *Science, Technology, and Human Values* (Summer 1980), 5.

21. John Henahan, in Metzger, *Science in the Newspaper*, pp. 3–5. "Goodbye to Gore," *Time*, February 21, 1972, pp. 64–65. A typical statement was Jeremy Bernstein, "Science Education for the Non-Scientist," *American Scholar*, 52 (1982–1983), 7–12. The market could not support all of the magazines. *SciQuest* in 1982

sold out to *Discover* because the advertising revenue was inadequate to sustain it. "American Chemical Society Annual Report," *Chemical and Engineering News*, April 12, 1982, p. 45. *Science 86* [*Science 80*] folded in 1986.

22. See especially Shramm and Wade, "Knowledge and the Public Mind;" Jon D. Miller, *The American People and Science Policy: The Role of Public Attitudes in the Policy Process* (New York: Pergamon Press, 1983), pp. 111–115. There was some evidence that many children began to lose interest in science at the point at which mathematics becomes crucial to mastery, at about the eighth grade level; Alex F. Perrodin, "Children's Attitudes toward Elementary School Science," *Science Education*, 50 (1966), 214–218.

23. Odom Fanning, "The Editor, the Scientists, and the Taxi Driver All Urge More Science News," *Quill* (May 1954), 10, 14. Stephen R. Graubard, "Nothing to Fear, Much to Do," *Daedalus*, 112 (1983), 242. Cecily Cannan Selby, "Turning People on to Science," *Physics Today* (July 1982), 96. Some of the social structures involved in the impact of education on popular understanding are explored in the literature surveyed by Jon D. Miller and Thomas M. Barrington, "The Acquisition and Retention of Scientific Information," *Journal of Communication* (Spring 1981), 178–189. An interesting attempt of educators to fit education to popularization is found in efforts in the literature for a couple of decades before midcentury to define how biology appeared in the public press so that biology teaching could prepare students to read what they might expectably find in the mass media. If carried through, the emphasis would, of course, have been on applied science: "Human Biology; Health and Disease; Animal Biology; Foods and Nutrition; and Plant Biology;" in that order. See especially Charles W. Finley and Otis W. Caldwell, *Biology in the Public Press* (New York: The Lincoln School of Teachers College, 1923), and W. Edgar Martin, "A Chronological Survey of Published Research Studies Relating to Biological Materials in Newspapers and Magazines," *School Science and Mathematics*, 45 (1945), 543–550. Recent research on science publics and on the critical nature of teacher attitudes is alluded to below in this chapter.

24. *School Science and Mathematics* took its present title in 1905. E.g., Robert H. Carleton, *The NSTA Story: A History of Ideas, Commitments, and Actions* (Washington: National Science Teachers Association, 1976).

25. R. Will Burnett, "Circles, Pendulums, and Progress in Science Education," *Journal of Research in Science Teaching*, 2 (1964), 33–42. Sidney Rosen, "A Century of High-School Science," *Science Teacher*, 23 (1956), 324. See in general Alan M. Voelker and Charles A. Wall, "Historical Documents of Significance to Science Educators: A Bibliographical Listing," *Science Education*, 57 (1973), 111–119.

26. Benjamin C. Gruenberg, "Science and the Layman," *Scientific Monthly*, 40 (1935), 450–457. Jane Oppenheimer, "Science and the Private Mind" (manu-

script report to the Rockefeller Foundation, 1951 [copy kindly lent by the author]). Oppenheimer after an extensive survey concluded that the U.S. was still better off in adult science education than other Western countries, which suffered a similar neglect of the subject. See also Ralph A. Beals and Leon Brody, *The Literature of Adult Education* (New York: American Association for Adult Education, 1941), pp. 180–184.

27. Fletcher C. Scott, "The Battle of the Curriculum in the Space Age," *Adult Education*, 8 (1958), 113–123, is a good example of the lack of attention to the subject in adult education literature; Palmer Wright, "Science for the Non-Scientist," *Adult Education*, 11 (1960), 19–22. One curious and partial exception may have been the Elderhostel program, in which senior citizens participated in Chautauqua-like residence study programs; by the mid-1980s, 13.5 percent of the courses were in science, virtually all in the traditional natural sciences.

28. Particularly cogent summaries of the literature on the history of science education include John H. Woodburn and Ellsworth S. Obourn, *Teaching the Pursuit of Science* (New York: The Macmillan Company, 1965), pp. 167–260; Katharine Ulrich Isenbarger et al., eds., *A Half Century of Science and Mathematics Teaching* (Oak Park, IL: Central Association of Science and Mathematics Teachers, Inc., 1950); and Rodger W. Bybee, "The New Transformation of Science Education," *Science Education*, 61 (1977), 85–93.

29. Bybee, "The New Transformation," p. 88. Tyree G. Minton, "The History of the Nature-Study Movement and Its Role in the Development of Environmental Education" (doctoral diss., University of Massachusetts, 1980), pp. 108–110. L. H. Bailey, *The Nature-Study Idea, Being an Interpretation of the New School-Movement to Put the Child in Sympathy with Nature* (New York: Doubleday, Page & Company, 1903), p. 5. Orra E. Underhill, *The Origins and Development of Elementary-School Science* (Chicago: Scott, Foresman and Company, 1941), pp. 155–214. Wayne E. Fuller, *The Old Country School: The Story of Rural Education in the Middle West* (Chicago: University of Chicago Press, 1982), pp. 221–223. E.g., "Nature Study in Education," *Popular Science News*, 36 (1902), 210. Dora Otis Mitchell, "A History of Nature-Study," *Nature-Study Review*, 19 (1923), 305–321.

30. Edward Gardinier Howe, *Systematic Science Teaching: A Manual of Inductive Elementary Work for All Instructors* (New York: D. Appleton and Company, 1894), especially pp. xvii, 207.

31. Much of this enthusiasm can be followed not only in the *Nature-Study Review*, *Natural History*, and similar magazines but in official publications of any number of organizations throughout the twentieth century. To some extent the enthusiasm made nature study vulnerable; Gerald S. Craig et al., "A Program for Teaching Science," *31st Yearbook of the National Society for the Study of Education* (Bloomington, IL: Public School Publishing Co., 1932), pp. 14–23, found that among other untenable claims of advocates was that learning to feed squirrels

contributed to students' learning to value truth and develop moral uprightness. David I. Macleod, *Building Character in the American Boy: The Boy Scouts, YMCA, and Their Forerunners, 1870–1920* (Madison: The University of Wisconsin Press, 1983), pp. 233–247, found that nature appreciation and nature study did not come into camping programs until well after the turn of the century.

32. Woodburn and Obourn, *Teaching the Pursuit of Science*, pp. 185–198; Sidney Rosen, "A History of the Physics Laboratory in the American Public High School," *American Journal of Physics*, 22 (1954), 194–204; Sidney Rosen, "The Rise of High-School Chemistry in America (to 1920)," *Journal of Chemical Education*, 33 (1956), 627–633. Edward A. Krug, *The Shaping of the American High School* (New York: Harper & Row, 1964), gives the ideal curriculums, pp. 59, 61, and much evidence of the variability of actual practice.

33. Jerome C. Isenbarger and John C. Mayfield, "The Biological Sciences," in Isenbarger, *A Half Century*, pp. 80–125; Otto B. Christy, *The Development of the Teaching of General Biology in the Secondary Schools* (Nashville: George Peabody College for Teachers, 1936); Paul DeHart Hurd, *Biological Education in American Secondary Schools, 1890–1960* (Washington: American Institute of Biological Sciences, 1961); Bruno A. Casile, "An Analysis of Zoology Textbooks Available for American Secondary Schools before 1920" (doctoral diss., University of Pittsburgh, 1953); Sidney Rosen, "The Origins of High School General Biology," *School Science and Mathematics*, 59 (1959), 473–489; Philip Pauly, "The Appearance of Academic Biology in Late Nineteenth-Century America," *Journal of the History of Biology*, 17 (1984), 369–397.

34. Hurd, *Biological Education*, especially chap. 4. Paul Johnson Fay, "The History of Science Teaching in American High Schools" (doctoral diss., The Ohio State University, 1930), pp. 166–198. Ira C. Davis et al., "The Physical Sciences," in Isenbarger, *A Half Century*, pp. 127–128. Krug, *Shaping of the American High School*, pp. 414–417.

35. Hanor A. Webb, "How General Science Began," *School Science and Mathematics*, 59 (1959), 421–430. Fay, "The History of Science Teaching," pp. 396–408. George W. Hunter and Walter G. Whitman, *Civic Science in the Home* (New York: American Book Company, 1921). N. J. Quickstad, "Some Phases of the General Science Problem," *General Science Quarterly*, 1 (1917), 155, 160; John Dewey, "Method in Science Teaching," *General Science Quarterly*, 1 (1916), 3, and *General Science Quarterly* in general. The "everyday science" approach had antecedents in the nineteenth century, such as object lessons, but this familiar approach was now employed at the high-school level, tending to replace the disciplinary training that had been appropriate for an elite group. Edward A. Krug, *The Shaping of the American High School, 1920–1941* (Madison: The University of Wisconsin Press, 1972), especially pp. 88–104, discusses the general context.

36. Otis W. Caldwell, "Considerations Which Led to the Proposal of a Six-

Year Science Sequence," National Education Association *Addresses and Proceedings*, 1923, pp. 851–852.

37. Fay, "The History of Science Teaching," pp. 178–196. Underhill, *The Origins and Development*, chap. 6, especially pp. 220–225. Davis, "The Physical Sciences," pp. 156–163.

38. See previous note. Hanor A. Webb and John J. Didcoct, *Early Steps in Science* (New York: D. Appleton and Company, 1924), p. ix. See in general Isenbarger, *A Half Century*.

39. A good summary is Charles A. Wall, "An Annotated Bibliography of Historical Documents in Science Education," *Science Education*, 57 (1973), 297–317. Fay, "The History of Science Teaching," pp. 352–354. Herbert S. Zim, *Science Interests and Activities of Adolescents* (New York: Ethical Culture Schools, 1940). Rodger W. Bybee, "Toward a Third Century of Science Education," *American Biology Teacher*, 39 (1977), 340–341. Elliot R. Downing, "A New Interpretation of the Functions of High-School Science," *Journal of Higher Education*, 4 (1933), 366. Paul DeHart Hurd, "A Critical Analysis of the Trends in Secondary School Science Teaching from 1895–1948" (doctoral diss., Stanford University, 1949), pp. 31, 36–40. John Morgan Flowers, Jr., "A Study of Selected Viewpoints Pertaining to Science Education in the United States" (doctoral diss., Duke University, 1960), pp. 64–101. A contemporary denunciation of life adjustment was Stewart Scott Cairns, "Mathematics and the Educational Octopus," *Scientific Monthly*, 76 (1953), 231–240. Concern about higher education paralleled that about the schools; see, e.g., Earl J. McGrath, ed., *Science in General Education* (Dubuque: Wm. C. Brown Company, 1948). In all of this discussion of change, it is necessary to bear in mind the caution of Larry Cuban, *How Teachers Taught: Constancy and Change in American Classrooms, 1890–1980* (New York: Longman, 1984), that actual practice in teaching changed in perhaps only a minority of classrooms.

40. Seymour Trieger, "New Forces Affecting Science in the Elementary School," *Science and Children* (October 1963), 22. J. Myron Atkin, "The Government in the Classroom," *Daedalus*, 109 (1980), 86–89.

41. One notable change in the school textbooks even before the new curriculum was the reappearance of the educational goal of persuading students to become scientists. This was a striking feature, for example, in Glenn O. Blough, *It's Time for Better Elementary School Science* (Washington: National Science Teachers Assocation, 1958), a transitional document following Sputnik in which cultivating young scientists was placed under the heading "Meeting Individual Differences."

42. William R. Ogden, "A Chronological History of Selected Objectives for the Teaching of Secondary School Chemistry in the United States during the 1918–1972 Period, as Reflected in Periodical Literature" (EDRS Document, 1974); William R. Ogden and Janis L. Jackson, "A Chronological History of Selected Objectives for the Teaching of Secondary School Biology in the United

States during the 1918–1972 Period, as Reflected in the Periodical Literature" (EDRS Document, 1976). Textbooks reflected a similar trend. See in general Flowers, "A Study of Selected Viewpoints," pp. 98–115; Hurd, *Biological Education*, chap. 8.

43. See especially Philip W. Jackson, "The Reform of Science Education: A Cautionary Tale," *Daedalus*, 112 (1983), 143–166. *Theory into Action . . . in Science Curriculum Development* (Washington: National Science Teachers Association, 1964), p. 17. This general approach also owed a debt to Piagetian developmental psychology. Martin Mayer, *Where, When, and Why: Social Studies in American Schools* (New York: Harper & Row, 1963), pp. 163–181.

44. See especially the perceptive work of Hayden, "A History of the 'New Math.'"

45. Arnold B. Grobman, *The Changing Classroom: The Role of the Biological Sciences Curriculum Study* (Garden City: Doubleday & Company, 1969), p. 290.

46. William Charles Kyle, Jr., "A Meta-Analysis of the Effects on Student Performance of New Curricular Programs Developed in Science Education Since 1955" (doctoral diss., University of Iowa, 1982), shows that the new programs were effective, especially in biology and physics, and that they developed a favorable attitude toward science in students taught by teachers trained in the new methods. Clearly the negative feelings were the product of other forces, not least of which was no doubt bureaucratic resistance and natural conservatism. See also Hayden, "A History of the 'New Math,'" and Jackson, "The Reform of Science Education."

47. Jackson, "The Reform of Science Education." Gerald S. Craig, "Children and Science," *Science Education*, 40 (1956), 167. Bybee, "The New Transformation of Science Education," pp. 90–91. Examples include Lauren B. Resnick, "Mathematics and Science Learning: A New Conception," *Science*, 220 (1983), 477–478; Marshall D. Herron, "Nature of Science: Panacea or Pandora's Box," *Journal of Research in Science Teaching*, 6 (1969), 105–107; Thomas D. Troy and Karl E. Schwaab, "A Decade of Environmental Education," *School Science and Mathematics*, 82 (1982), 209–216; D. Sadara, "Attitudes toward Science of Nonscience Major Undergraduates: Comparison with the General Public and Effect of a Science Course," *Journal of Research in Science Teaching*, 13 (1976), 79–84; John S. Rigdon, "Editorial: Creativity Lost," *American Journal of Physics*, 46 (1978), 1209; Frank Press, "The Fate of School Science," *Science*, 216 (1982), 1055. Sam Blanc, "A Topical Analysis of High School Biology Textbooks," *Science Education*, 41 (1957), 209.

48. Mary Budd Rowe, "Science Education: A Framework for Decision-Makers," *Daedalus*, 112 (1983), 126–127.

49. The mass media will be taken up below. A contemporary statement was I. Bernard Cohen, "The Education of the Public in Science," *Impact of Science on Society*, 3 (1952), especially 94–95. Robert H. Maybury et al., "Science and

Games: Learning through Structured Play," *Impact of Science on Society*, 32 (1982), 393–491, suggests the range of popularizing media available. A cogent recent summary of research is Margareta Cronholm and Rolf Sandell, "Scientific Information: A Review of Research," *Journal of Communications* (Spring 1981), 85–96.

50. E.g., Frank Eyerly, "Editors and the Arts," *ASNE Bulletin* (December 1969), 5–9; "Press Determines Public Issues," *Editor and Publisher*, January 1, 1977, p. 13; John Hulteng, "Any Ideas in the Paper?" *Nieman Reports* (April 1960), 15.

51. See, for example, Waldemar Kaempffert, "Popularizing Science," and E. H. McClelland, "Selecting Books for a Technical Department," in Louis R. Wilson, ed., *The Practice of Book Selection* (Chicago: University of Chicago Press, 1940); "A List of One Hundred Popular Books in Science," *Journal of the Washington Academy of Sciences*, 11 (1921), 353–366; "The Second Revised Edition of the Academy's List of One Hundred Popular Books in Science," *Journal of the Washington Academy of Sciences*, 15 (1925), 353–358; Arthur E. Bostwick, "Scientific Reading in a Public Library," *Popular Science Monthly*, 61 (1902), 524–527. Indications of books available can be found in the *Cumulative Book Index*.

52. See, for example, Alexander Marshack, "How Kids Get Interested in Science," *Library Journal*, 83 (1958), 1253–1255; Annette M. Woodlief, "Science," in M. Thomas Inge, ed., *Concise Histories of American Popular Culture* (Westport, CT: Greenwood Press, 1982), p. 360. *Scientific Book Club Review* (January 1936), unpaginated. See similarly, Badash, "Radium," p. 149. Jennie Mohr, *A Study of Popular Books on the Physical Sciences* (New York: [Columbia University doctoral diss.], 1942). A good example of the genre is the *Popular Science Library*, edited by Garrett P. Serviss, which began with seventeen volumes in 1922 and lasted until 1948, with emphasis on the physical sciences at first and then, at the end, on human sciences also, in a separate set.

53. See in general Frank Luther Mott, *A History of American Magazines, 1885–1905* (Cambridge, MA: Harvard University Press, 1957), pp. 2–9; Matthew D. Whalen and Mary F. Tobin, "Periodicals and the Popularization of Science in America, 1860–1910," *Journal of American Culture*, 3 (1980), 195–200; La Follette, "Authority, Promise, and Expectation;" Matthew D. Whalen, "Science, the Public, and American Culture: A Preface to the Study of Popular Science," *Journal of American Culture*, 4 (1981), 20–21. James Steel Smith, "America's Magazine Missionaries of Culture," *Journalism Quarterly*, 43 (1966), 449–458.

54. "Two Remarks Concerning the 'Monthly,'" *Popular Science Monthly*, 59 (1901), 511.

55. See, for example, Arthur E. Bostwick, "Science in Periodical Literature," *Library Journal*, 54 (1929), 927–932; Memdouh Mehmed Mazloum, "The Popularizing of Scientific Material for Magazine Publication" (master's thesis, University of Wisconsin, 1931).

56. See, for example, Edward Weeks, "The Place of Magazines in America,"

Quill (September 1962), 14–16; Paul H. Oehser, review of Ratcliff, ed., *Science Yearbook of 1946*, in *Scientific Monthly*, 63 (1946), 480–481; Jerome Ellison and Franklin T. Gosser, "Non-Fiction Magazine Articles: A Content Analysis Study," *Journalism Quarterly*, 36 (1959), 28–34. Whalen, "Science, the Public," p. 21, comments on the special function of *Science Digest* in bridging science and scientism. W. S. DeLoach, "The Scientific Articles in a Popular Magazine," *Science Education*, 25 (1941), 273–274, found *Life* devoting just over 2 percent of its pages to science.

57. See, for example, Donald D. Zahner and Armand N. Spitz, "'The Review of Popular Astronomy,'" *Review of Popular Astronomy* (January-February 1961), 3. Robert Root and Christine V. Root, "Magazines in the United States: Dying or Thriving?" *Journalism Quarterly*, 41 (1964), 15–22.

58. "Editorial," *American Naturalist*, 32 (1898), 49–51. Curvin H. Gingrich, "*Popular Astronomy*: The First Fifty Years," *Popular Astronomy*, 51 (1943), 1–18.

59. Philip E. Damon, in *Scientific American* (July 1948), 1–2. A useful summary is "Piel, Gerard," *Current Biography*, 1959, 361–362. "Gerard Piel: President-Elect of the AAAS," *Science*, 225 (1984), 385–387. Ann Roberta Larson, "Subjects and Literary Style in *Newsweek*, *Scientific American*, and *Today's Health* Science Stories in 1959 and 1969" (master's thesis, University of Texas, 1972), especially pp. 73–112.

60. "Making Culture Pay," *Time*, January 14, 1974, pp. 28–29. "Time for *Discover*," *Science*, 208 (1980), 577. Broad, "Science Magazines." Bennett, "Science Hits the Newsstand." D. H. Michael Bowen, "Why SciQuest?" *SciQuest* (April 1979), 2. Pradal, *The Literature of Science Popularisation*, p. 28.

61. Roger Allen Myers, "The Training of Science News Reporters" (doctoral diss., The Ohio State University, 1979), contains good coverage of modern bibliography. Major contemporary discussions that invite comparison included "Scientists and the Press," *Bulletin of the Atomic Scientists*, 9 (1953), 328–340, and Friedman, Dunwoody, and Rogers, *Scientists and Journalists*.

62. As someone observed, how could anyone have sensationalized the news about atomic physics anyway? See Rhees, "A New Voice," and see, too, for example, the summary of much of the literature in Krieghbaum, *Science and the Mass Media*. A perceptive contemporary account is Arthur J. Snider, "Covering Science in the Age of Sputnik," *Nieman Reports* (October 1958), 9–12. Watson Davis, "Science, the Press, and Intellectual Advance," *Vital Speeches*, 3 (1937), 207. Watson Davis, "Science and the Press," *Annals of the American Academy of Political and Social Science*, 219 (1942), 100–106. Richard V. Reeves, "A Survey of Science Reporting in Representative American Newspapers" (master's thesis, Boston University, 1950), especially pp. 7, 25. The kinds of problems persisting at midcentury are described in David E. Davis et al., "Unscientific Reporting," *Science*, 116 (1952), 125.

63. "Science and the Press," *Nation*, 133 (1931), 590. "'Something Called Fission': Science in the Press," *Nieman Reports* (April 1947), 11. Raymond John Foley, "The Presentation of Atomic Energy by a Group of Selected Magazines" (master's thesis, University of Missouri, 1949).

64. G. G. Simpson, "The Case History of a Scientific News Story," *Science*, 92 (1940), 148–150.

65. "Dr. Mayo's Appreciation," *Editor and Publisher*, October 24, 1931, p. 36. William K. Stuckey, "The University Science Writer: Investigative Reporter, Matchmaker, Free Lancer," *Nieman Reports* (September 1966), 11–14. Examples include Austin H. Clark, "Science and the Press," *Science*, 68 (1928), especially 92–93; Austin H. Clark, "Science and the Newspaper Press in the United States," *Nature*, 135 (1936), 239–240; "Science Gathering in Cleveland Treated as Major News Event," *Editor and Publisher*, January 10, 1931, p. 18; H. Ellis Mott, "Science Writers Probe News with Scientists," *Editor and Publisher*, January 18, 1947, p. 52; "O'Neill Asks Different Attitude on Science," *Editor and Publisher*, December 16, 1944, p. 48. A good positive summary is David Perlman, "Science and the Mass Media," *Daedalus*, 103 (1974), 207–222.

66. Harvey Maitland Watts, "The Weather vs. the Newspapers," *Popular Science Monthly*, 58 (1901), 382. See n. 10. T.D.A. Cockerell, "Aspects of Modern Biology," *Popular Science Monthly*, 73 (1908), 540. "Dailies Advised to Establish Science Beat," *Editor and Publisher*, December 30, 1944, p. 51. Austin H. Clark, quoted in L. N. Diamond, "Interpreting Science to the Public," *Scientific Monthly*, 40 (1935), 372. A particularly apt example of flattery is Leona Baumgartner, "Decisive Role of the Science Reporter," *Nieman Reports* (July 1956), 20–21, since she was, as a wise public servant, used to manipulating the press; most scientists were probably rather more unwitting in their efforts to win the journalists over.

67. "Magazine Science," *Popular Science Monthly*, 63 (1903), 185. Rhees, "A New Voice," especially p. 48. Hillier Krieghbaum, "Scientists on Science News," *Nieman Reports* (January 1954), 25–27. Some reporters eventually stood up against demands of scientists to review stories for accuracy; for an example of this controversy, see James W. Tankard, Jr., and Michael Ryan, "The Right of Review: Error Check or Censorship?" *Quill* (May 1973), 20–22.

68. See, for example, William E. Ritter, "Science and the Newspapers," *Science*, 67 (1928), 279–286; Ralph Coghlan, "The Need for Science Writing in the Press," *Scientific Monthly*, 62 (1946), 538–540. Earl Ubell, "Science in the Press," *Journalism Quarterly*, 10 (1963), 293, observed that "like lichens clinging to some Arctic rock, science and science writing live together in the 20th century helping each other to survive." F. Barrow Colton, "Some of My Best Friends Are Scientists," *Scientific Monthly*, 69 (1949), 160.

69. Lee Z. Johnson, "Status and Attitudes of Science Writers," *Journalism Quarterly*, 34 (1957), 247–251. Bruce J. Cole, "Trends in Science and Conflict

Coverage in Four Metropolitan Newspapers," *Journalism Quarterly*, 52 (1975), 465–471. Phillip J. Tichenor, "Teaching and the 'Journalism of Uncertainty,'" *Journal of Environmental Education* (Spring 1979), 5–6. Joye Patterson, "The Journalism of Uncertainty," *Environmental Education* (Spring 1979), 2–3. June Goodfield, *Reflections on Science and the Media* (Washington: American Association for the Advancement of Science, 1981). Rhees, "A New Voice for Science," especially pp. 30–32, 87–88, has analyzed the early stages through which science writers took on scientists' values.

70. Arthur J. Snider, "A Science Writer Has His Problems, Including the Habits of Scientists," *Quill* (October 1955), 14–16. Alton L. Blakeslee, "President's Letter," *NASW Newsletter*, March 1, 1955, p. 4. Michael Ryan and Sharon L. Dunwoody, "Academic and Professional Training Patterns of Science Writers," *Journalism Quarterly*, 52 (1975), 239–246, 290. Sharon Dunwoody, "The Science Writing Inner Club: A Communication Link Between Science and the Lay Public," *Science, Technology, and Human Values* (Winter 1980), 14–22. Dunwoody notes that the further the writer from the center of the club, the less favorable the writing toward science. Typical accounts include Hillier Krieghbaum, "NASW History," *NASW Newsletter*, December 1, 1952, pp. 8–11. Arthur J. Snider, "Covering Science in the Age of Sputnik," *Nieman Reports* (October 1958), 9–12. David Dietz, "Science, Newspapers, and the Future," *Quill* (July 1966), 12–17; Frank Carey, "A Quarter Century of Science Reporting," *Nieman Reports* (June 1966), 7–10; Everette E. Dennis and James McCartney, "Science Journalists on Metropolitan Dailies," *Journal of Environmental Education* (Spring 1979), 9–15; "Science of Reporting," *Time*, December 27, 1963, pp. 32–33. Cole, "Trends in Science." Carla Marie Rupp, "Apollo-Soyuz Mission: 'Round the World," *Editor and Publisher*, July 26, 1975, pp. 9, 26, reported that the only stories unfavorable to NASA originated with reporters who were not part of the group at Houston. Krieghbaum, *Science and the Mass Media*, can now be supplemented with Victor McElheny, in Metzger, *Science in the Newspaper*.

71. Hillier Krieghbaum, "The Background and Training of Science Writers," *Journalism Quarterly*, 17 (1940), 18.

72. The classic study is David Manning White, "The 'Gate Keeper': A Case Study in the Selection of News," *Journalism Quarterly*, 27 (1950), 383–390. William L. Laurence, "How to Know Nothing about Everything," *Saturday Review of Literature*, March 5, 1949, p. 9.

73. Herbert B. Nichols, "Abstracts for the Press," *Scientific Monthly*, 65 (1947), 405–407. Kenneth G. Johnson, "Dimensions of Judgment of Science News Stories," *Journalism Quarterly*, 40 (1963), 315–322. Allan Mazur, "Media Coverage and Public Opinion on Scientific Controversies," *Journal of Communication* (Spring 1981), 106–109, shows how the famous "sociobiology debate" was largely contrived by a very small media campaign, not entirely unlike the Scopes

trial. Neal O. Hines, "Atomic Energy and the Press: Two Years after Hiroshima," *Journalism Quarterly*, 24 (1947), 315–322. Hillier Krieghbaum, "Two Gemini Space Flights in Two Metropolitan Dailies," *Journalism Quarterly*, 43 (1966), 120–121. One of the most amusing instances came during the extraordinary publicity that editors gave to psychical research during the 1930s; when proponents were successful in portraying it as ordinary science, the gatekeepers lost interest in the subject, and it dropped out of the media to a substantial extent, a result that skeptical scientists had been unable to achieve through public statements; see Seymour H. Mauskopf and Michael R. McVaugh, *The Elusive Science: Origins of Experimental Psychical Research* (Baltimore: Johns Hopkins University Press, 1980), especially pp. 155–168.

74. E.g., Carroll J. Glynn and Albert R. Tims, "Sensationalism in Science Issues: A Case Study," *Journalism Quarterly*, 59 (1982), 126–131. Cole, "Trends in Science"; Tichenor, "Teaching and the 'Journalism of Uncertainty.'" Burkett, "There's More Going On," pp. 17–18. Recent history of the encounter of scientists with the press is vividly evoked in Rae Goodell, *The Visible Scientists* (Boston: Little, Brown and Company, 1977), especially pp. 120–121 ("What's a Nice Scientist Doing in a Place like the Press?").

75. See, for example, Jane Kutz, "Federal Agencies Label Science Writing Superficial," *Editor and Publisher*, June 24, 1978, p. 25. J. A. Udden, "Science in Newspapers," *Popular Science Monthly*, 84 (1914), 483–489.

76. Oppenheimer, "Science and the Private Mind," found lectures exemplary for popularizing. John Tebbel, "Chautauqua: A Nostalgic Salute," *Saturday Review*, January 11, 1969, p. 123.

77. See, for example, Henry Crew, "The Exposition of Science," *Scientific Monthly*, 35 (1932), 231, 233–238; Margaret Baker, "Make It a Hobby," *Adult Education Journal*, 5 (1946), 85–89; Anne W. Branscomb, "Knowing How to Know," *Science, Technology, and Human Values* (Summer 1981), 7.

78. Behnke, "Cultural Trends." Barnouw, *The Sponsor*, which see on radio and television generally. Austin H. Clark, "Science and the Radio," *Scientific Monthly*, 34 (1932), 268–272. Neil B. Reynolds and Ellis L. Manning, eds., *Excursions in Science* (New York: Whittlesey House, 1939), is one collection. A late example is the collection edited by James Stokely, *Science Marches On* (New York: Ives Washburn, 1951). Both the AAAS and the American Chemical Society were still producing educational radio programs in the 1980s. An incisive summary is Sharon M. Friedman, "The Journalist's World," in Friedman, Dunwoody, and Rogers, *Scientists and Journalists*, pp. 34–35.

79. John E. Lodge, "How Popular Science Is Put on the Screen," *Popular Science* (December 1936), 34–36, 131. L. A. Handel, *Hollywood Looks at Its Audience: A Report of Film Audience Research* (Urbana: University of Illinois Press, 1950), p. 170. Nathan Reingold, "Metro-Goldwyn-Mayer Meets the Atom Bomb," in

328 *Notes to Pages 202–204*

Terry Shinn and Richard Whitley, eds., *Expository Science: Forms and Functions of Popularisation* (Dordrecht: D. Reidel Publishing Company, 1985), pp. 229–245, indicates that the issues in 1946–1947 were essentially irrelevant to popularizing more than images.

80. For example, see Robert M. Yoder, "TV's Shoestring Surprise," *Saturday Evening Post*, August 21, 1954, pp. 30, 90–92; E. G. Sherburne, Jr., "Science on Television: A Challenge to Creativity," *Journalism Quarterly*, 40 (1963), 300–305. Krieghbaum, *Science and the Mass Media*, passim. Perlman, "Science and the Mass Media," pp. 216–218. Marcel C. La Follette, "Science on Television: Influences and Strategies," *Daedalus*, 111 (1982), 183–197, especially 185.

81. La Follette, "Science on Television." Jack Lyle, "Why Adults Do or Do Not Watch Educational Television," *Journal of Broadcasting*, 5 (1961), 325–334. "They Want Culture, but Won't Watch It," *Broadcasting*, March 6, 1961, p. 46. Gladstone, "Commentary: Remarks on the Portrayal of Scientists," pp. 4–9. See the summary in Branscomb, "Knowing How to Know," p. 8. Makers of a 1980 TV science show found that even with the best sponsorship and intentions they still had to deal with attitudes rather than "lengthy explanations," and the producers had great problems in trying to meet the expectations of the audience, which of course took precedence over intellectual content; see Constance Holden, "Science Show for Children Being Developed on TV," *Science*, 202 (1978), 730–731; "Teaching the Scientific ABCs," *Time*, January 21, 1980, p. 79.

82. "Scientific Intelligence," *Sugar Molecule* (October 1947), 1–2.

83. Heywood, "Scientists and Society," especially p. 7. C. R. Orcutt, "Popularizing Science," *Science*, 35 (1912), 776–777. "The Vision of a Blind Man," *Popular Science Monthly*, 88 (1916), viii. The new editor, interestingly enough, was none other than Waldemar Kaempffert, later doyen of the "science writers." This change from nature to mechanics was not limited to the United States. Henry de Varigny, reporting "Science News from France," *Popular Science News*, 29 (1895), 29, testified, "Since the bicycle has come into existence, most young men who willingly had some sport with boats and horses, have given it up, and the bicycle is their queen. Some book sellers also greatly complain; they say that as the people give up walking, they no longer buy natural history books, and no longer care to pick up flowers or animals and inquire about their names and habits." Philip J. Pauly, "The World and All That Is in It: The National Geographic Society, 1888–1918," *American Quarterly*, 31 (1979), 517–532, describes the outstanding exception, an organization taken over by amateurs who let the public participate not by doing science but by contributing to the support of explorers whose findings the amateurs could then read about in the *National Geographic*.

84. See especially W. Stephen Thomas, *The Amateur Scientist: Science as a Hobby* (New York: W. W. Norton and Company, 1942), chap. 2.

85. Thomas, *The Amateur Scientist*, which grew out of the American Philo-

sophical Society's Philadelphia-area inquiry, will be mentioned again later in this section. See, for example, Paul Ammon Maxwell, *Cultural Natural Science for the Junior High School: Objectives and Procedures* (Baltimore: Williams and Wilkins, 1932). "Cultural" refers to leisure time pursuits of cultured people. Zim, *Science Interests*. W. Stephen Thomas, "Report of the Committee on Education and Participation in Science," American Philosophical Society *Yearbook*, 1940, p. 327.

86. Amateurs found their activities less rewarding in a professional milieu. Textbooks tend to build up expectations, noted a writer in "Make-Shift Apparatus," *Popular Science News*, 29 (1895), 167, by describing the great discoveries made in the past with simple apparatus. "We hope our young friends," he continued, "will . . . not be discouraged because they fail to accomplish, with inferior apparatus and tools, things which can be done only with the very best appliances. Neither should they be discouraged because they do not at first succeed in using their tools with the ease and skill which older hands have acquired." Obviously the more one compared with professionals, the more discouraging amateur science.

87. Katharine B. Claypole, "With the Microscopists at Detroit," *Popular Science News*, 24 (1890), 146–147. John Harley Warner, "'Exploring the Inner Labyrinths of Creation': Popular Microscopy in Nineteenth-Century America," *Journal of the History of Medicine and Allied Sciences*, 37 (1982), 29–33. Walter B. Hendrickson, "Science and Culture in the American Middle West," *Isis*, 52 (1961), 357–371. *Journal of Adult Education*, 11 (1939), 454–455. W. Stephen Thomas, "Report of the Committee on Education and Participation in Science," American Philosophical Society *Yearbook*, 1941, p. 273.

88. C. H. Nettels, "Science Topics That Are of Interest and Use to Adults," *Science Education*, 15 (1931), 139–145. Robert P. Shaw, "The Layman Wants to Know," *Scientific Monthly*, 45 (1937), 143. And in general, Tobey, *The Ideology*. La Follette, "Authority, Promise, and Expectation," found that in 1910 the category "scientist" included inventors, engineers, and explorers; half a century later these groups had dropped out, but social scientists were more often included.

89. G. Ray Funkhouser, "Levels of Science Writing in Public Information Sources," *Journalism Quarterly*, 46 (1969), 721–726. *The Scientific American* strategy was to have scientists write and lay persons edit and to target the technical audience. "Decade-Old 'Scientific American' Sells 'Gone Highbrow' Readership," *Advertising Age*, May 5, 1958, pp. 3, 6.

90. This insulation of specialists from each other was recognized as early as 1905 by William E. Ritter, "Organization in Scientific Research," *Popular Science Monthly*, 67 (1905), 49–53. "The Aim of Science Conspectus," *Science Conspectus*, 4 (1914), unpaginated. The point is spelled out clearly in David Shakow and David Rapaport, *The Influence of Freud on American Psychology* (New York: International Universities Press, 1964), p. 11.

91. *American Scientist* had formerly been the *Sigma Xi Quarterly*, and as will be noted below, to some extent the new guise helped it, along with the new *Scientific American*, to replace the defunct *Scientific Monthly*. William Bennett, "The Medium Is Large, but How Good Is the Message?" in Friedman, Dunwoody, and Rogers, *Scientists and Journalists*, pp. 121–122.

92. Joye Patterson, Laurel Booth, and Russell Smith, "Who Reads about Science?" *Journalism Quarterly*, 46 (1969), 599–602. See chapter 6, below. Donald L. Shaw and Paul Van Nevel, "The Informative Value of Medical Science News," *Journalism Quarterly*, 44 (1967), 548. John Henahan, in Metzger, *Science in the Newspaper*, p. 5.

93. Larson, "Subjects and Literary Style."

94. Greta Jones, Ian Connell, and Jack Meadows, *The Presentation of Science by the Media* (Leicester: University of Leicester, Primary Communications Research Centre, 1978), p. 1.

95. "The editor cannot overemphasize the desirability of writing for SM in a popular but dignified manner," wrote editor F. L. Campbell as late as "The Brownstone Tower," *Scientific Monthly*, 66 (1948), 179. Warren Weaver, ed., *The Scientists Speak* (New York: Boni & Gaer, 1947). An example of the way this genre persisted, exemplifying good popularization by leading academics, is Eugene H. Kone and Helene J. Jordan, eds., *The Greatest Adventure: Basic Research That Shapes Our Lives* (New York: The Rockefeller University Press, 1974). Frank Carey, "Reporting Science," *Science*, 115 (1952), 409–412.

96. Bostwick, "Science in Periodical Literature," p. 927. "There are those among us, especially in university work, who, in one breath lament the layman's lack of interest in scientific matters and in the next, urge the academic ostracism of any of their colleagues who attempt to create such an interest by writing 'popular' articles or books on scientific subjects," observed anatomist William Walter Greulich, in a review of Scheinfeld, *Women and Men,* in *American Journal of Physical Anthropology*, 3 (1945), 208.

97. Sharon Dunwoody, "Factors Influencing Scientists as Journalistic Sources" (EDRS Document, 1982). A detailed modern study is Bernard H. Gustin, "Charisma, Recognition, and the Motivation of Scientists," *American Journal of Sociology*, 78 (1973), 1119–1134. As noted above, sometimes writing in the *Scientific American* or similarly prestigious media could bring exceptional professional recognition.

98. Leroy M. Carl, "Oil and Water: Journalism and Science Can Mix," *Quill* (March 1970), 24–26, told of his teaching students science content in a journalism course. Wesley C. Mitchell, "The Public Relations of Science," *Science*, 90 (1939), 605. Patterson, "The Journalism of Uncertainty," p. 3. Cf. William E. Dick, "Science and the Press," *Impact of Science on Society*, 5 (1953), 170–173. M. T. O'Keefe, "The Mass Media as Sources of Information for Doctors," *Journalism Quarterly*, 47 (1970), 95–100.

99. W. D. Lewis, in Bertha M. Clark, *An Introduction to Science* (New York: American Book Company, 1915), p. 7. Bentley Glass, "Renascent Biology: A Report on the AIBS Biological Sciences Curriculum Study," *School Review*, 70 (1962), 41.

100. Ogden and Jackson, "A Chronological History," p. 9. Hurd, "A Critical Analysis," p. 9. Fay, "The History of Science Teaching," pp. 351–352. Audrey B. Champagne and Leopold E. Klopfer, "A Sixty-Year Perspective on Three Issues in Science Education," *Science Education*, 61 (1977), 431–452. This change persisted even when the new science curriculums were coming in, according to William E. Brownson and Joseph J. Schwan, "American Science Textbooks and Their Authors, 1915 and 1955," *School Review*, 71 (1963), 170–180. William R. Ogden, "An Analysis of the Authorship of Articles Dealing With the Objectives of Secondary School Chemistry Teaching, 1918–1967," *Science Education*, 58 (1974), 181–184.

101. Austin H. Clark, "What Science Owes the Public," *Scientific Monthly*, 23 (1926), 52.

102. Bryant Kearl and Richard D. Powers, "Estimating Understanding of Scientific Terms," *Journalism Quarterly*, 38 (1961), 221–223. G. Ray Funkhouser and Nathan Maccoby, "Communicating Specialized Science Information to a Lay Audience," *Journal of Communication*, 21 (1971), 58–71. Reeves, "A Survey of Science Reporting," p. 30. Francis D. Curtis, *Investigations of Vocabulary in Textbooks of Science for Secondary Schools* (Boston: Ginn and Company, 1938), concluded that much of the difficulty in texts grew out of inept choice of inappropriate vocabulary rather than science terms or science content. Gina Kolata, "A Math Image Problem," *Science*, 232 (1986), 1087–1088, uncovered a delightful instance of inept attempts at popularizing by mathematicians, including a pamphlet for the general public in which the contents assumed a familiarity with mathematical concepts that easily led to well-taken satire.

103. Raymond J. Tarleton, "Accuracy and Comprehension in Science News Writing," *Journalism Quarterly*, 30 (1953), 69–71. Phillip J. Tichenor, Clarice N. Olien, Annette Harrison, and George Donohue, "Mass Communication Systems and Communication Accuracy in Science News Reporting," *Journalism Quarterly*, 47 (1970), 673–683. Benjamin C. Gruenberg, "A Study of Indoctrination in Science Teaching," *Science Education*, 14 (1930), 621–634. D. Sadara, "Attitudes toward Science of Non–Science Major Undergraduates: Comparison with the General Public and Effect of a Science Course," *Journal of Research in Science Teaching*, 13 (1976), 79–84. James W. Tankard, Jr., and Michael Ryan, "News Source Perceptions of Accuracy of Science Coverage," *Journalism Quarterly*, 51 (1974), 219–225, 234. Donald J. Schmidt, "A Test on Understanding Science: A Comparison among Several Groups," *Journal of Research in Science Teaching*, 5 (1968), 365–366. This incident is recounted in McClelland, "Selecting Books for a Technical Department," pp. 159–160. A later incident, involving *Science Digest*,

is described by Warner Clements, "Editors and Crank Science," *Skeptical Inquirer* (Summer 1981), 76.

104. John E. Bowers and Keith R. Stamm, "Science Writing Techniques and Methods," *Journal of Environmental Education* (Spring 1979), 26. Hillier Kriegh-baum, ed., *When Doctors Meet Reporters* (New York: New York University Press, 1957), p. 65.

105. G. Ray Funkhouser and Nathan Maccoby, "Tailoring Science Writing to the General Audience," *Journalism Quarterly*, 50 (1973), 226. Eugene Rabinowitch, quoted in John Troan, "Science Reporting—Today and Tomorrow," *Science*, 131 (1960), 1194. Michael Ryan, "Attitudes of Scientists and Journalists toward Media Coverage of Science News," *Journalism Quarterly*, 56 (1979), 18–26, 53. Benjamin T. Brooks, "The Interpretation of Research," *Scientific Monthly*, 26 (1928), 411.

106. Ryan, "Attitudes of Scientists." Goodfield, *Reflections on Science and the Media*, pp. 20–21. The actual influence of media emphases on general science textbooks was documented in Maitland P. Simmons, "Changing Conceptions of Dominant Problems Relating to Major Topics in General Science Textbooks," *Journal of Experimental Education*, 6 (1938), 399–405.

107. Tobey, *The American Ideology*; Tobey (p. 103) cryptically dates the end of popular science as before World War I, when the press ignored exciting develop-ments in physics. David J. Rhees, "'Making the Nation Chemically Conscious': The Popularization of Chemistry, 1914–1940" (unpublished paper presented at History of Science Society Meetings, Chicago, December 1984), has explored the rich institutional and social context of this pioneer effort.

108. A recent survey is Carol L. Rogers, "The Practitioner in the Middle," in Friedman, Dunwoody, and Rogers, *Scientists and Journalists*, pp. 42–54. The American Association for the Advancement of Science first developed a year-round public relations office after the disruptions of meetings in 1970; *APA Monitor* (March 1971), 3.

109. H.E. Howe, "The Awakening in Science," *Scientific Monthly*, 21 (1925), 637: "The desire of the modern scientist to have the non-technical public ac-quainted with his work is one of the striking differences between to-day and yes-terday." Edwin E. Slosson, "Science for the Million," *NEA Addresses and Proceed-ings*, 62 (1924), 754–761. Sharon Dunwoody and Byron T. Scott, "Scientists and the Press: Are They Really Strangers?" (EDRS Document, 1979). Sharon Dun-woody and Michael Ryan, "Public Information Persons as Mediators Between Scientists and Journalists," *Journalism Quarterly*, 60 (1983), 647–656.

110. Dunwoody and Ryan, "Public Information Persons." Tobey, *The Ameri-can Ideology*. Rhees, "'Making the Nation Chemically Conscious,'" especially ex-plores the blurring of popularization into public relations. The early issues of the *NASW Newsletter* contain numerous comments that show the discomfiture of the science writers with the confusion between press agentry and science writing.

111. La Follette, "Authority, Promise, and Expectation," especially pp. 280–281.

112. Thomas H. Maugh II, "The Media: The Image of the Scientist is Bad," *Science*, 200 (1978), 37. Allan Mazur, "Public Confidence in Science," *Social Studies of Science*, 7 (1977), 123–125 (and Mazur has published other studies of a similar kind, especially "Commentary: Opinion Poll Measurement of American Confidence in Science," *Science, Technology, and Human Values* [Summer 1981], 16–19). A recent summary is National Science Board, *Science Indicators: The 1985 Report* (Washington: Government Printing Office, [1986]), pp. 142–154. A classic paper is Alvin M. Weinberg, "In Defense of Science," *Science*, 167 (1970), 141–145. Walter Hirsch, *Scientists in American Society* (New York: Random House, 1968), pp. 38–49, summarizes findings to that date. "More Good Than Bad," *Science*, 228 (1985), 1294, reported a study showing the television image of scientists to be ambivalent and another showing the science image to consist of products rather than science or scientists. Insights into the confusion of science with bureaucracy and its impact on perceptions of science can be found in Henry Milner, "Scientific Authority: A Critical Reappraisal of the Role of Science and Technology in Contemporary American Society" (doctoral diss., Carleton University, 1976). In part of course the monolithic image of science in the twentieth century was a reflection of the essentially Platonic ideal of science developed especially in the late nineteenth and early twentieth centuries; see Whalen, "Science, the Public," p. 17; David A. Hollinger, *Morris R. Cohen and the Scientific Ideal* (Cambridge, MA: The MIT Press, 1975).

113. Modern literature with extensive citations includes Lorelei R. Brutsh, "Avoidance of Science and Stereotypes of Scientists," *Journal of Research in Science Teaching*, 16 (1979), 237–241; Renato A. Schibeci and Irene Sorensen, "Elementary School Children's Perceptions of Scientists," *School Science and Mathematics*, 83 (1983), 14–19; Patricia M. Schwirian, "On Measuring Attitudes toward Science," *Science Education*, 70 (1968), 172–179; Patricia M. Schwirian and Barbara Thomson, "Changing Attitudes toward Science: Undergraduates in 1967 and 1971," *Journal of Research in Science Teaching*, 9 (1972), 253–259; Jeffrey G. Reitz, "The Flight from Science Reconsidered: Career Choice of Science and Engineering in the 1950's and 1960's," *Science Education*, 57 (1973), 121–134; Amitai Etzioni and Clyde Nunn, "The Public Appreciation of Science in Contemporary America," *Daedalus*, 103 (1974), 191–205. In fact of course attitudes correlated with social class; the higher the class, the more favorable toward science. Simon Newcomb, "Exact Science in America," *North American Review*, 119 (1874), 286–308. Freeman H. Quimby, "Unpopular Science," *Science*, 119 (1954), 162–163.

114. Kenneth Prewitt, "The Public and Science Policy," in Marcel Chotkowski La Follette, ed., *Quality in Science* (Cambridge, MA: The MIT Press, 1982), pp. 82–99. Jon D. Miller, Robert W. Suchner, and Alan M. Voelker, *Citizenship in an*

334 Notes to Pages 215–216

Age of Science: Changing Attitudes among Young Adults (New York: Pergamon Press, 1980). Miller, *The American People and Science Policy*, especially pp. 39–47; Daniel Yankelovich, "Changing Public Attitudes to Science and the Quality of Life: Edited Excerpts from a Seminar," *Science, Technology, and Human Values* (Spring 1982), 24–25. Jon D. Miller and Thomas M. Barrington, "The Acquisition and Retention of Scientific Information," *Journal of Communication* (Spring 1981), 178–189. A complicating factor is described in Barbara J. Culliton, "Science's Restive Public," *Daedalus*, 107 (1978), 147–156.

115. Edwin E. Slosson, "Science and Pseudo-Science," *Scientific Monthly*, 18 (1924), 216–219. Francis B. Sumner, "The New Dogmatism," *Scientific Monthly*, 45 (1937), 348. A good, typical statement is Walter Lowrie, "A Meditation on Scientific Authority," *Theology Today*, 2 (1945), 302: "Belief in the infallibility of science is itself a sort of credulity in view of the fact that in a single generation . . . almost every science has undergone a thorough transformation." Tobey, *The American Ideology of National Science*, pp. 96–132.

116. The outstanding example, much discussed, was P. W. Bridgman, "The New Vision of Science," *Harper's Magazine*, 158 (1929), 443–451. A good account of the initial impact is Carter, *The Other Side of the Twenties*. See, for example, Herbert Dingle, "Knowledge without Understanding," *Atlantic Monthly*, 160 (1932), 116–124; Walter Sullivan, ed., *Science in the Twentieth Century* (Danbury, CT: Grolier Educational Corporation, 1978), p. 78. *New York Times*, quoted in *Science*, 81 (1935), 47.

117. Compare, for example, Henry Smith Williams, *Miracles of Science* (New York: Harper & Brothers, 1913), and Wendt, *Science for the World of Tomorrow*. W. S. Franklin, "Popular Science," *Science*, 17 (1903), 10. Wright, "Science for the Non-Scientist," p. 19. Patrick Young, quoted in Sharon M. Friedman, "The Journalist's World," in Friedman, Dunwoody, and Rogers, *Scientists and Journalists*, p. 21. The cultural context of this development is described in Michael L. Smith, "Selling the Moon: The U.S. Manned Space Program and the Triumph of Commodity Scientism," in Richard Wightman Fox and T. J. Jackson Lears, eds., *The Culture of Consumption: Critical Essays in American History, 1880–1980* (New York: Pantheon Books, 1983), pp. 177–209.

118. Victor E. Levine, "Why We Should Be More Interested in Nutrition," *Scientific Monthly*, 22 (1926), 19. Howard E. Gruber, "Science as Doctrine or Thought? A Critical Study of Nine Academic Year Institutes," *Journal of Research in Science Teaching*, 1 (1963), 127. A startling demonstration of the separation of science from science products appeared in the survey carried out by Margaret Mead and Rhoda Métraux, "Image of the Scientist among High-School Students: A Pilot Study," *Science*, 126 (1957), 384–390, which revealed that young people favored science in abstract terms but not the work or people connected with science (they did not, for example, want to marry scientists).

119. Joseph F. Patrouch, Jr., "Mystery Stories, Science Fiction, and the Scientific Method" (unpublished paper presented at the meetings of the Popular Culture Association, Toledo, 1969). Patrouch contrasts science fiction with the mystery story, in which scientific thinking is the basis of the genre. Thomas D. Clareson, "The Scientist as Hero in American Science Fiction, 1880–1920," *Extrapolation*, 7 (1965), 18–28. Walter Hirsch, "The Image of the Scientist in Science Fiction: A Content Analysis," *American Journal of Sociology*, 63 (1958), 506–512. Stephen Tonsor, "The Image of Science and Technology in Utopian and Science Fiction Literature," *Modern Age*, 20 (1976), 86–93. Michelle Herwald, "Anticipating the Unexpected: *Amazing Stories* in the Interwar Years," in Catherine L. Covert and John D. Stevens, eds., *Mass Media between the Wars: Perceptions of Cultural Tension, 1918–1941* (Syracuse: Syracuse University Press, 1984), pp. 39–53. Dale Beyerstein, "Skepticism, Close-Mindedness, and Science Fiction," *Skeptical Inquirer* (Summer 1982), 50–51. I am not here, of course, attempting to use science fiction as more than an illustrative side eddy; the subject needs much study, as suggested particularly in Linda Fleming, "The American SF Subculture," *Science-Fiction Studies*, 4 (1977), 263–271.

120. Whalen, "Science, the Public." Oscar Cargill, "Science and the Literary Imagination in the U.S.," *College English*, 13 (1951), 90–94. I. Bernard Cohen, *Science, Servant of Man: A Layman's Primer for the Age of Science* (Boston: Little, Brown and Company, 1948), p. 7.

121. George Comstock and Heather Tully, "Innovation in the Movies, 1939–1976," *Journal of Communication* (Spring 1981), 97–105.

122. Quoted in Sharon M. Friedman, in *Science in the Newspaper*, p. 19. J. S. Sorenson and D. D. Sorenson, "A Comparison of Science Content in Magazines in 1964–65 and 1969–70," *Journalism Quarterly*, 50 (1973), 101.

123. W. C. Van Deventer, "Organization of a Basic Science Course," *Science Education*, 30 (1946), 201. See, for example, Thomas E. J. Keena, "Interpreting Science Is Our Job Too," *Masthead* (Summer 1958), 28–32. Harold C. Urey, quoted in Ralph Coghlan, "The Need for Science Writing in the Press," *Scientific Monthly*, 62 (1946), 540.

124. Alexander Frazier, "The 'New' Science: Shall *We* Decide What to Teach?" *Science Education*, 30 (1946), 230. Eugene Rabinowitch, "Science Popularization in the Atomic Age," *Impact of Science on Society*, 17 (1967), 107–113. Nancy Pfund and Laura Hofstadter, "Biomedical Innovation and the Press," *Journal of Communication* (Spring 1981), 138–154. John Lear, "The Trouble with Science Writing," *Columbia Journalism Review* (Summer 1970), 30. Robert M. Hutchins, "Doing What Comes Scientifically," *Center Magazine* (January 1969), 56. Of course this muddling was not new in the twentieth century any more than it had been in the nineteenth, but the extent of it made the more recent decades distinctive.

125. Historical references are in Nancy Barnett Hamilton, "The Scientific Lit-

eracy of Seniors in Urban, Suburban, and Rural High Schools in Kentucky" (master's thesis, The Ohio State University, 1965), chaps. 1–2. Herbert J. Walberg, "Scientific Literacy and Economic Productivity in International Perspective," *Daedalus*, 112 (1983), 1 (the whole issue is devoted to scientific literacy). James B. Conant, "Foreward," in I. Bernard Cohen and Fletcher G. Watson, eds., *General Education in Science* (Cambridge, MA: Harvard University Press, 1952), p. xiii. Branscomb, "Knowing How to Know," pp. 5–9. Other examples include "The NSTA Conferences on Scientific Literacy," *Science Teacher* (May 1968), 30–32; and Donald R. Daugs, "Scientific Literacy—Re-Examined," *Science Teacher* (November 1970), 10–11. Daniel E. Koshland, Jr., "Scientific Literacy," *Science*, 230 (1985), 391.

126. See particularly Albert F. Eiss and Mary Blatt Harbeck, *Behaviorial Objectives in the Affective Domain* (Washington: National Science Supervisors Association, 1969). Kenneth Prewitt, "Scientific Illiteracy and Democratic Theory," *Daedalus*, 112 (1983), 49–64. Jon D. Miller, "Scientific Literacy: A Conceptual and Empirical Review," *Daedalus*, 112 (1983), 29–48.

127. See, for example, A. B. Arons, "Achieving Wider Scientific Literacy," *Daedalus*, 112 (1983), 91–122.

128. E. N. Transeau, "Passing of the Teleological Explanation," *School Science and Mathematics*, 13 (1913), 371. "What Is the Scientific Attitude?" *Forum*, 79 (1928), 769–771. An example of the close connection between attitude education and fighting superstition is Otis W. Caldwell, "Science—Truth or Propaganda," *School Science and Mathematics*, 33 (1933), 30–33.

129. Morton White, *Social Thought in America: The Revolt against Formalism* (2nd ed., Boston: Beacon Press, 1957). David A. Hollinger, "The Problem of Pragmatism in American History," *Journal of American History*, 67 (1980), 88–107, discusses popular as well as technical faces of this stance. See, for example, the list of references on science as process and method in Charles C. Adams, "Selected References on the Relation of Science to Modern Life," *New York State Museum Bulletin*, 322 (1940), 81–85.

130. Casile, "An Analysis of Zoology Textbooks." Further information was developed from a large sample of various textbooks. Hurd, "A Critical Analysis of the Trends," especially p. 347. George W. Hunter and Walter G. Whitman, *Civic Science in the Home* (New York: American Book Company, 1921), pp. 16–18. Philosophers were of course soon upset because they denied that there was "a" scientific method (see chapter 6), but such doubts showed up only as another of the certainties of science that popularizers later surrendered. Gordon Otto Besch, "The Evolution of Some Major Concepts in Science Education" (doctoral diss., The Ohio State University, 1969), p. 78.

131. E.g., Robert A. Millikan, "The Problem of Science Teaching in the Secondary Schools," *School Science and Mathematics*, 25 (1925), 966–975; Elliot R.

Downing, "Does Science Teach Scientific Thinking?" *Science Education*, 17 (1933), 87–89. Victor H. Noll, "The Habit of Scientific Thinking," *Teachers College Record*, 35 (1933), 1–9; Victor H. Noll, "Teaching the Habit of Scientific Thinking," *Teachers College Record*, 35 (1933), pp. 202–212. Ira D. Garard, "The Scientific Method and the Popular Mind," *Education*, 54 (1933), 129–134. Tunis Baker, "Teaching the Scientific Method to Prospective Elementary School Teachers," *Science Education*, 29 (1945), 79–82. Oreon Keeslar, "The Elements of Scientific Method," *Science Education*, 29 (1945), 273–278, is a good example of content.

132. Hurd, "A Critical Analysis," p. 31. J. Wayne Wrightstone, "Correlation of Natural Science Beliefs and Attitudes with Social and Intellectual Factors," *Science Education*, 18 (1934), 10. Robert L. Ebel, "What Is the Scientific Attitude?" *Science Education*, 22 (1938), 1–5, 75–81. The idea of teaching the scientific attitude of course did not die out, but it was overshadowed by other concerns; in a well-known botany textbook, for example, the concept was strongly urged not only in the 1930s but at least briefly in the 1960s, though in the latter period in a context emphasizing research: Edmund W. Sinnott, *Botany: Principles and Problems* (3rd ed., New York: McGraw-Hill Book Company, 1935), pp. xvii–xix; Edmund W. Sinnott and Katherine S. Wilson, *Botany: Principles and Problems* (6th ed., New York: McGraw-Hill Book Company, 1963), pp. 12–13. A good example of the negatives in a general book is Frederick Barry, *The Scientific Habit of Thought: An Informal Discussion of the Source and Character of Dependable Knowledge* (New York: Columbia University Press, 1927), pp. 45–46 and passim.

133. For example, A. B. Champagne and L. E. Klopfer, "A Sixty-Year Perspective on Three Issues in Science Education," *Science Education*, 61 (1977), 442–444. Gray, *The Advancing Front of Science*, pp. 334–335. Haym Kruglak, "The Scientific Method and Science Teaching," *School and Society*, 69 (1949), 201. Bertha E. Slye, "Science Developments of Importance to Teachers," *Yearbook, National Science Teachers Association*, 1944, p. 23.

134. Edward A. Purcell, Jr., *The Crisis of Democratic Theory: Scientific Naturalism and the Problem of Value* (Lexington: University Press of Kentucky, 1973). Hurd, "A Critical Analysis," passim. Ernest Nagel, "The Methods of Science: What Are They? Can They Be Taught?" *Scientific Monthly*, 70 (1950), 22. Marvin D. Solomon, "Studies in Mental Rigidity and the Scientific Method," *Science Education*, 36 (1952), 240–247. Woodburn and Obourn, *Teaching the Pursuit of Science*, chap. 3. See, for example, J. T. Morrisey, "An Analysis of Studies on Changing the Attitude of Elementary Student Teachers toward Science and Science Teaching," *Science Education*, 65 (1981), 155–177; Ralph E. Martin, Jr., *The Credibility Principle and Teacher Attitudes toward Science* (New York: Peter Lang, 1984).

135. Gerard Piel, "Science, Censorship, and the Public Interest," *Nieman Reports* (April 1957), 30.

136. See, for a good example, Joseph Mayer, *The Seven Seals of Science: An*

Account of the Unfoldment of Orderly Knowledge and Its Influence on Human Affairs (New York: The Century Co., 1927). Anonymous, quoted in Sharon M. Friedman, in *Science in the Newspaper*, p. 19.

137. The figures in Goodell, *The Visible Scientists*, functioned differently from the old-fashioned men of science; see below. John L. Tildsley, "Teaching Science as a 'Way of Life,'" *Journal of Chemical Education*, 8 (1931), 672. Joseph B. Fish, "Science as a Way of Life," *Bulletin of High Points* (May 1929), 29–34. The astronomer Harlow Shapley, "Status Quo or Pioneer? The Fate of American Science," *Harper's Magazine*, 191 (1948), 312, likewise spoke of "science as a basic way of life," but other scientists tended not to articulate this idea. Obviously the educators' embracing science ideals a generation or so later was a form of cultural lag.

138. Patterson, "A Q Study of Attitudes of Young Adults." Jay Tepperman, "The Research Scientist in Modern Fiction," *Perspectives in Biology and Medicine*, 3 (1960), 547, complained, "All kinds of educators, scientists, philosophers, and ordinary taxpayers appear to be writing to the newspapers in very large numbers with a bewildering variety of rigidly held opinions on how we can beat the Communists in the egghead production race." Friedman, Dunwoody, and Rogers, *Scientists and Journalists*, contains essentially an examination of the 1980s activity. Carl J. Sindermann, *The Joy of Science: Excellence and Its Rewards* (New York: Plenum Press, 1985), pp. 238–251, does include popularizing as one of four public areas in which successful scientists could and did function, but his emphasis on politics and policy represented a remarkable secularizing of the religion of science.

139. Larson, "Subjects and Literary Style," points out that the later *Scientific American* was distinctive from general audience publications in that the editors did not noticeably embrace journalistic fads such as space, ecology, etc.

140. See, for example, Norman W. Storer, "The Coming Changes in American Science," *Science*, 142 (1963), 464–467. Peter S. Buck and Barbara Gutmann Rosenkrantz, "The Worm in the Core: Science and General Education," in Everett Mendelsohn, ed., *Transformation and Tradition in the Sciences: Essays in Honor of I. Bernard Cohen* (Cambridge: Cambridge University Press, 1984), pp. 371–394, detail how, in the mid-twentieth century, disciplinary claims of individual sciences tended to undermine attempts to include science as such in general education efforts at the college level.

141. A good example is Mayer, *Seven Seals of Science*. In his current research, David Rhees is developing the idea that in the United States the history of science served the same public motives as did popularization.

142. See, for example, James Bryant Conant, "The Scientific Education of the Layman," *Yale Review*, 36 (1946), 15–36. I. Bernard Cohen, "The Education of the Public in Science," *Impact of Science on Society*, 3 (1952), 67–100. The literature on the two-cultures debate is too extensive for review here; the point is the attempt to move science into a "culture" context different from the "civilization" of the late nineteenth century.

143. Stephen Brush, "Should the History of Science Be Rated X?" *Science*, 183 (1974), 1164–1172. Goodell, *The Visible Scientists*. Leading scientists battled sometimes against McCarthyism rather than superstition; e.g., Kirtley F. Mather, "The Problem of Anti-Scientific Trends Today," *Science*, 115 (1952), 533–537; and the symposium "The Scientist in American Society," *Scientific Monthly*, 78 (1954), 129–141.

144. See, for example, Frank Trippett, "Science: No Longer a Sacred Cow," *Time*, March 7, 1977, pp. 72–73.

145. *Discover* and *Science 80* were the only new magazines that made a special effort to debunk even pseudoscience; see Kendrick Frazier, "Exploring the Fringes of Science," *Skeptical Inquirer*, 9 (1984–1985), 101. See the discussion of skepticism per se in chapter 6.

Chapter 6: The Pattern of Popularization and the Victory of Superstition

1. Although from a different perspective, a very brief parallel summary, with a comparative note, appears in June Goodfield, *Reflections on Science and the Media* (Washington: American Association for the Advancement of Science, 1981), pp. 2–8. A similar change, but with a different time frame, is described in Kurt Bayertz, "Spreading the Spirit of Science: Social Determinants of the Popularization of Science in Nineteenth-Century Germany," in Terry Shinn and Richard Whitley, eds., *Expository Science: Forms and Functions of Popularisation* (Dordrecht: D. Reidel Publishing Company, 1985), pp. 209–227.

2. Knight Dunlap, "Antidotes for Superstitions Concerning Human Heredity," *Scientific Monthly*, 51 (1940), 225.

3. The functional equivalent of commercial exploitation and superstition is evident in the shift of the focus of attack from superstition to hucksters in the *American Journal of Public Health*, for example, between the 1920s and the 1950s.

4. William Wells Newell, "Current Superstitions Collected from the Oral Tradition of English Speaking Folk," *American Folklore Society Memoirs*, 1896, p. 4. E. T. Bell, *Debunking Science* (Seattle: University of Washington Bookstore, 1930), p. 17. A particularly choice example is W. E. Forsythe, "Things to Forget in Health Teaching," *Journal of Health and Physical Education* (March 1934), 18–19, 67. A more general cultural setting is in Daniel J. Boorstin, *The Americans: The Democratic Experience* (1973; repr. New York: Vintage Books, 1974), pp. 525–555.

5. Pseudoscience has been treated extensively as such by scholars; see, for example, R.G.A. Dolby, "Reflections on Deviant Science," in *Sociological Review Monograph*, 27 (1979), 9–47, especially 19–38; *Virginia Tech Center for the Study of Science in Society, Working Papers in Science and Technology* (April 1983) ["The Demarcation Between Science and Pseudo-Science"]; Marsha P. Hanen, Margaret J.

Osler, and Robert G. Weyant, eds., *Science, Pseudo-Science and Society* (Waterloo, Ontario: Wilfrid Laurier University Press, 1980). The fight against pseudoscience has a particularly rich history in the health field; James Prim[e]rose, *Popular Errours; or, the Errours of the People In Physick*, trans. Robert Wittie (London: Nicholas Bourne, 1651), was a well-known example often cited by writers who were concerned about superstition. Otis W. Caldwell and Gerhard E. Lundeen, "Students' Attitudes regarding Unfounded Beliefs," *Science Education*, 15 (1931), 246–266. Pseudoscience is also taken up later in this chapter in connection with magical appearances.

6. Paul Kurtz, "News of the Committee," *Skeptical Inquirer* (Fall 1978), 3–4; Paul Kurtz, "From the Chairman," *Skeptical Inquirer* (Spring 1981), 2–4; Kendrick Frazier, "Exploring the Fringes of Science," *Skeptical Inquirer*, 9 (1984–1985), 98–105; and the *Skeptical Inquirer* generally. A general account is in Douglas R. Hofstadter, *Metamagical Themas: Questing for the Essence of Mind and Pattern* (New York: Basic Books, 1985), chap 5.

7. Frederick A. Bushee, "Science and Social Progress," *Popular Science Monthly*, 79 (1911), 251. Joseph Jastrow, ed., *The Story of Human Error* (New York: D. Appleton-Century, 1936), represents the full development of this view of popularizing and includes as contributors many eminent scientists.

8. Ronald E. Martin, *American Literature and the Universe of Force* (Durham: Duke University Press, 1981), pp. 85–86, provides one intellectual context.

9. Much of the moral context is explored in James Turner, *Without God, Without Creed: The Origins of Unbelief in America* (Baltimore: Johns Hopkins University Press, 1985), passim. David A. Hollinger, "Inquiry and Uplift: Late Nineteenth-Century American Academics and the Moral Efficacy of Scientific Practice," in Thomas L. Haskell, ed., *The Authority of Experts: Studies in History and Theory* (Bloomington: Indiana University Press, 1984), pp. 142–156, provides an intellectual history of how romantic interest in nature was transformed into emphasis on the scientific method and moralism.

10. See, for example, Joan Shelley Rubin, "'Information, Please!': Culture and Expertise in the Interwar Period," *American Quarterly*, 35 (1983), 499–517. The author of an editorial, "Ancient and Modern Superstition," in *Popular Science Monthly*, 42 (1893), 411, commented: "Truths of science [should be] . . . welcomed and honored, not alone for the mastery they give over the outward world but for the clearer light they throw upon questions of moral obligation."

11. "The Public Interest in Science," *Modern Medicine*, 2 (1920), 710. Philip J. Pauly, "The World and All That Is in It: The National Geographic Society, 1888–1918," *American Quarterly*, 31 (1979), 517–532, emphasizes the editorial policy of the influential *National Geographic* to present facts for the sake of facts, without a context but in "particularistic detail." I shall discuss below Michael Schudson, *Discovering the News: A Social History of American Newspapers* (New York: Basic Books, 1978).

12. See, for example, Charles M. Radding, "Superstition to Science: Nature, Fortune, and the Passing of the Medieval Ordeal," *American Historical Review*, 84 (1979), 968. [N. Sargent], "Introductory Remarks," *Mechanics' & Farmers' Magazine of Useful Knowledge*, 1 (1830), 4.

13. *Harper's Weekly*, 1 (1857), 14.

14. Jennie Mohr, *A Study of Popular Books on the Physical Sciences* (New York: [Columbia University doctoral dissertation], 1942), p. 7. J. L. Crammer, "Popularization of Science through Cheap Books," *Illinois Libraries*, 31 (1949), 394.

15. Stratton D. Brooks, "The Demand for Science Teachers," *School Science*, 1 (1901), 53. Jessie Williams Clemensen, "Vitalizing High School Science through the Learning Process," *Science Education*, 19 (1935), 49. F. C. Robinson, "Education of and Co-Operation with the General Public in Health Work," *Public Health Papers and Reports*, 31 (1905), 123. Carl J. Potthoff, "Teaching Correctness of Thinking in Matters of Health," *American Journal of Public Health*, 35 (1945), 1036. [National Analysts, Inc.], "A Study of Health Practices and Opinions—Final Report" (Conducted for Food and Drug Administration, Department of Health, Education, and Welfare, Contract No. FDA 66–193, June 1972), pp. xv–xvi. I. Bernard Cohen, "For the Education of the Layman," *New York Times Book Review*, September 7, 1947, p. 32. Leon E. Trachtman, "The Public Understanding of Science Effort: A Critique," *Science, Technology, and Human Values* (Summer 1981), 12. An official report of the American Association for the Advancement of Science in 1952 referred to the need to "put science back together"; "The American Association for the Advancement of Science Faces Its Social Responsibilities," *Impact of Science on Society*, 3 (1952), 49.

16. Herbert Brucker, *The Changing American Newspaper* (New York: Columbia University Press, 1937), chap. 1; the quotation is, of course, a classic from the history of journalism. Daniel Lawrence O'Keefe, *Stolen Lightning: The Social Theory of Magic* (New York: Continuum, 1982), p. 477. Paul F. Lazarsfeld and Robert K. Merton, "Mass Communication, Popular Taste, and Organized Social Action," in Lyman Bryson, *The Communication of Ideas: A Series of Addresses* (New York: Harper & Brothers, 1948), pp. 95–118.

17. R. B. Lindsay, "Survival of Physical Science," *Scientific Monthly*, 74 (1952), 140.

18. Modern Studies include Katie Broberg, "Scientists' Stepping Behavior as Indicator of Writer's Skill," *Journalism Quarterly*, 50 (1973), 766–767; Susan Cray Borman, "Communication Accuracy in Magazine Science Reporting," *Journalism Quarterly*, 55 (1978), 345–346. Criticism of the snippet format was of course not new; Simon Newcomb, "Exact Science in America," *North American Review*, 119 (1874), 307, denounced science appearing as "fugitive items, hardly more interesting or important than the column of daily clippings of one short sentence each which has become a feature of our newspapers."

19. Calvin Pryluck, Charles Teddlie, and Richard Sands, "Meaning in Film/

Video: Order, Time, and Ambiguity," *Journal of Broadcasting*, 26 (1982), 685, connect the inference of meaning with the "Kuleshov experiment," in which film viewers produced differing interpretations of their own to the same stimulus presentations. Even William H. Allen, "Surveying Science Stories," *SIPIscope* (January-February 1985), 14–15, with a public affairs bias found the fact dominance distressing.

20. I. Bernard Cohen, "The Education of the Public in Science," *Impact of Science on Society*, 3 (1952), 94. See the comments in "Erikson Speaks Out," *Newsweek*, December 21, 1970, p. 85.

21. "Preface," *Science Record*, 1873, p. 3. For example, Edward R. Murrow, "Why Should News Come in 5-Minute Packages?" *Nieman Reports* (June 1959), 23–24; plus many more general critiques of television civilization that need not be detailed here. Robert G. Dunn, "Science, Technology, and Bureaucratic Domination: Television and the Ideology of Scientism," *Media, Culture, and Society*, 1 (1979), 343–354, for example, discusses within a tendentious context the "fetishization of fact" as well as the reduction of scientism to myth in television dramas.

22. Geoffrey Harpham, "Time Running Out: The Edwardian Sense of Cultural Degeneration," *Clio*, 5 (1976), 299. George E. Axtelle, "Why Teach Science?" *Science Education*, 34 (1950), 163. The implications are explored in Robert G. Dunn, "Science, Technology, and Bureaucratic Domination: Television and the Ideology of Scientism," *Media, Culture, and Society*, 1 (1979), 343–354, and Carl Gardner and Robert Young, "Science on TV: A Critique," in P. Bennett et al., eds., *Popular Television and Film* (London: BFI Publishing, 1981), pp. 171–196. Stephen B. Withey, "Public Opinion about Science and Scientists," *Public Opinion Quarterly*, 23 (1959), 386, found that the attributes of science stories in newspapers that most appealed to mid-twentieth-century readers included (1) actuality—not hope for the future, (2) specificity—not abstraction or theorizing, (3) relevance to one's own circumstances (as, findings about molecules might affect the gas mileage of one's car), and (4) colorful and exciting headlines. People recognized for decades that undesirable social effects flowed from the fragmentary and aimless popularization that misrepresented science and that might have been avoided by classic popularization. In the "two cultures" controversy, for example, many critics of science, such as Alan D. Perlis, "Science, Mysticism, and Contemporary Poetry," *Western Humanities Review*, 29 (1975), 210–212, portrayed science as merely factual. Or in the world of public policy, the opponents of water fluoridation found it easy to confuse the public with health "facts"; see, for example, Morris Davis, "Community Attitudes toward Fluoridation," *Public Opinion Quarterly*, 23 (1960), 474–482.

23. Everett Dean Martin, *Psychology and Its Use* (Chicago: American Library Association, 1926), pp. 12–13. "Popular Appreciation of Scientists," *Nation*, 74 (1902), 46. See, for example, Malachi Martin, "The Scientist as Shaman,"

Harper's (March 1972), 54–61; Paul A. Carter, *Another Part of the Twenties* (New York: Columbia University Press, 1977), chap. 4. Warren Susman, *Culture as History: The Transformation of American Society in the Twentieth Century* (New York: Pantheon Books, 1984), p. xxvii, provides context.

24. See, for example, "Medicine's Seven Greatest Mysteries," *Look*, February 1, 1949, pp. 86–87; Mrs. Bloomfield Moore, "A Newton of the Mind. The Propeller of Keely's Air-Ship Described," *New Science Review*, 1 (1894), 33–50. Henry H. Bauer, *Beyond Velikovsky: The History of a Public Controversy* (Urbana: University of Illinois Press, 1984). Isaac Asimov, *The New Intelligent Man's Guide to Science* (New York: Basic Books, 1965), pp. 15–16. While Asimov's work was itself to some extent contaminated by mid-twentieth-century standards, he nevertheless was distinctly superior in intention as well as better in execution than many congeners. See also comments on magic below in this chapter.

25. David J. Rhees, "A New Voice for Science: Science Service under Edwin E. Slosson, 1921–29" (master's thesis, University of North Carolina, 1979). The founders of Science Service did have in mind a high-class magazine of popularization, but it never came to fruition, and since the model would probably have been the *National Geographic*, the problem of disconnected facts might well not have been solved even by the fulfilling of such aspirations. George W. Gray, *The Advancing Front of Science* (New York: Whittlesey House, 1937), p. vii. Gray was a writer.

26. See, for example, H. T. Wilson, *The American Ideology: Science, Technology, and Organization as Modes of Rationality in Advanced Industrial Societies* (London: Routledge & Kegan Paul, 1977), especially chap. 2; Otto Friedrich, "There are oo Trees in Russia: The Function of Facts in Newsmagazines," *Harper's* (October 1964), 59–65.

27. Victor Cohn, "Are We Really Telling the Truth About Science?" *Quill* (December 1965), 13. *Popular Science News*, 19 (1885), 127. In "Science Quacks," *Popular Science News*, 30 (1896), 230, the editors noted that unless errors are constantly pointed out, ignorant novices will continue to claim wonderful discoveries and ideas, "long since abandoned as untenable and worthless."

28. See, for example, James L. Crouthamel, "James Gordon Bennett, the *New York Herald*, and the Development of Newspaper Sensationalism," *New York History*, 54 (1973), 294–316. Catherine Fichten, "Scientist Denies Astrology Breakthrough! Or, Beware of the Press," *APA Monitor* (May 1984), 5; this is a particularly useful account because the author discusses her helplessness in seeking remedies.

29. See, for example, Alan Hunsaker, "Enjoyment and Information Gain in Science Articles," *Journalism Quarterly*, 56 (1979), 617–619; Warren Francke, "An Argument in Defense of Sensationalism: Probing the Popular and Historiographical Concept," *Journalism History*, 5 (1979), 70–73; Howard W. Blakeslee, "Scien-

tific Men and the Newspapers," *Science*, 81 (1935), 591, and Waldemar Kaempffert, "Scientific Men and the Newspapers," *Science*, 81 (1935), 640.

30. Robert B. McCall and S. Holly Stocking, "Between Scientists and Public," *American Psychologist*, 37 (1982), 989–990. Memdouh Mehmed Mazloum, "The Popularizing of Scientific Material for Magazine Publication" (master's thesis, University of Wisconsin, 1931), especially pp. 65–66. Evart G. Routzahn, "Public Health Education," *American Journal of Public Health*, 27 (1937), 79, in giving advice on getting health items into the newspapers, noted that when handouts were ignored, inquiry revealed that they were too long—that space was at a premium and only brief copy could be published.

31. Schudson, *Discovering the News*. Silas Bent, "A Mirror for Editors," *Virginia Quarterly Review*, 10 (1934), 374–390, testified to the influence of the journalistic model on other media.

32. Richard S. Musser, Jr., "Newspaper Treatment of Alfred C. Kinsey's Sexual Research" (master's thesis, Indiana University, 1974), shows that people learned about Kinsey's work primarily through opinion pieces rather than factual reporting of what Kinsey actually said. Gilman Ostrander, *American Civilization in the First Machine Age: 1890–1940* (New York: Harper & Row, 1970), p. 232. John W. Garberson, "Magazine Market Demand for the Factual Article," *Journalism Quarterly*, 24 (1947), 32–33. Frederick Lewis Allen, *Only Yesterday, An Informal History of the Nineteen-Twenties* (1931; repr. New York: Harper & Row, 1964), especially pp. 155–160. Krieghbaum, *Science and the Mass Media*, p. 55, commented on the difficulties of arousing more than transient interest in science items. More recently, students of the media conceptualized science in terms of the way in which the mass media set the agenda for science information to be attended to by the public; see, for example, Margareta Cronholm and Rolf Sandell, "Scientific Information: A Review of Research," *Journal of Communication* (Spring 1981), 92.

33. Richard A. Kallan, "The Noncritical Posture of American Print Journalism," *Journal of Popular Culture*, 15 (1981), 116–124. "Superstitious America," *Scientific American*, 114 (1916), 658. Barry Singer and Victor A. Benassi, "Occult Beliefs," *American Scientist* (January-February 1981), 49–55. Substantial documentation is in Curtis D. MacDougall, *Superstition and the Press* (Buffalo, NY: Prometheus Books, 1983). Gaye Tuchman, "Objectivity as Strategic Ritual: An Examination of Newsmen's Notions of Objectivity," *American Journal of Sociology*, 77 (1972), 660–679, offers analysis. As late as 1982, Kendrick Frazier, "How to Cover 'Psychics' and the Paranormal," *ASNE Bulletin* (April 1982), 16–19, was still trying to correct this obvious flaw in journalism.

34. Daniel J. Boorstin, *The Image: A Guide to Pseudo Events in America* (1961; repr. New York: Atheneum, 1973). William R. Oates, "Social and Ethical Content in Science Coverage by Newsmagazines," *Journalism Quarterly*, 50 (1973), 680–684. Stephen J. Whitfield, "From Publick Occurrences to Pseudo-Events: Journalists and Their Critics," *American Jewish History*, 72 (1982), 74–81, summa-

rizes much recent history of this criticism. One of the most notorious incidents in the science field was "K-Day," when a Kinsey report was released; "K-Day," *Time,* August 31, 1953, p. 52. T. J. Jackson Lears, "From Salvation to Self-Realization: Advertising and the Therapeutic Roots of the Consumer Culture, 1880–1930," in Richard Wightman Fox and T. J. Jackson Lears, eds., *The Culture of Consumption: Critical Essays in American History, 1880–1980* (New York: Pantheon Books, 1983), pp. 21–22.

35. Boorstin, *The Image.* Hillier Krieghbaum, "Dr. Barnard as a Human Pseudo-Event," *Columbia Journalism Review* (Summer 1968), 24–25. An insightful account is Carter, *Another Part of the Twenties,* chap. 4. "Tesla, the Wonder Worker, Tells Why He Turned Vegetarian," *New York Magazine of Mysteries,* 1 (1901), 23. Martin, "The Scientist as Shaman." Rae Goodell, *The Visible Scientists* (Boston: Little, Brown and Company, 1977). Mohr, *A Study of Popular Books,* p. 47, remarked on a transitional work, Bernard Jaffe, *Outposts of Science: A Journey to the Workshops of Our Leading Men of Research* (New York: Simon & Schuster, 1935), "It is worth contemplating whether the technique used by Jaffe is adaptable to the communication of science to the layman." I. Daniel Turkat, "Television Psychologists and Therapeutic Set," *Psychology: A Journal of Human Behavior* (May 1977), 65–68.

36. William Bennett, "The Medium Is Large, but How Good Is the Message?" in Sharon M. Friedman, Sharon Dunwoody, and Carol L. Rogers, eds., *Scientists and Journalists: Reporting Science as News* (New York: The Free Press, 1986), pp. 127–128, draws similar conclusions. Goodell, *The Visible Scientists.* See, for example, Donald M. Hausdorff, "They Laughed When Einstein Went to the Blackboard," *University College Quarterly,* 11 (1965), 3–7. I have not dealt with obvious political motivation in the media, which for example led certain mid-twentieth-century publications to discover physicist Edward Teller. Rubin, "'Information Please!'" describes the process of deterioration of cultural authorities in general. The bizarre extreme came as the spokespersons for science in public discourse became the science publicists and science journalists more than the scientists themselves, although in some cases, such as that of the celebrity publisher of the new *Scientific American,* Gerard Piel, the public and science were both well served. In discussing science education, Stephen R. Graubard, "Nothing to Fear, Much to Do," *Daedalus,* 112 (1983), 239, concluded, "Science is treated almost as a mystery, a luxury that one chooses or refuses without serious loss to oneself."

37. "TV Affecting News Columns," *Broadcasting,* October 3, 1960, p. 68, is an early comment. Herbert J. Walberg, "Scientific Literacy and Economic Productivity in International Perspective," *Daedalus,* 112 (1982), 17, summarized the evidence of a negative correlation between television viewing and science learning. Robert Pittman, quoted in Margot Hornblower, "The Age of Video," *Columbus Dispatch,* June 8, 1986, p. 5G.

38. See, for example, in addition to material presented in previous chapters,

the classic F. J. Ingelfinger, "Hygeia on the TV Screen," *New England Journal of Medicine*, 286 (1972), 541–542; and Greta Jones, Ian Connell, and Jack Meadows, *The Presentation of Science by the Media* (Leicester: University of Leicester Primary Communications Research Center, 1978); Herbert J. Gans, *Deciding What's News: A Study of CBS Evening News, NBC Nightly News, Newsweek, and Time* (New York: Pantheon Books, 1979). When Leo Rosten, "The Intellectual and the Mass Media: Some Rigorously Random Remarks," *Daedalus*, 89 (1960), 333–346, for example, set out to refute many of the criticisms, he did not meet the problem of format, and he did not accommodate the problems of commercial interest and crowding out of anything good by the bad. Neil Postman, *Amusing Ourselves to Death: Public Discourse in the Age of Show Business* (New York: Viking Penguin Inc., 1985), especially p. 16.

39. Stephen H. Schneider, "Both Sides of the Fence: The Scientist as Source and Author," in Friedman, Dunwoody, and Rogers, eds., *Scientists and Journalists*, pp. 216–217, found that even the most carefully constructed stories would ultimately be distorted as they passed through the media. See, for example, Alexander Klein, "The Challenge of the Mass Media," *Yale Review*, 39 (1950), 675–691; Gaye Tuchman, *Making News: A Study in the Construction of Reality* (New York: Free Press, 1978); Clyde Z. Nunn, "Readership and Coverage of Science and Technology in Newspapers," *Journalism Quarterly*, 56 (1979), 27–30; Percy H. Tannenbaum, "Communication of Science Information," *Science*, 140 (1963), 579–583; Lois Ruskai Melina, "An Experimental Study of Reader Response to a Science Page in a Newspaper" (master's thesis, The Ohio State University, 1976); Perry Garfinkel, "Psychic Pulps: Giving the People What They Want," *New York*, December 27, 1976, pp. 57–58; Celeste Huenergard, "Study Says Reporters Are Cynical, Arrogant, Isolated," *Editor and Publisher*, May 22, 1982, pp. 14, 36; Paul Block, Jr., "Who Blows the Whistle?" *ASNE Bulletin*, October 1, 1962, pp. 3–4. Heywood, "Scientists and Society," p. 103. Otto Struve, "Fifty Years of Progress in Astronomy," *Popular Astronomy*, 51 (1943), 481. " 'Something Called Fission': Science in the Press," *Nieman Reports* (April 1947), 11. Arnold J. Meltsner, "The Communication of Scientific Information to the Public: The Case of Seismology in California," *Minerva*, 17 (1979), 331–354.

40. See, for example, Philip J. Tichenor, Clarice N. Olien, Annette Harrison, and George Donohue, "Mass Communication Systems and Communication Accuracy in Science News Reporting," *Journalism Quarterly*, 47 (1970), 673–683; Barbara E. Rasmussen, "Academic Engineers and Science Writers: A Survey of Attitudes and Experiences" (master's thesis, University of West Virginia, 1981), especially pp. 3, 42. Kathleen Joan Goldman, "An Analysis of Science Reporters' Views of Scientists as Sources" (master's thesis, California State University, Northridge, 1978), especially pp. 68, 70–72.

41. Charles W. Finley and Otis W. Caldwell, *Biology in the Public Press* (New

York: Lincoln School of Teachers College, 1923); a summary of this line of work is in W. Edgar Martin, "A Chronological Survey of Published Research Studies Relating to Biological Materials in Newspapers and Magazines," *School Science and Mathematics*, 45 (1945), 543–550. See Marcel C. La Follette, "Science on Television: Influences and Strategies," *Daedalus*, 111 (1982), 183–197, especially 194. The journalistic influence of course went into even the more or less respectable popularization aimed at the sci-tech community; see, for example, James E. Oberg and Robert Sheaffer, "Pseudoscience at Science Digest," *Zetetic* (Fall/Winter 1977), 41–44.

42. There are competent descriptions of the American consumer culture, and I cannot in a discussion of popularizing science go into detail. See especially Susman, *Culture as History*. Other recent general commentators include Stewart Ewen, *Captains of Consciousness: Advertising and the Social Roots of the Consumer Culture* (New York: McGraw-Hill Book Company, 1976); Fox and Lears, *The Culture of Consumption*, and Roland Marchand, *Advertising the American Dream: Making Way for Modernity, 1920–1940* (Berkeley: University of California Press, 1985), especially chap. 5. Frank George, ed., *Science Fact: Astounding and Exciting Developments That Will Transform Your Life* (New York: Sterling Publishing Company, 1978).

43. Quentin James Schultze, "Advertising, Science, and Professionalism, 1885–1917" (doctoral diss., University of Illinois, 1978), especially pp. 30–32. *Nation*, 1905, quoted in Christopher P. Wilson, "The Rhetoric of Consumption: Mass-Market Magazines and the Demise of the Gentle Reader, 1880–1920," in Fox and Lears, *The Culture of Consumption*, p. 50. Fred W. Decker, "Scientific Communications Should Be Improved," *Science*, 125 (1957), 101–105, emphasizes, with specific instances, ways in which isolated facts and conflicting authorities combined with commercial interests to corrupt communication of science to the public. "Letter from the Editor," *Modern Medicine*, February 1, 1951, p. 14. Iago Galdston, "The Problem of Motivation in Health Education," in *Motivation in Health Education: The 1947 Health Education Conference of the New York Academy of Medicine* (New York: Columbia University Press, 1948), p. 19, denounced advertising "facts, near-facts and nowhere-near-facts." See also previous note.

44. See, for example, the "Personal Computers" segment in the "Science Times" section of the *New York Times*, beginning July 6, 1982.

45. See, for example, Ralph Edwards, "Indoctrination: A Respectable Technique in Health Education," *Journal of Health—Physical Education—Recreation* (January 1963), 44–45, 66. Edward A. Moree, "Public Health Publicity: The Art of Stimulating and Focussing Public Opinion," *American Journal of Public Health*, 6 (1916), 278. Don S. Kirschner, "'Publicity Properly Applied': The Selling of Expertise in America, 1900–1929," *American Studies*, 19 (1978), 65–78. See in general Marchand, *Advertising the American Dream*.

46. At one point, the American Medical Association was essentially endorsing products that were advertised in an AMA publication.

47. There were many examinations of the untruthfulness of advertisers; Rita S. Rosenberg, "An Investigation of the Nature, Utilization, and Accuracy of Nutritional Claims in Magazine Food Advertisements: An Analysis and Evaluation of the Nutritional Statements Made in Food Advertisements Over a Fifty Year Period" (doctoral diss., New York University, 1955), pp. 26–28, summarizes research on the first half of the twentieth century; and that study can be supplemented with such reports as Peter Morell, *Poisons, Potions, and Profits: The Antidote to Radio Advertising* (New York: Knight Publishers, 1937), and Michael L. Geis, *The Language of Television Advertising* (New York: Academic Press, 1982); other examples of course are in James Harvey Young, *The Medical Messiahs: A Social History of Health Quackery in Twentieth-Century America* (Princeton: Princeton University Press, 1967). The 1960s critics of advertising were diverted into arguments about literal truthfulness and missed the issues of social and cultural impact; see, for example, "Truth and Taste in Advertising—1960," *Printer's Ink*, November 27, 1959, pp. 23–34. Erik Barnouw, *The Sponsor: Notes on a Modern Potentate* (Oxford: Oxford University Press, 1978), especially pp. 83–91, puts deception in a much broader context. The improvements in advertising standards recorded by Rosenberg, "An Investigation of the Nature," Otis Pease, *The Responsibilities of American Advertising: Private Control and Public Influence, 1920–1940* (New Haven: Yale University Press, 1958), and others did not in the end result in more truthful intent or effect. Instead, the more "respectable" advertisers developed their own world, which even limited to puffery subverted a naturalistic, antisuperstitious way of thinking. See n. 42 above on culture, and, for example, Lucille Hollander Blum, "Health Information Via Mass Media: Study of the Individual's Concepts of the Body and Its Parts," *Psychological Reports*, 40 (1977), 991–999. Herbert Jack Rotfeld, "Advertising Deception, Consumer Research, and Puffery: An Inquiry into Puffery's Power and Potential to Mislead Consumers (doctoral diss., University of Illinois, 1978), concludes that substantial numbers of consumers were misled by puffery (which appears to be "unprovable"), that the intent to mislead was present, and that even relatively sophisticated consumers were deceived and affected.

48. See, for example, Herbert E. Krugman, "The Impact of Television Advertising: Learning without Involvement," *Public Opinion Quarterly*, 29 (1965), 349–356; Ivan L. Preston and Storen E. Scharbach, "Advertising: More than Meets the Eye?" *Journal of Advertising Research* (June 1971), 19–24; John C. Maloney, "Curiosity versus Disbelief in Advertising," *Journal of Advertising Research*, 2 (1962), 2–8; Jonathan Price, "Now a Few Words about Commercials," *Esquire*, October 24, 1978, pp. 102–110. Compare the admittedly unusual dissent, Robert H. Moser, "The New Seduction," *JAMA*, 230 (1974), 1564. Michael R. Real,

"Media Theory: Contributions to an Understanding of American Mass Communications," *American Quarterly*, 32 (1980), 238–258, summarizes literature that emphasizes the implicit rather than explicit messages of the media, and Marchand, *Advertising the American Dream*, pp. 115–116 and passim, provides a historical dimension.

49. See, for example, Edna M. Kech et al., "Evaluation of Commercial Advertising," *American Journal of Public Health*, 38 (1948), 109–112 (appendix); Gertrude I. Duncan and Frederick H. Lund, "The Validity of Health Information Gained through Radio Advertising," *Research Quarterly*, 16 (1945), 102–105. Charles E. Lewis and Mary Ann Lewis, "The Impact of Television Commercials on Health-Related Beliefs and Behaviors of Children," *Pediatrics*, 53 (1974), 431–435. Blanche M. Trilling, "A Twenty-Five Year Perspective on Physical Education Needs," *Journal of Health and Physical Education* (May 1935), 3. *Saturday Evening Post*, March 2, 1940, p. 36. A. T. Poffenberger, "The Conditions of Belief in Advertising," *Journal of Applied Psychology*, 7 (1923), 2. T. J. Jackson Lears, "Some Versions of Fantasy: Toward a Cultural History of American Advertising, 1880–1930," *Prospects*, 9 (1984), 349–405. The organized skeptics described above did not take on advertising pseudoscience as such.

50. Marchand, *Advertising the American Dream*, especially pp. xxi, 1, 160–163.

51. See, for example, Dallas W. Smythe, "What TV Programming is Like," *Quarterly of Film, Radio, and Television*, 7 (1952), 25–31. As Michael Schudson, *Advertising, The Uneasy Persuasion: Its Dubious Impact on American Society* (New York: Basic Books, 1984), points out, the intentions of the advertisers were very frequently not carried out, or only ineffectively so. Such a conclusion does not in any way contradict the evidence gathered by many researchers showing the powerful cultural effects of advertising; as Lears, "Some Versions of Fantasy," in his historical analysis of advertising shows, copywriters and commercial authorities often held conscious values very different from those they propagated. William R. Catton, Jr., "Changing Cognitive Structure as a Basis for the 'Sleeper Effect,'" *Social Forces*, 38 (1960), 348–354, shows that the mass media have effects that are very great but cannot be measured simplistically. Bruce H. Westley, "Communication and Social Change," *American Behavioral Scientist*, 14 (1971), 719–743. John L. Caughey, "Artificial Social Relationships in Modern America," *American Quarterly*, 30 (1978), 70–89, shows how the television world furnished profoundly influential social relationships.

52. The parallels between O'Keefe, *Stolen Lightning*, especially pp. 349–457 and 478–502, and Marchand, *Advertising the American Dream*, especially chap. 10 and pp. 11–13, 356–358, from which the examples are taken, are striking; my summary does not do justice to the subtleties of either account.

53. Lears, "Some Versions of Fantasy," identifies the trend from factual argument in advertising to addressing imagined aspirations in consumers, various fan-

tasies that may or may not have been conscious. Marchand, *Advertising the American Dream*, documents the process in detail. Paul Rand Dixon, quoted in Rotfeld, "Advertising Deception," p. 17.

54. Treffie Cox, J. S. McCollum, and Ralph K. Watkins, "Science Claims in Magazine Advertising," *Science Education*, 22 (1938), 14; Bob Bullock et al., "Science and Superstition Minicourse" (EDRS Document 124381, 1974); and, for example, Mary Swartz Rose, "Belief in Magic," *Journal of the American Dietetic Association*, 8 (1933), 489–503; and "Simeon Stylites," "Advertising Witchcraft," *Christian Century*, February 10, 1954, p. 169. The parallels between skeptics opposed to superstition and those opposed to advertising claims were of course equally striking. O'Keefe, *Stolen Lightning*, pp. 473–474, comes close to making the general point, but he is restricted by taking "magic" literally rather than more functionally so as to encompass advertising.

55. Schudson, *Advertising*, especially pp. 222–233. See, for example the uses made of modeling theory in Peter Ester and Richard Winett, "Toward More Effective Antecedent Strategies for Environmental Programs," *Journal of Environmental Systems*, 11 (1981–1982), 201–222, and Mark Costanzo et al., "Energy Conservation Behavior: The Difficult Path from Information to Action," *American Psychologist*, 41 (1986), 521–528. Joseph Agassi, "Towards a Rational Theory of Superstition," *Zetetic Scholar*, 1 (1978), 107–120. Raymond Williams, *Problems in Materialism and Culture* (London: Verso Editions and NLB, 1980), pp. 186–189, described modern advertising as magic. Lears, "Some Versions of Fantasy," pp. 397–398, objects that advertising contains too many unreconciled elements to serve functionally as magic in a culture. The issue rather is magical thinking, not the institution. Again, superstition, which embodies only a general approach—although of course including much magical thinking—is, like advertising, as Lears points out, distinctively fragmented.

56. A clear case of withdrawal (in this case leaders of the AAAS) is noted in [John E. Pfeiffer], "President's Page," *NASW Newsletter*, December 1, 1955, pp. 7–8, and *NASW Newsletter* (March 1956), 10–12, when the AAAS refused to undertake a program for the general public but announced intentions of restricting any such program to the type of audience that read the *Scientific American*. In more recent years, of course, the AAAS moved vigorously into the area of popularization. Edwin G. Boring to Marjorie Van de Water, May 19, 1943, quoted in James H. Capshew, "Military Text and Professional Context: Psychology for the Fighting Man and World War II" (paper presented at the History of Science Society Meetings, Pittsburgh, October 1985). See, for example, Lyell D. Henry, Jr., "Unorthodox Science as a Popular Activity," *Journal of American Culture*, 4 (1981), 6–9. Jeffrey H. Goldstein, ed., *Reporting Science: The Case of Aggression* (Hillsdale, NJ: Lawrence Erlbaum Associates, 1986), contains some accounts of the forces

that made some scientists attempt to regain some control over the publicizing of their own work, at least.

57. Francis B. Sumner, "The New Dogmatism," *Scientific Monthly*, 45 (1937), 348. James R. Angell, *Popular and Unpopular Science: Elihu Root Lectures of Carnegie Institution of Washington on the Influence of Science and Research on Current Thought* (Washington: Carnegie Institution of Washington, 1935), p. 10. S. B. Barnes and R. G. A. Dolby, "The Scientific Ethos: A Deviant Viewpoint," *Archives européennes de sociologie*, 11 (1970), 3–25, point out that programmatic statements—and presumably awareness—flourished in the context of the warfare between science and mysticism.

58. Wallace R. Brode, "Who Speaks For Science?" *Topic*, 11 (1966), 34.

59. Peter J. Kuznick, "The Science Popularizers' Dilemma: The Battle over the Presentation of Science at the 1939 New York World's Fair" (paper presented at the meetings of the Organization of American Historians, Los Angeles, April 1984); Robert W. Rydell, "The Fan Dance of Science: American World's Fairs in the Great Depression," *Isis*, 76 (1985), 525–542. For example, Morris Fishbein, *Shattering Health Superstitions: An Explosion of the False Theories and Notions in the Field of Health and Popular Medicine* (New York: Horace Liveright, 1930). Frank A. Smith et al., "Health Information during a Week of Television," *New England Journal of Medicine*, 286 (1972), especially 519.

60. An example of attempting to teach the scientific spirit is Carl William Gray, Claude W. Sandifur, and Howard J. Hanna, *Fundamentals of Chemistry* (2nd ed., Boston: Houghton Mifflin Company, 1924), pp. 4–5. Hayden, "History of the New Math," p. 65.

61. Rhees, "A New Voice for Science"; the quote is from p. 39. Edwin E. Slosson, *Chats on Science* (New York: The Century Co., 1924), pp. 4–5.

62. William Bateson, quoted in R. D. Harvey, "The William Bateson Letters at the John Innes Institute," *Mendel Newsletter* (November 1985), 9. The irony of specialization was that even when the group appeared that opposed credulity, it was segregated from science because it was a specialized group; see, for example, the discussion in Hofstadter, *Metamagical Themas*, especially p. 95.

63. In a highly organized society, failure of nerve was not unique to the scientists; Sidney Hook, "The New Failure of Nerve," *Partisan Review*, 10 (1943), 2–23. R. S. Mulliken, "Science and the Scientific Attitude," *Science*, 86 (1937), 66. Stephen Toulmin, "Science and Our Intellectual Tradition," *Advancement of Science*, 20 (1963), 29–30. Roger J. Lederer and Barry Singer, "Pseudoscience in the Name of the University," *Skeptical Inquirer* (Spring 1983), 57–62, describe the results of the failure of nerve: outrages within higher education against which academic scientists did not move effectively even though there were local institutional means to do so. Roy Ringo, "The Justification of Science to Scientists,"

Bulletin of the Atomic Scientists (March 1975), 29–33, described the failure of nerve even in the policy area.

64. Gene Weltfish, "Science and Prejudice," *Scientific Monthly*, 61 (1945), 211. Conway Zirkle, "Our Splintered Learning and the Status of Scientists," *Science*, 121 (1955), 516.

65. A. J. Goldforb, "Medical and Other Sciences," *Science*, 71 (1930), 77–81. Edward Shils, "Mass Society and Its Culture," *Daedalus*, 89 (1960), especially 289, 300. Frederick S. Hammett, "Integration in Science Teaching," *Scientific Monthly*, 62 (1946), 430–431. Gerard Pelletier, in *Civilization and Science—In Conflict or Collaboration?* (Amsterdam: Elsevier, 1972), p. 53. William Bevan, "The Sound of the Wind That's Blowing," *American Psychologist*, 31 (1976), 482. Peter S. Buck and Barbara Gutmann Rosenkrantz, "The Worm in the Core: Science and General Education," in Everett Mendelsohn, ed., *Transformation and Tradition in the Sciences: Essays in Honor of I. Bernard Cohen* (Cambridge: Cambridge University Press, 1984), pp. 371–394, detail how in the mid-twentieth century, specialist disciplinary claims of individual sciences tended to undermine attempts to include science as such in general education efforts at the college level.

66. Kimball Young, "The Need of Integration of Attitudes among Scientists," *Scientific Monthly*, 18 (1924), 291. See, for example, *New York Times*, February 23, 1971, p. 40, and June 22, p. 22. *APA Monitor* (August 1983), 2, and (March 1985), 15; the controversy can be followed in earlier issues of the same journal.

67. David Gerrold, quoted in Thomas H. Maugh II, "The Media: The Image of the Scientist Is Bad," *Science*, 200 (1978), 37. The organized skeptics were of course specialists acting in the name of skepticism, not science. Alvin M. Weinberg, "Science in the Public Forum: Keeping It Honest," *Science*, 191 (1976), 341, documents the corrupting influence of political interests. Joseph Haberer, "Politicization in Science," *Science*, 178 (1972), 713–724.

68. An authoritative account of this movement is Ronald L. Numbers, "The Creationists," in David C. Lindberg and Ronald L. Numbers, eds., *God and Nature: Historical Essays on the Encounter between Christianity and Science* (Berkeley: University of California Press, 1986), pp. 391–423; and similarly Ronald L. Numbers, "Creationism in 20th-Century America," *Science*, 218 (1982), 538–544. Roger Lewin, "A Response to Creationism Evolves," *Science*, 214 (1981), 635–638. There is no intention here of failing to recognize the brave souls who did fight "creation science" on scientific rather than civil libertarian grounds; the point is, however, how little support they got from scientific colleagues. Thomas F. Gieryn, George M. Bevins, and Stephen C. Zehr, "Professionalization of American Scientists: Public Science in the Creation/Evolution Trials," *American Sociological Review*, 50 (1985), 392–409, interpret the scientific presentations as attempts to establish the boundaries of an economic interest group as much as science. Extended discussion of other examples—such as the physical scientists

who so frequently mistook their own expertise and got involved with psychic phenomena, or antivivisectionist technicians—belongs in another place.

69. Shils, "Mass Society and Its Culture." Jon D. Miller, *The American People and Science Policy: The Role of Public Attitudes in the Science Process* (New York: Pergamon Press, 1983), especially pp. 77–78. Daniel Yankelovich, "Changing Attitudes to Science and the Quality of Life: Edited Excerpts from a Seminar," *Science, Technology, and Human Values* (Spring 1982), 25.

70. For example, Kirschner, "'Publicity Properly Applied,'" especially pp. 76–77. Also see comments in chapter 5.

71. See, for example, James E. Brinton and L. Norman McKown, "Effects of Newspaper Reading on Knowledge and Attitudes," *Journalism Quarterly*, 38 (1961), 186–195; "Survey Shows Freshman Shift on Careers, Values," *Science*, 219 (1983), 822. There was of course conflicting evidence about how much popularizing and what kind of popularizing campaigns had what kind of social effects; see, for example, James W. Swinehart and Jack W. McLeod, "News about Science: Channels, Audiences, and Effects," *Public Opinion Quarterly*, 24 (1960), 589; Edward J. Robinson, "Analyzing the Impact of Science Reporting," *Journalism Quarterly*, 40 (1963), 306–314; Rodolfo N. Salcedo, Hadley Read, James F. Evans, and Ana C. Kong, "A Successful Information Campaign on Pesticides," *Journalism Quarterly*, 51 (1974), 91–95, 110.

72. See especially the wise observation in Michael M. Sokal, "James McKeen Cattell and American Psychology in the 1920's," in Josef Brozek, ed., *Explorations in the History of Psychology in the United States* (Lewisburg, PA: Bucknell University Press, 1984), p. 275. For example, M. Timothy O'Keefe, "The Mass Media as Sources of Medical Information for Doctors," *Journalism Quarterly*, 47 (1970), 95–100; Donald L. Shaw and Paul Van Nevel, "The Informative Value of Medical Science News," *Journalism Quarterly*, 44 (1967), 548. The *Scientific American* by the 1980s was issuing a basic medical updating service, *Scientific American Medicine*, for physicians to help them keep up with developments in the field of medicine.

73. William Bennett, "Science Goes Glossy," *The Sciences* (September 1979), 11. See, for example, the "Letter from the Editor," *Modern Medicine*, January 1, 1951, p. 15.

74. Anne Roe, *The Making of a Scientist* (New York: Dodd, Mead & Company, 1953). Edwin E. Slosson, *Creative Chemistry Descriptive of Recent Achievements in the Chemical Industries* (New York: The Century Co., 1919).

75. See, for example, David Bakan, "John Broadus Watson (1878–1958)," *Psychological Reports*, 7 (1960), 81–82. The classic discussion of the hero problem is Brush, "Should the History of Science Be Rated X?"

76. Ann Roberta Larson, "Subjects and Literary Style, In *Newsweek*, *Scientific American*, and *Today's Health* Science Stories in 1959 and 1969" (master's thesis, University of Texas, 1972), p. 147. G. T. W. Patrick, "The New Optimism," *Popu-*

lar Science Monthly, 82 (1913), 493. Watson Davis, "Science Parades the Front Pages," *Quill* (October 1934), 10. Bill Meyers, "The Advance of Science," *Washington Journalism Review* (November 1981), 37. *New Yorker,* March 31, 1951, p. 68. The comment was: "Well! We can have a good night's sleep now!" Cramp, "Popular Magazines as Medical Advisors," p. 157, points out that writers used the personal pronoun to publicize wonder drugs at midcentury so that they were relevant to "you," not the world of science.

77. Earl James McGrath, "Science in General Education," *Scientific Monthly,* 71 (1950), 118. The elements in this forward-looking theme in constant scientific discovery have not, to my knowledge, been analyzed systematically. Aside from "new hope" and the promise of a future, the certainty that gaps in knowledge will be filled—and the suspense of waiting—are certainly important. Michael Gossop, "News as a Drug: It Relieves Anxiety," *Journalism Studies Review* (July 1982), 16, notes that bad news can be habit forming; but so can good news of the constantly expanding findings and products of science. Robert L. Bishop, "Anxiety and Readership of Health Information," *Journalism Quarterly,* 51 (1974), 40–46, found that anxious people were extremely eager to read reassuring health stories.

78. John S. Rigden, "Creativity Lost," *American Journal of Physics,* 46 (1978), 1209. William Bennett, "Science Hits the Newsstand," *Columbia Journalism Review* (January-February 1981), 55. In 1962, in a high-quality and revealing example, John Rader Platt, *The Excitement of Science* (Boston: Houghton Mifflin Company, 1962), added, to intellectual excitement, interest in the personalities of science and tended to follow journalistic sensationalism; his book is remarkably free of traditional negative enthusiasms. Peggy Thompson, "A TV Series Starring Science," *American Education* (March 1980), 6–13, found that at least one audience was still receptive to contextualized science: children who otherwise thought science was tedious and boring responded to attempts to put the world into a scientific perspective.

79. There were of course departments that carried the now-obsolete term, such as "Science for the Citizen," and it appeared sometimes in historical articles. One exceptional article did appear in 1984: "Leon M. Lederman, "The Value of Fundamental Sciences," *Scientific American* (November 1984), 40–47.

80. See, for example, Daniel S. Greenberg, "Let's Hear It for Science," *Columbia Journalism Review* (July-August 1974), 16–23.

81. See note 58 above.

82. Joseph Jastrow, "Belief and Credulity," *Educational Review,* 23 (1902), 29. See, for example, the touching confession of new hope writer Edith M. Stern, "Medical Journalism—With and without Upbeat," *Saturday Review,* January 7, 1954, pp. 9–10, 36. John Morgan Flowers, Jr., "A Study of Selected Viewpoints Pertaining to Science Education in the United States" (doctoral diss., Duke Uni-

versity, 1960), pp. 4–5, points out that where once demystifying the world had given science the popular role of combatting fear (fear on which superstititon, of course preyed), in the atomic bomb–Sputnik era, science was the source of fear. Obviously in such a context an optimistic message from popularizers fulfilled with the products of science a role once played by knowledge and the process of discovery.

83. Such labeling was not possible in a mass culture in which, as Dwight Mac-Donald points out in "A Theory of Mass Culture," in Bernard Rosenberg and David Manning White, eds., *Mass Culture: The Popular Arts in America* (New York: The Free Press, 1957), p. 66, the adult and child audiences lost differentiation. Robert K. Merton, *The Sociology of Science: Theoretical and Empirical Investigations*, ed. by Norman W. Storer (Chicago: University of Chicago Press, 1973), pp. 264–266, long ago pointed out the symbolic function of skepticism in science as he discussed "Public Hostility toward Organized Skepticism."

84. The organized skeptics of the late 1970s and after were not identified, except often individually, as scientists; the initial organizing took place not at meetings of a scientific group but at those of the American Humanist Association.

85. See, for example, Agassi, "Towards a Rational Theory," p. 116; Leo Marx, "Reflections on the Neo-Romantic Critique of Science," *Daedalus*, 107 (1978), 61–74. Haskell, *The Authority of Experts.* See also Dorothy Nelkin, "Threats and Promises: Negotiating the Control of Research," *Daedalus*, 107 (1978), 196–197, and other essays in this issue. John C. Burnham, "American Medicine's Golden Age: What Happened to It?" *Science*, 215 (1982), 1474–1482. No attempt is made here to describe in detail the common phenomenon of those who criticized faulty thinking, emotionalism, and error finding themselves under attack for being "intolerant." Nor are the parallels to the phenomena described by Jeffrey Herf, *Reactionary Modernism: Technology, Culture, and Politics in Weimar and the Third Reich* (Cambridge: Cambridge University Press, 1984), explored.

86. Edward S. Holden, "The Conflict of Religion and Science," *Popular Science Monthly*, 65 (1904), 289. Lancelot Hogben, *Science for the Citizen: A Self-Educator Based on the Social Background of Scientific Discovery* (New York: Alfred A. Knopf, 1938), pp. ix–x.

87. See, for example, J. E. Teder, "A Prophylaxis for Emotional Thinking," *Science Education*, 18 (1934), 171–174; Wilbur L. Beauchamp, *Instruction in Science* (Washington: Government Printing Office, 1933, U. S. Office of Education Bulletin no. 17), especially pp. 11–12.

88. Edward Shils, "Anti-Science," *Minerva*, 9 (1971), 442–443. J. R. Ravetz, *Scientific Knowledge and Its Social Problems* (Oxford: Clarendon Press, 1971), p. 390. The civilization idea was of course implicitly part of the target in the attack on the behavioral and social sciences noted in chapter 3. Murray G. Murphey, "On the Relation between Science and Religion," *American Quarterly*, 20 (1968),

275–295, for example, treated science as just another belief system—the same relativistic model that had been so devastating to religion. The issue of the style of science was referred to in chapter 1, and it was relevant quite aside from the two-cultures debates.

89. Robert Ray Haun, "Changes within the Decade," in idem, ed., *Science in General Education* (Dubuque, IA: Wm. C. Brown Company, 1960), p. 5. Singer and Benassi, "Occult Beliefs," p. 54 (an inconsequential spelling error has been corrected silently). David A. Hollinger, *Morris R. Cohen and the Scientific Ideal* (Cambridge, MA: The MIT Press, 1975), and elsewhere describes the high point of and assault on the ideal of science among intellectuals.

90. See, for example, Michael J. Mahoney, *Scientist as Subject: The Psychological Imperative* (Cambridge, MA: Ballinger Press, 1977), pp. 170–171.

91. Ironically, a number of philosophers of science whose technical works were perhaps misunderstood did on occasion take public stands themselves. The philosophers' impact is essentially the same as that described in Brush, "Should the History of Science Be Rated X?" Sindermann, *The Joy of Science*, pp. 4–6, affirmed, "There is a state of mind, an approach to problem-solving, that is common to scientific obvservation," and he included in it objectivity and controls, suggesting that the potential for a traditional viewpoint was far from dead in the 1980s.

92. A wise, well-informed general comment is Edward Shils, "Faith, Utility, and the Legitimacy of Science," *Daedalus*, 103 (1974), 1–15.

Index

patent medicines. *See* nostrums
Patrick, G.T.W., 257
Patrouch, Joseph F., Jr., 216
Pattison, Granville Sharp, 138, 145
Pauling, Linus, 238
Peale's Museum, 128, 138
Pearson, Karl, 168
Peck, William G., 167
Pendray, G. Edward, 197
personalities. *See* journalism,
  celebrities
philosophers of science, 260–261
photography, 164, 203
phrenology, 86, 142, 150
Physical Culture. See Macfadden,
  Bernarr
physical geography, 136, 158, 183,
  185
physics (including natural philosophy), 133, 140, 183, 184, 187, 209,
  215
Physics Today, 179, 206, 224
physiology. *See* hygiene instruction
Piel, Gerard, 222, 345n36
political aspects of science popularization, 105, 108–109, 241, 253, 258,
  345n36
pop science. *See* folk science
Popular Astronomy, 193, 231
Popular Mechanics, 191
Popular Psychology, 106
Popular Psychology Guide, 99, 103
Popular Science Monthly, 30, 31, 34, 35,
  37, 41, 43, 55, 129, 132, 152, 159,
  160, 163, 166, 168, 172, 191, 193,
  197, 198, 203, 205, 207, 220, 232,
  239
Popular Science News, 40, 159, 165,
  167, 168, 172, 203, 235, 243
popularization by non-scientists, 7,

31, 37, 208–212, 226, 236–237,
  240–241, 248–250
popularization by scientists, 22,
  33–34, 205–206, 207–208, 226,
  234–237, 247–249, 251–254,
  257–259, 261–262. *See also* men of
  science
popularization of health, 48, 72–84,
  226, 243, 244; early nineteenth century, 48–51; late nineteenth century,
  52–56; early twentieth century,
  56–62; 1930s, 62–65; mid-twentieth century, 65–67; after midcentury, 67–69, 178
popularization of psychology, 258;
  new psychology, 89–90; beginning
  of twentieth century, 92–94; 1920s,
  95–97; 1930s, 97–100; World War II
  and after, 100–103; midcentury,
  103–106; late twentieth century,
  106–108, 114–115
popularization of science, 3–8, 31–44,
  226–229, 254–256, 259–262,
  263n1, and passim in Chapters 4, 5,
  and 6; definition of, 33–35, 37–38,
  179–180; patterns in, 5–6, 85,
  127–128, 144, 226; two tiers, 152,
  154, 179; first half of nineteenth
  century, 128–151; intensity in first
  half of nineteenth century, 144; second half of nineteenth century,
  151–169; intensity in second half of
  nineteenth century, 159–161; intensity in twentieth century, 171–178.
  See also audience and appeal
population, social changes in, 35, 36
positivism, 15–16, 80, 162–169,
  269n47. *See also* Baconianism
Postman, Neil, 240
Potthoff, Carl J., 230

Powell, John Wesley, 25
Practical Psychology, 93
practicality of science, 139, 140–141,
 143–144, 146–148, 150–151, 168,
 183–184, 217–218. *See also* products of science; progress; technology
Pradal, Jean, 194
pragmatism, 220, 222
pre-Socratic philosophers, 13
products of science, 62, 64, 70,
 81–84, 105–106, 107–108, 109,
 203, 215–218, 220, 223, 225, 260;
 popularized science as product, 239
progress, 25–26, 143–144, 150–151,
 162–163, 164–166, 167, 171, 216,
 217, 225, 227, 232, 244–245,
 256–257
Protestantism, 14–15, 23. *See also*
 religion
pseudoevent. *See* journalism
pseudoscience, 18, 339–340n5. *See
 also* error
psychology: academic, 87–89, 91, 98,
 100–101, 106, 112–113; applied,
 86–87, 95–97, 102, 108, 110;
 clinical identity, 99, 102–106; fragmentation, 95–96, 109–110, 114; in
 health popularization, 66–67; popular not distinctive in nineteenth century, 85–87; textbooks, 110,
 112–113, 299n69. *See also* audience
 and appeal; popularization of
 psychology
*Psychology—Health! Happiness! Suc-
 cess!,* 96, 99
Psychology Today, 106–107, 108, 115,
 178, 193, 238, 253
psychopathological thinking, 20, 222,
 267n31. *See also* superstitition, as
 deviant

public health movement, 57–61, 64,
 66, 68. *See also* sanitarians
public relations, 73–74, 104–105,
 108, 197, 209, 212–214, 218, 225,
 238, 259, 291n12, 333n112
pupil development, 65, 185, 187–188

radio, 36, 58, 77, 98, 174, 175, 188,
 201. *See also* mass media
Rafinesque, Constantine, 131
Ravetz, J. R., 35
Reader's Digest, 63, 76, 189, 191, 239
reductionism, 9, 27, 54, 82, 90–91,
 93, 98, 112, 164–166, 214, 225, 254
Reese, David, 142
Reid, Whitelaw, 159
religion: confused with superstition,
 18–19, 21, 90–91, 149–150; underlying motive for interest in popular
 science, 41–42; warfare against science, 12–15, 259. *See also* Protestantism; Roman Catholicism;
 warfare of science against
 superstition
religion of science, 21–29, 111–112,
 154, 163–169, 223, 225, 226, 232,
 247, 250, 255, 258, 260–262,
 269n42
Rensselaer Polytechnic Institute, 133
Rhees, David J., 249
Rice, Thurman B., 72
Robinson, Edward S., 113
Robinson, F. C., 230
Robinson, James Harvey, 110
Roe, Anne, 256
Rogers, Carl, 104
Roman Catholicism, 14–15. *See also*
 religion
Rosa, E. B., 166
Rosen, Sidney, 16, 133